Drug Courts

Drug Courts

A New Approach to Treatment and Rehabilitation

James E. Lessenger, MD, FACOEM
Consultant in Occupational Medicine,
Solano County, Benicia, California, USA

Glade F. Roper, JD
Judge, Superior Court of California, Tulare County,
Porterville, California, USA

Editors

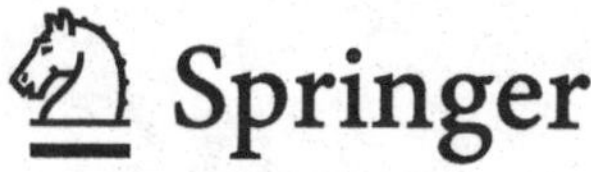

James E. Lessenger, MD, FACOEM
Consultant in Occupational Medicine
Solano County
Benicia, CA 94510
USA

Glade F. Roper, JD
Judge
Superior Court of California
Tulare County
Porterville, CA 93267
USA

ISBN: 978-1-4419-2442-1 e-ISBN: 978-0-387-71433-2

Printed on acid-free paper.

9 8 7 6 5 4 3 2 1

springer.com

Foreword

I've done them all, and I'm not talking about stage, screen, and television. I stopped taking drugs in the 1970s and stopped smoking in the 1980s. I ceased drinking in the 1990s when I needed a liver transplant and my doctors told me they wouldn't do it if I continued drinking. So, I stopped, got the transplant, and became a friend of Bill W. Stopping was the best thing I ever did, second to marrying Maj.

My substance abuse started, like most people's, in high school through peer pressure. It progressed while I was on the stage and in the Air Force, where alcohol was the drug of choice. The problem continued as I worked in motion pictures where the day ended with drinks. When I finally made it big in television, I was drinking a case of champagne a day.

I tell myself that I did this because of my insecurities about being at the top, but it also tasted good. Looking back and having read some of the things in this book, I realize that I have the addictive personality and the genetic predisposition to be a substance abuser. All that was necessary was a situation in which I was near drugs and had peer pressure to get me going. In the end, peer pressure is what made me stop—that, and liver failure. I was seven years clean and sober when I received a call from a friend putting me in touch with a judge in Porterville, California, who wanted me to speak at a graduation. Two things came to mind: what kind of graduation, and where is Porterville?

Judge Roper talked to me on the phone and sent me some materials about a new program for criminal drug users called *Drug Court*. He sent me newspaper articles and information about the program and what it means to the graduates. I was immediately taken by the enthusiasm of the judge, who clearly believed in what he was talking about. My good friend, Dallas Taylor, had spoken at a previous graduation and urged me to go.

So I went to the graduation. Quite frankly, I expected to see a couple dozen addicts in a small meeting room telling about their experiences, something like an Alcoholics Anonymous meeting. Instead I was led to a large auditorium and a crowd of 1,600 people who cheered when 150 or so men and women walked down the aisle and sat on the stage.

To my left sat a uniformed highway patrol captain and members of the legal, law enforcement, and political communities, including a state senator and the mayors of every city in the county. A member of the Board of Supervisors read a proclamation. I saw a video presentation showing the before and after photos of the graduates and heard two of them tell their stories. I thought I had it bad. These people had been arrested, imprisoned, and enslaved to their drugs. At least I didn't have to go to jail as part of my recovery.

I soon realized that this was no hug-a-thug program for wayward abusers. This was a tough program of recovery from drugs and criminal offenses that was administered by a tough judge and carefully monitored by probation officers and counselors. If someone wanted a break in this program, he had to earn it.

At the graduation, Judge Roper told me that the drug court was in danger because of budget cuts. There are always budget cuts and the government program that wins out is the one with the most vocal constituency, so I volunteered to help.

With the aid of an able photographer, I made a public service announcement in Porterville. We drove around town with Dr. Lessenger, Rick McIntire, who ran the drug testing program, and several graduates. We visited the orange orchard where one family, a husband and wife who are now graduates, lived for nine months because all of their welfare money went into shooting crank into their veins. We visited a machine shop where the husband now works as a foreman and master welder and where he proudly showed me his top-notch welds. His wife is an outstanding substance abuse counselor. They had just purchased a new home and drive nice cars. While waiting in the shop, Dr. Lessenger and the graduate constructed a rough spread sheet showing the enormous savings to the taxpayers from the drug court—money saved by getting people off welfare, off disability, out of the jails and prisons, and into jobs. The savings are so great that we cannot afford to not have a drug court.

Judge Roper and Dr. Lessenger sent me an article that they had published, and I arranged to have it made available free of charge on the Internet to anybody who wants it. This article showed how the program is divided into phases and requires participants to find employment, engage in 12 Step meetings, and submit to ongoing drug testing—definitely not a hug-a-thug program.

About a year later, Judge Roper stood for office. Several low-ranking law enforcement officers and ultraconservative politicians opposed him on the grounds that he was too easy on drug offenders. Judge Roper won handily, and, through watching the campaign from a distance and reading more about drug courts and substance abuse, something became clear.

Drug courts were created by the judges. It is a response by the judges to the failure of the criminal justice system to deal with drug-related crimes. It was the judges who saw the impossible problem of chaos in the criminal drug justice system and did something about it. The legislative branch couldn't have dreamed up this program because they were blind to the problems of prison overcrowding and were afraid of being accused of being soft on crime. The executive branch—the President and governors—didn't realize that the courts and prisons had become a turnstile where people accused of drug offenses were recycled back to the streets, sometimes the same day. They were also invested in decades of failed programs and were afraid of being accused of being soft on crime or easy on drug users. The judges, who were free to change a broken system, stepped into the breach and created the only really effective criminal drug program in the history of the country. They did it with help from all segments of society, but it was the judges who took the political heat.

This book covers politics, policy, supportive services, and program funding for drug courts; the physiology and sociology of drug addiction; strategies for effective probation and for administering rewards and sanctions; and the treatment and rehabilitation of addicts. I congratulate Dr. Lessenger and Judge Roper on a prodigious effort and wish the readers well in operating their own drug courts. It is time, energy, and money well spent that reduces crime and saves money and lives.

Larry Hagman
Ojai, California, 2006

Preface

This book is for those who are operating or wishing to create a drug court, physicians who will frequently see people who are drug court clients, judges, prosecutors, treatment providers, defense attorneys, probation officers, case managers, and coordinators currently working in a drug court.

Drug courts are for nonviolent, drug-driven criminal offenders and are a judicial response to a system failure. The criminal justice systems on three continents have failed to control criminal drug use through incarceration and counseling. The courts have become revolving doors where drug offenders are arrested, processed, and returned to the streets, often within the same day, only to offend again. Alternatively, offenders are incarcerated for long periods of time. For these people, prison becomes a training ground for violent, criminal behavior. Drug courts evolved as a solution to this situation.

Drug courts use the coercive powers of the court to leverage the therapeutic abilities of drug testing and mental health professionals. What clients really want and need is a workable path to sobriety and the resulting social and psychological benefits.

Like any other disease, addiction will not automatically respond to a standard treatment. Every person is unique and will react differently to external forces and influences. Some people die from an infected hangnail, whereas others can fall from an airplane and survive. The suggestions in this book are not foolproof, and, despite our best efforts, some people will be resistant to treatment and will die in the throes of their addiction. Others will respond with miraculous changes and gain a state of happy, sustained productivity. Some will respond to treatment and cease drug abuse but maddeningly will return to drugs just when they appear to have achieved sustained sobriety. Like oncology, treatment of addicts is not for the faint of heart or those who cannot abide frustration. One must be ready for multiple relapses.

One of the pleasant surprises we encountered in writing this book was that so many people were willing to spend time and effort in writing chapters to support the drug court movement. Many of them expressed their enthusiasm in being associated with the first book for a movement that is a viable alternative to failure. Because we have so many contributors involved in this book, the reader may encounter some differences of opinion. We have retained them to stimulate thought and discussion and to recognize that there are various ways to accomplish the same goal. The opinions in this book are those of the individual contributors; we may not agree with all of them, but we found them to be enlightening, well conceived, and worth consideration. We wish to thank the contributors for their help and encouragement.

A special tribute goes to the judges who created Drug Court and who contributed to this book, especially Judge Stanley Goldstein, who helped pioneer the system and was the first drug court judge. In order to make a systemic change in a broken system, many judges took great political risks in starting drug courts.

We want to thank Rob Albano, our editor at Springer SBM, for his enthusiasm and encouragement. Chieko Hara did an excellent job taking photographs for the book. We are grateful to Amber Roper Brown, Court Roper, and Ernest Lessenger for computer and editorial assistance.

Most important, we want to thank our wives, Leslie Lessenger, PhD, and Glena Roper, JD, for their support, editorial input, and manuscript review.

James E. Lessenger, MD, FACOEM
Glade F. Roper, JD
November 2006

Contents

Contributors

Cheryl L. Asmus MA, PhD
Research Associate, Psychology, Colorado State University, Fort Collins, CO 80538, USA

Karl Auerbach, MD
Assistant Professor, Department of Environmental Medicine (Occupational Medicine Division), University of Rochester, Rochester, NY 14642, USA

Ira J. Chasnoff, MD
Professor of Clinical Pediatrics, University of Illinois Hospital, Children's Research Triangle, Chicago, IL 60601, USA

Denise E. Colombini, MA
Drug Court Director, Colorado Eighth Judicial District, Ft. Collins, CO 80525, USA

James M. Gaither, MD
Fairbanks Hospital, Indianapolis, IN 46256, USA

James P. Gray, JD
Judge, Superior Court, Santa Ana, CA 92701, USA

Helen Harberts, MA, JD
Special Assistant District Attorney, Butte County District Attorney, Oroville, CA 95965, USA

Heather R. Hayes, MEd, LPC
Counselor, Consultant, Interventionist, Private Practice, Cumming, GA 30040, USA

Cary N. Heck, PhD
Assistant Professor, Department of Criminal Justice, University of Wyoming, Laramie, WY 82070, USA

Edward L. Hendrickson, MS, LMFT, LSATP
Adjunct Faculty, Virginia Technical University, Alexandria, VA 22304, USA

Anne M. Herron, MS CRC, CASAC, NCAC II
Director, Division of State and Community Assistance, Center for Substance Abuse Treatment, Substance Abuse and Mental Health Services Administration, Rockville, MD 20852, USA

Nikita B. Katz, MD, PhD
Director, Sed Tamen Sum Foundation, Senior Lecturer in Neurology, INR/Biomed, Inc., Concord, CA 94520, USA

Olga A. Katz, MD, PhD
Clinical Instructor of Neurology, Jefferson Medical College, Neurology and Neurophysiology Associates, PC, Philadelphia, PA 19107, USA

Timothy J. Kelly, MD
Fairbanks Hospital, Indianapolis, IN 46256, USA

Lucy J. King, MD
Professor Emeritus, Psychiatry, Indiana University School of Medicine, Indianapolis, IN 46202, USA

Kathy R. Lay, PhD
Assistant Professor, School of Social Work, Indiana University, Indianapolis, IN 46220, USA

James E. Lessenger, MD, FACOEM
Consultant in Occupational Medicine, Solano County, Benicia, CA 94510, USA

Richard L. McIntire, BS
Owner, Global Testing Services, Porterville, CA 93257, USA

Steven Mandel, MD
Clinical Professor of Neurology, Jefferson Medical College, Neurology and Neurophysiology Associates, PC, Philadelphia, PA 19107, USA

Douglas B. Marlowe, JD, PhD
Director of Law and Ethics Research and Adjunct Associate Professor of Psychiatry, Treatment Research Institute, University of Pennsylvania, Philadelphia, PA 19106, USA

Hitoshi Nakaishi, MD, DMSc
Chief Executive Officer of YNMedical Co. Ltd., Former Lecturer of University of Tsukuba, Suginami-Ku, Tokyo 167-0031, Japan

Noosha Niv, PhD
Department of Psychiatry and Biobehavioral Sciences, David Geffen School of Medicine at UCLA, Los Angeles, CA 90095, USA

Dee S. Owens, MPA
CAI(Certified ARISE Interventionist), Director, Alcohol and Drug Information Center, Division of Student Affairs, Indiana University, Bloomington, IN 47406, USA

Bert Pepper, MD
Clinical Professor of Psychiatry, New York University College of Medicine, New York, NY 10956, USA

Julie M. Queler, BBA
Director, Orchid Recovery Center for Women, Palm Springs, FL 33461, USA

Dennis A. Reilly, JD
Director, Brooklyn Treatment Court, Kings Supreme Court, Second Judicial District, Brooklyn, NY 11201, USA

Glade F. Roper, JD
Judge, Superior Court of California, Tulare County, Porterville, CA 93267, USA

Aaron Roussell, BA
Department of Sociology, University of Wyoming, Laramie, WY 82070, USA

S. Alex Stalcup, MD
Medical Director, New Leaf Treatment Center, Lafayette, CA 94549, USA

Jerri E. Thompson, ICADC-II, SAP
Co-Owner, Recovery Resources and Director and Coordinator of Women's Services, A Solution thru Treatment, Education and Prevention, Inc. (ASTEP), Visalia, CA 93291, USA

Rick A. Thompson, ICADC-II, SAP
Co-Owner, Recovery Resources and CEO, A Solution thru Treatment, Education and Prevention, Inc. (ASTEP), Visalia, CA 93291, USA

Ronald R. Thrasher, PhD
Visiting Assistant Professor, Sociology Department, Oklahoma State University, Deputy Chief of Police, Stillwater, OK 74078, USA

1 Introduction to Drug Courts

Glade F. Roper

To understand the nature and purpose of drug courts, it is important to know the events and policy actions that led to the movement and the philosophical basis behind it. This chapter discusses the history of the drug abuse problem in the United States, the effects of the drug problem on the criminal justice system, and the judicial response. It explores the concept and principles behind drug courts, and looks at the Tulare County, California, program and lessons learned in starting a drug court.

A Short History of Drug Abuse in the United States

The United States has suffered three drug epidemics with profound consequences to the criminal justice system. This section discusses the three phases of the history of illegal drug use in the United States.

The First Phase

The first phase, from 1885 to 1925, started with opium and morphine, which were prescribed freely as pain relievers. Major pharmaceutical companies advertised products containing heroin, cocaine, and codeine as refreshing drinks, children's pain relievers, and cough suppressants. When it became apparent that opiate addiction was becoming widespread, physicians turned to cocaine, which was touted as a nonaddictive cure that Sigmund Freud called a "magical drug" (1).

In 1900, public health officials estimated that 250,000 Americans, about 1 in 300, were addicted to opiates, and that 200,000 were addicted to cocaine. Congress responded by passing the Harrison Narcotics Act of 1914 and other laws controlling the import of opium and coca products and their dissemination by pharmacists and physicians. At the same time, local governments passed ordinances against opium dens and cocaine joints. President Taft dubbed this effort a "War on Drugs" (1).

Publicly funded rehabilitation clinics were established, but very little was known about addiction or how to treat it. By 1925, heroin had become illegal in the United States, and half of the prisoners in the federal penitentiary at Leavenworth, Kansas (717 of 1,482), were narcotics law violators. Government interdiction was apparently successful, and by the early 1940s illegal drugs were hard to find and heavily diluted when sold. By the onset of World War II, illegal drugs had virtually disappeared from the United States (1).

The Second Phase

The second wave of drugs swept over the United States between 1950 and 1970 as a badge of status and nonconformity. Heroin use seeped from the inner city slums into middle-class homes, while superstar musicians sang about the joys of using marijuana, LSD, and cocaine. Beatniks and hippies established a counterculture embracing drug use as a rebellion against mainstream society. Federal and state governments responded with laws prohibiting the distribution, possession, and use of many different types of drugs. Law enforcement agencies were expanded, and narcotics task forces were formed. Mandatory minimum sentences for drug offenders were established. Congressman Hale Boggs of Louisiana authored legislation that mandated 2- to 5-year sentences for first-time offenders, 5 to 10 years for second-time offenders, and 10 to 20 for third-time offenders. President Eisenhower declared a second war on drugs in 1954, and the mandatory minimum sentences for drug possession were increased again to 2 to 10 years for a first-time offense, 5 to 20 years without parole for the second offense, and 10 to 40 years without parole for the third offense (1,2).

Increasing demand for drugs fueled the supply, and European sources joined traditional Oriental suppliers of opiates, while South American farmers flooded the United States with cocaine. Mobsters like Lucky Luciano made millions of dollars in the narcotics trade. The infamous French Connection distributed tons of heroin into the United States during the 1950s and 1960s, despite the best efforts to stop the flow by the Federal Bureau of Narcotics, the Central Intelligence Agency, the Federal Bureau of Investigation, the U.S. Customs Service, and numerous state law enforcement agencies. The Bureau of Drug Abuse Control and the Bureau of Narcotics and Dangerous Drugs were created (1,2).

During the Nixon years, governments had contradictory policies about the drug problem. The use of marijuana became a minor offense in many states, and federal mandatory sentences for possession of marijuana were removed. However, upon learning of the high incidence of heroin use among soldiers serving in Vietnam, many of whom continued to use after their discharge, President Nixon declared drug abuse "the number one domestic concern." Nixon created in 1973 the U.S. Drug Enforcement

Administration to enforce federal drug laws. For the first time, the federal government made a serious effort at treatment of addicts with the establishment of the White House Special Action Office for Drug Abuse Prevention, which was headed by a treatment specialist. Little was done to interdict the flow of drugs from foreign countries (1,2).

As drug use continued to grow, invading cities and causing welfare rolls to burgeon, experimentation in treatments expanded. Distribution of the synthetic opiate methadone showed promise to some researchers, whereas other experts denounced it as nothing more than legalized addiction and a mere resting point on the road to continued heroin use. Though scattered and ineffective, official attention to heroin addiction produced positive results. In 1973, heroin use declined for the first time in 6 years. As the hippie movement waned in the late 1960s, use of psychedelic drugs also declined (1–3).

The Third Phase

The latest epidemic began around 1980 with the reemergence of cocaine as a fashionable recreational drug and a new method to use it by smoking, called *free basing*. Increasing knowledge about addiction revealed that cocaine, far from providing a nonaddictive, relaxing diversion, is highly addictive, particularly when inhaled. Laboratory animals have been shown to voluntarily use cocaine to the exclusion of all other activities, including eating and sleeping, until they die (4). Exploding cocaine use proved lucrative to Colombian drug cartels. The Drug Enforcement Administration estimated in 1980 that Florida's illegal drug trafficking was a $7 billion business, surpassing tourism in dollars and making Miami substantially less attractive to tourists (5). In the spring of 1980, Fidel Castro authorized 125,000 Cubans to travel by boat to the United States, including over 7,000 criminals released from Cuban prisons. The influx of foreign drug users caused criminal drug activity to burgeon in Florida (1).

On the West Coast, methamphetamine use proliferated, and it rapidly became the drug of choice. Easy to manufacture in a small garage or mobile home and comparatively inexpensive, crank, or meth, rapidly outstripped the more expensive cocaine, heroin, and psychedelic drugs, which required more elaborate operations to manufacture. Although meth produces a high similar to that of cocaine, it lasts for hours rather than minutes (1).

Legislatures again turned to increasingly harsh mandatory minimum sentences. Although new diagnostic techniques such as positron emission tomography brain scans continued to demonstrate that addicted brains have different physical characteristics from unaddicted brains and that addiction can be appropriately designated a disease or disorder, popular misunderstanding about addiction drove legislatures to treat drug use as a criminal rather than a public health issue. The perception that government could punish addicts out of drug use prevailed (1,2).

Effects on Law Enforcement and the Judicial System

Law enforcement agencies had all they could handle in arresting and prosecuting drug offenders in Dade County, Florida, and the court and penal systems were inadequate to handle the flood of convicted drug criminals. The situation was the same throughout the United States. President Reagan designated narcotics an official threat to our national security. Congress created the Office of National Drug Control Policy in 1988. There was no place to incarcerate defendants once they had been convicted, resulting in the release of prisoners after they had served days or weeks of their long sentences (6). Associate Chief Judge Herbert Klein of Florida's Eleventh Judicial Circuit (6) explained:

> Putting more and more offenders on probation just perpetuates the problem. The same people are picked up again and again until they end up in the state penitentiary and take up space that should be used for violent offenders.

Criminal court judges became frustrated at committing the same drug offenders to jail over and over, each time seeing them in increasingly deteriorated physical condition. Placement in court-ordered treatment facilities achieved some results, but such facilities were also inadequate to handle the tide of convicted addicts. A single failure to comply with the prescribed treatment frequently resulted in revocation of probation and return to custody, which often meant release because of jail overcrowding.

The Judicial Response

Recognizing the futility of the existing system, some judges sought changes that would break the criminality–addiction vortex. One possible alternative was decriminalizing the use and possession of drugs. Support for this alternative was the recognition that the pharmaceutical cost of producing drugs is about 2% of the street price, with the 98% markup due to illegality. Proponents of decriminalization argued that decreasing the cost of drug use from hundreds or thousands of dollars per day to $5 or $10 per day would eliminate the need for addicts to steal and prostitute and would disempower criminal gangs and cartels that flourish in the underground drug market. They also pointed out that treatment has been shown to be five to seven times more effective at decreasing drug use than prosecution and incarceration, meaning that we could decriminalize drug use, reduce our resources dedicated to the war on drugs by half or more, provide drug treatment centers with the balance, and have a much greater impact on drug abuse (7,8).

Other observers advocated taxing drug sales to raise revenue for drug treatment. Still others advocated "dumping piles of drugs in the streets and letting anyone who wants them to kill themselves and good riddance." This comment was made by a friend of the author's who, although somewhat extreme in his approach, is by no means alone in his viewpoint.

Some judges have simply refused to participate further in drug cases, citing conscientious objection to imposing decades-long or lifetime sentences for addicts. Some have taken the extreme position of resigning from office rather than imposing mandatory minimum sentences (9).

Continuing budget constraints have made construction of new jails and prisons difficult, while the advisability of constructing them has been actively debated. An increasingly strong voice contends that the policy of incarcerating addicted people is not only unacceptably costly but also poor social policy. Many social critics question whether additional prisons should be built because nonviolent addicts are housed with violent antisocial offenders, causing the addicts to become educated in violent criminal behaviors (10,11).

As the cost of incarceration increased and the cost of new construction of penal facilities became prohibitive, corrections officials tried other methods of punishment, including home arrest, electronic monitoring, day reporting, and work release. Judges have also made unsupervised referrals to addiction treatment facilities. Although these actions marginally relieved the pressure on penal facilities, their value in either punishing or rehabilitating offenders is questionable. Many prisoners were released to relieve overcrowding long before they completed their sentences (11,12).

A major drawback of unsupervised referrals to addiction treatment facilities was the lack of a rapid feedback loop to the judge. It was common for months to pass before it came to the judge's attention that an offender had absconded from the facility.

For a judge, it is unacceptable to sentence repeat offenders to a year in custody only to have them released after a few weeks and immediately rearrested on new charges. Such early releases send the message to drug and alcohol addicts that there are no consequences for undesirable behavior and, in fact, may reinforce the very behavior society is attempting to extinguish. The revolving door of justice for drug use undermines the integrity of and public confidence in the criminal justice system.

Rather than abandoning the value of the criminal court system in interdicting drug use, judges and prosecutors in Florida conceived the idea of combining the coercive power of the criminal justice system with rehabilitative treatment. Coerced treatment has been found to be as effective in reducing drug use as voluntarily sought treatment (2). Most drug addicts are unhappy with their lives and want to quit using drugs but do not know how to do so. Drug treatment courts are not only humanely appealing to judges constitutionally charged with fair treatment of offenders but personally satisfying as they see positive, observable changes in offenders who achieve abstinence, become employed, reunite with their families, complete their educations, and resume normal lifestyles. As a result, drug courts have proliferated. The first drug court began in Miami in 1989. By 1999, over 470 drug courts were functioning across the nation with another 200 in the planning stages. By 2005, over 1,600 drug courts were operational, and almost 500 more were being organized (13).

Concept of Drug Court

Although specific methods vary, all drug courts use the same basic approach. Addicted offenders are identified and assessed for amenability to treatment. Certain classes of offenders are excluded because of the nature of their charges. For example, defendants with a history of sex offenses, violent offenses, possession of illegal or dangerous weapons, or with an extensive nondrug-related criminal history are generally excluded. Most drug courts do not accept defendants charged with sale of drugs or possession of drugs for sale; however, it should be noted that because of the high cost of drugs, most drug users are also drug sellers. Many drug courts have successfully dealt with offenders who have been convicted of selling small quantities of drugs to support their own drug addiction.

Instead of incarceration, offenders are referred to treatment programs and closely supervised by court personnel. Offenders may be referred prior to entering a plea, or they may be sent to treatment as a term of probation after pleading guilty. They are tested frequently for drug use, and sanctions are imposed for deviation from the treatment program. The judge is a critical part of the process, and most drug courts require the participants to return to court to report on their progress. In addition to negative sanctions for violations, positive rewards are presented for milestones of progress. Treatment providers, probation officers, county addiction personnel, or specialized drug court caseworkers closely supervise the clients.

The success and benefits of a specialized court process for nonviolent, drug-addicted offenders are well documented. Numerous studies have demonstrated that when drug offenders are incarcerated after conviction, recidivism is the norm rather than the exception. According to a U.S. Department of Justice study, 50.47% of drug offenders were rearrested for a new offense within 3 years of release from custody. By 1994, that number had grown to 66.7%. Almost every penal facility in the country has exceeded its maximum designed capacity, as drug arrests and convictions increased over 10 times between 1980 and 1996 (14).

Drug courts have demonstrated lower recidivism rates. Although with a wide variance in reported results, almost every study of drug courts has shown reduced recidivism in drug court participants both during and after participating in a drug court as compared with incarceration (5,15).

Although the success of drug courts has been remarkable, the cost of implementing them is always a challenge. Placing offenders in treatment programs saves the cost of incarceration, but the treatment, usually a fraction of the cost of jail or prison, must be financed. For example, in

California it costs approximately $26,000 to incarcerate one person for a year in the state prison system, while the cost of a year in a county jail varies between $12,500 and $40,000. Effective treatment for a year can cost as little as $3,000. Testing and supervision are critical elements of drug court, and each incurs a significant cost (16,17).

Drug Court Principles

There are seven principles on which drug courts are based:

1. Retaining the participant in treatment through the pain of withdrawal.
2. Helping the participant overcome fear, craving, and shame.
3. Providing modulated and immediate sanctions.
4. Discriminating between behavior and addiction symptoms.
5. Providing a system of rewards.
6. Understanding that whether an act constitutes a punishment or a reward depends on the perception of the recipient.
7. Dismissing charges as a reward.

Retaining the Participant in Treatment Through Withdrawal

Although treatment of addicts is effective, the pain of withdrawal from drug use in the early stages of recovery from addiction is so intense that most people will avoid it by returning to drug use unless coerced to remain in treatment. In drug court, a judge has the power to impose significant sanctions sufficient to coerce people to remain in treatment. The judge, prosecutor, defense counsel, probation department, and addiction treatment providers contribute their skills to craft a treatment program that will nurture and support the person seeking recovery while providing sufficient structure and guidance through the difficult path to recovery.

Overcoming Fear, Craving, and Shame

Addiction has physical, emotional, and psychological consequences, all of which trigger dysphoria when drug use ceases. Dysphoria is an intolerable state of anxiety, depression, and discomfort that demands action to alleviate the undesirable feelings. Dysphoria is an inherent defense mechanism of all animals that provides a physiologic drive to resolve the undesirable state. It is generally associated with processes that will ensure survival. For example, hunger or thirst creates a demand for food or water to eliminate the dysphoria. A person in a compelling state of hunger will think of little else except how to obtain food to eliminate the hunger.

When the natural survival processes go awry, serious, debilitating conditions result. For example, one of the most serious problems facing the

United States today is obesity. Most overweight people recognize their obvious condition and desperately desire to remedy it. Millions of dollars are spent on various methods to help people lose weight; most of these yield no results. The logical answer is simple: eat less. Yet when faced with the compelling hunger associated with eating less, most people succumb and eat until the hunger is satisfied. No amount of self-berating guilt, shame, or desire will counteract the compulsion of acute hunger for many people.

A drug user who attempts to stop using drugs will suffer intense cravings similar to acute hunger. The cravings are overpowering and intolerable and in some instances will be accompanied by physical pain, particularly in the case of withdrawal from opiates and alcohol. Most people will seek to escape the intense adverse effects of withdrawal if they possibly can. The most obvious and readily available method of doing so is to return to illicit drug use, a response with which they are familiar that has proved satisfactory in the past.

Studies have shown that the minimum dose–response time for recovery is 3 months of treatment. Those receiving less than 3 months of treatment derive no measurable benefit (18). Those remaining in treatment the longest were the most likely to reduce or eliminate drug abuse after treatment. The intensity of withdrawal cravings will attenuate over time, although they may unexpectedly come back with renewed intensity after a period of relative calm. A client who is strongly invested in treatment and who can seek the help of his or her trained counselor during times of acute craving is better able to withstand the cravings and apply abstinence techniques learned in treatment than one who is not presently involved in treatment.

The principal value of a drug court is the ability to encourage and pressure addicts to remain in treatment through periods of dysphoria. The most effective pressure is applied by sanctions or punishments that, while undesirable themselves, also serve as a reminder of the more significant and longer punishments that will result from abandoning treatment and returning to drug use. Rewards for adhering to the treatment and recovery plan have been shown to be much more effective at retaining people in treatment than have punishments (18).

Humans are imbued with an inherent fight or flight or stress response to frightening or threatening stimuli. A person who seeks recovery but succumbs to severe cravings and returns to illegal drug use will immediately suffer feelings of guilt and shame. Shame in particular seems to contribute to an inability to refrain from continued drug use (19). The failure to refrain from drug use, followed by feelings of guilt, shame, and fear, will provoke the flight response, and drug court participants will be inclined to flee rather than to appear in court to face undesired consequences. This flight response can be very powerful, even overwhelming, especially when combined with cravings and pain from withdrawal. Past experience with punishment in courtrooms has taught many addicts that it is much easier to flee than to return to court and face the frightening prospects of punishment from the judge along with more cravings (18).

It is necessary for a drug court judge to understand the overpowering fear and craving experienced by those in early recovery and to understand that most addicts cannot simply stop using drugs. Although there are many and varied definitions of addiction, they all include elements of uncontrollable, compulsive drug-seeking behavior and use, even in the face of extremely negative health and social consequences (20). Simply stated, if a drug user can quit when the consequences of drug use become too undesirable, they are not addicted.

Although drug courts can benefit unaddicted offenders by persuading them to stop using drugs, most nonaddicted people will cease using drugs when faced with the undesirable consequences imposed by the traditional criminal justice system. It is the addicted persons, those who are unable to stop using drugs despite a burning desire to do so, who are most benefited by a drug court. Many have desperately tried time after time to cease their drug use as they observed their own physical, emotional, spiritual, mental, and social deterioration but have been unable to do so. Often they have been afforded access to addiction treatment but were unable to force themselves to remain in treatment long enough to benefit from it. Those remaining in treatment longer are less likely to return to drug use (21).

Modulated and Immediate Sanctions

The most important function of drug courts is the ability to impose appropriately modulated sanctions within a short period of time. An appropriately modulated response is critically important. Judges are frequently faced with the unpleasant task of either crushing a defendant with a heavy sentence or imposing an excessively light punishment or no punishment at all. The ability to use a range of sanctions allows a response commensurate with the violation that will neither leave the participant feeling that there is no consequence for undesirable behavior nor that he was treated with unfair severity. Excessively light responses breed continued violations; excessive severity that is perceived as unfair causes abandonment of the program.

An immediate response to any departure from the treatment protocol is important so that the client will associate the sanction with the undesirable behavior. Waiting weeks or months between the behavior and the response causes the participant to lose the connection and to associate the response with some later behavior or, even worse, with no behavior, leaving a feeling that the system is simply punishing for the sake of punishing.

A properly structured drug court will allow the treatment team to craft a response that is forceful enough to correct the problem but not so harsh as to cause the participant to flee or to give up. If an excessively harsh or otherwise inappropriate punishment is imposed, such as remanding a participant to jail for every drug use, an unaddicted person may be persuaded to stop using and to complete the treatment. An addicted person will likely sense the futility of continuing and run away. If every gain is lost with every misstep, no progress will be made.

Discriminating Between Behavior and Addiction Symptoms

It is important to distinguish between behavior violations and addiction symptoms. No one would seriously argue that a patient who goes to a physician for an infection should be terminated from treatment and punished if the first antibiotic prescribed does not cure the infection. The doctor would continue to work with a patient, trying various antibiotics or other treatments until the patient recovers as long as the patient is compliant with the treatment protocol. If the patient refuses to take pills or to change bandages, the physician would be justified in terminating the relationship. As long as the patient does what the doctor directs, however, it would be unthinkable to send the patient away just because the medicine does not cure the disease.

Similarly, if the participant in the drug court refuses to attend the counseling sessions, continues to live with other drug users, fails to test, or fails to attend scheduled court appearances, punishment is appropriate. If such behaviors continue, it would ultimately be appropriate to terminate the participant from the drug court. There is no reason to waste valuable and scarce resources on a client who will not comply with the treatment protocol. It is, however, unreasonable, unrealistic, and unethical to punish someone who is fully compliant with all drug court requirements but continues to suffer the symptoms of addiction, including drug use. Additional and more intensive treatment may be necessary, such as moving from outpatient to residential treatment. However, punishing a client who is following the program as instructed but does not respond to the treatment as desired will cause hostility, frustration, helplessness, and abandonment.

System of Rewards

Drug courts can foster continued involvement in treatment and recovery through a system of rewards. Although short-term changes in behavior can be enforced through punishments, for many people behavior will revert to the baseline when the punishments cease. There are also unwanted side effects from imposing punishments, such as hostility and resistance (22). Punishing effectively is an art that many lack, and attempts at punishment leave the client feeling angry, frustrated, hostile, and resentful. Punishment teaches only what not to do, not what should be done.

A more effective way to induce long-term changes in behavior is through a system of rewards. The most effective rewards are those inherent in the behavior, but artificial rewards can be used in the short term until inherent rewards are realized. The life of a clandestine, illegal drug user is horrible. One has only to enter *methamphetamine* into any Internet search engine to retrieve a host of horrific photographs showing extreme dental decay and oral infections, gaunt, frightening images of users who appear skeletal compared with photographs taken prior to drug use, and hideous examples of infected arms and faces clawed by addicts seeking to alleviate the sensation of insects crawling under their skin. Although repairing abscessed gums and removing broken, decayed teeth may take months, in general the health of drug users begins to improve markedly as soon as they cease drug use. Once the inherent rewards of abstinence manifest themselves, there is constant reaffirmation for remaining engaged in recovery. Until then, artificial rewards can assist many people to make it through the difficult withdrawal.

One of the reasons that participating in drug court has been so satisfying for judges is the stark contrast between their experience in repeatedly imposing punishments on the same people for the same offenses and their experience in seeing participants in drug court change to law-abiding, clean and sober people who are employed and happy. The traditional approach of punishment to stop drug use has been ineffective. If punishment were effective at stopping drug use, drugs would have been eradicated long ago. The combination of appropriate punishment and rewards for productive changes has rendered great results in drug courts.

A Punishment or a Reward Depends on the Perception of the Recipient

Whether an act by the judge constitutes a punishment or a reward depends on how the act is perceived by the recipient, not on the intent of the deliverer. What is intended as a punishment may be perceived as a reward, and an intended reward may be viewed as a punishment. For example, one young man who was sentenced to participate in the author's program was entitled to receive a special mug with the drug court logo on it for completing the first 6 months of treatment. He had complied with the requirements but had always appeared stoic, uninterested and somewhat resistant at review hearings. When the mug was offered to him as a reward, he said, with some hostility, "I don't want it, or any of the other things you hand out. I would just throw them away. I just want out of here, and you will never see me again as soon as I am done." He apparently perceived the small rewards offered as an insult rather than an encouraging reward. Ten months later at the community graduation ceremony, after he had completed the program, this same young man came to the author and said, with apparent sincerity, "I just wanted to thank you for helping me. I never told you in court, but I am very grateful for the opportunity to participate in the drug court and all you did for me." Although he was resistant to participate in the drug court, considering it a punishment, he came to consider it a reward after experiencing the benefits of sobriety.

Dismissal of Charges as a Reward

Many drug offenders will be attracted to a drug court by the potential of an ultimate reward, having the charges against them dismissed or expunged. This is not true of every potential participant, as many have lengthy criminal records and have spent years behind bars. However, a benefit for all participants, and a probable motivator to some degree, is the possibility of having their charges reduced, dismissed, or expunged after completing the drug court process.

Political ramifications differ in every jurisdiction, but, if it is politically palatable, it makes sense to provide some form of ultimate reward for those who complete the program successfully. The clients have made a difficult decision, struggled through withdrawal, and invested a great deal of time, money, and effort. They have saved the taxpayers thousands or tens of thousands of dollars and have reduced the probability that they will return with new charges. Yet these successful clients are now hampered in their desire to reintegrate into mainstream society by their criminal records, which impair their ability to obtain meaningful employment. It seems a small cost with great benefit to provide them with a way to eliminate or reduce the severity of their criminal record.

Expansion of Drug Courts

After the first bold step in Dade County, Florida, in 1989, the concept of drug courts spread with increasing rapidity. Two years later there were five drug courts, a number that doubled every year for the next 5 years. Over 100 new drug courts were added during the next 3 years, then almost 200 per year from 1999 to 2003. Nearly 500 new drug courts opened in 2004, with 500 more in the planning stages (13). One federal district court in New York has implemented a drug court.

Once the efficacy of the treatment court paradigm was demonstrated, translation to other criminal justice problems followed. Juvenile court systems, inundated with children who have been removed from their homes for neglect or abuse, became the next extension. When drug use by the parents is the root of the problem, there may be insufficient evidence to justify the filing of criminal charges, but the drug use must be addressed or the abuse and neglect will continue. Family or dependency drug courts allow the court to address the parents' addiction so that children can ultimately be returned to a stable, drug-free home. In addition, 357 juvenile drug courts help drug users or addicts under the age of 18 years escape the downward spiral of drug use before they have to face the adult criminal system.

According to the National Highway Traffic Safety Administration, there were 16,694 deaths from alcohol-related traffic crashes in 2004, with another 248,000 injured. Approximately 1.4 million drivers were arrested for driving under the influence of alcohol or some other drug in 2003. Of drivers involved in alcohol-related fatal crashes, 86% had a blood alcohol level of 0.08% or higher (23). Recognizing the serious threat intoxicated drivers pose to society, 176 jurisdictions have created special driving-under-the-influence courts to treat drivers convicted of driving while impaired by alcohol or some other drug.

Because over 600,000 prisoners are released from prison every year, many with serious, untreated drug addictions, reentry drug courts have been established to help them reintegrate into society. This concept is particularly valuable, because recently paroled people have a difficult time seeking employment and many have been denied any form of public assistance because of their criminal records. With no other form of sustenance, they turn to theft, prostitution, or drug sales to support themselves; they resume drug use to escape the unpleasant realities of life. Many have continued their drug use while imprisoned and have learned advanced criminal behaviors. Reentry drug courts can break the cycle of criminality and imprisonment, particularly if they assist with training in the life skills necessary to function in society.

Native American tribes have established tribal healing-to-wellness courts to assist members. These courts incorporate cultural values specific to the particular tribe to deal with substance abuse. Many reservations have been inordinately affected by substance abuse, and the healing-to-wellness courts can overcome cultural barriers in state-run criminal courts. Because they have sovereign status, tribes can implement the courts in a fashion that will not conflict with traditional customs and values.

Other "problem-solving courts" have been implemented to combine the power of a judicial or quasijudicial officer with treatment programs. Perpetrators of domestic violence, people with illegal weapons, compulsive gamblers, homeless persons, the mentally ill, habitually truant minors, and juveniles who engage in minor offenses have all been the subject of specialized courts that seek to address the root problem rather than simply impose punishment. Colorado State University and Indiana University have implemented special programs within their existing campus judicial systems to deal with thousands of university students who succumb to excessive alcohol and other drug use, derailing their academic careers and costing universities millions in lost tuition and fees every year. Rather than being terminated and expelled, offending students are sent to appropriate treatment and closely supervised.

All these problem-solving courts have shown results superior to the conventional approach of imposing a punishment and expecting the offender to translate the punishment into improved behavior. People caught in the descending spiral of destructive behaviors such as drug addiction, domestic violence, and theft frequently want to return to a state of normal, law-abiding behavior and to escape the enslavement of their addictions but do not know how. Years of drug use, a history of sexual or physical abuse, poverty, mental illness, and ignorance have taken a toll on their ability to make rational choices and decisions and to adapt their behavior to accepted social norms. Problem-solving courts can assist them with support, training, treatment, and incentives to achieve what they cannot do alone.

Lessons Learned in the Tulare County Program

Tulare County is located in California's rural, agriculture-rich San Joaquin Valley. It is one of the most productive agricultural counties in the nation. Much of the agriculture is dependent on migrant farm workers, many of whom live at a subsistence income level. Many residents live in poverty, and significant social problems challenge the county government. The rates of teenage pregnancy and unemployment are high, and a significant amount of money is expended on public assistance (24).

Beginning in 1990, Tulare County experienced a rapid increase in arrests for drug offenses, principally due to the influx of methamphetamine. It was comparatively easy to manufacture locally with readily available chemicals, as opposed to cocaine and heroin, which require importation of substances usually grown or manufactured outside the country. With an investment of $5,000, methamphetamine dealers can quickly turn a profit of up to $100,000. The addictive properties of methamphetamine rapidly ensnared thousands of people of all ages throughout the county. In increasing numbers, the courts sentenced drug offenders, many of whom were seriously addicted, to jail. As inmate populations grew, the jail facilities were unable to accommodate them, and prisoners were released early from their sentences. More serious offenders were sent to the state prison and returned to Tulare County on parole, usually to reoffend.

It became obvious to county judges that the standard practice of incarcerating addicts was a poor use of public funds. A meeting was held involving law enforcement, the judiciary, county government, and mental health officials; a judge and probation official from a neighboring county presented the concept of a drug court and provided convincing testimonials of its success. Many of those who attended the meeting were excited about the concept, and a series of planning meetings was held in which there was mixed support and opposition. Although there was a high level of support from the court, the probation department, local treatment providers, and the mental health department, there was vocal opposition from the district attorney's office and law enforcement. The general feeling was that no funds were available with which to implement the program.

It was the opinion of the judges that no additional judicial resources would be required because the defendants would either be involved in the drug court or proceed through the routine criminal process. If the drug court option induced only a few defendants to plead guilty without proceeding to jury trials, a large amount of court time and money would be saved. Probation officers assigned to each division of the court were willing to assume the additional burden of administering the program. The major obstacle was funding for drug treatment. Although the county alcohol and drug program administrators expressed support for the concept, they indicated they had no funds to contribute toward treatment.

Despite the existence of several alcohol-rehabilitation programs, there was little knowledge of treatment for nonalcohol drug addiction in the county. The owner of the local program for alcohol offenders proposed that participants be sent to this program, with modifications, and that they pay the cost of their treatment. At first this seemed unrealistic, as most people in the county with untreated addiction were thought to be destitute. The argument was made that if addicts are paying up to $200 per day for drugs, they could afford to pay $50 per week for treatment. The difficulty with this argument was that they were stealing, prostituting, or selling drugs to finance their own drug use, all of which the court wanted to eradicate. However, another treatment provider, himself in recovery, indicated that such behaviors are inconsistent with the process of recovery and that addicts would not steal, sell drugs, or prostitute to pay for recovery. Another judge with experience in a drug court laughed out loud when presented with that idea, saying, "Addicts are not going to waste their money from stealing on treatment!"

Many offenders had jobs and could be expected to use income that in the past had been used to buy drugs to pay for treatment. It was discovered later in a retrospective study that approximately 70% of the drug court clients had jobs at the time of their arrest and continued to work while in the program, many in state jobs (25).

With no other resources to draw on, the court was faced with the harsh reality of either starting the program by having participants pay for their own treatment or not having a drug court at all. Given those options, it seemed preferable to experiment with self-funded treatment rather than abandoning the concept entirely. With an uncertain future, the drug court began.

Potential participants were identified by the judges and referred to the probation officer for an interview in which the program was explained and background information about the defendant obtained. If the probation officer determined the defendant was interested in changing his or her life and embracing recovery and could pay the cost of treatment, the defendant was offered drug court. Formal terms of probation were signed that constituted an agreement to comply with the drug court requirements. The defendant was referred back to the judge and sentenced into the drug court.

Almost every participant was referred initially to an outpatient program. Several were determined to be unable to benefit from outpatient treatment and were referred to existing residential programs. Those who could not abstain from drug use after several weeks of outpatient treatment were also referred to residential treatment. Because of long waiting lists, participants referred to residential treatment were frequently required to wait in jail for several months until a bed became available. Experience showed that over 90% of participants who graduated were able to succeed with outpatient treatment.

The original program design consisted of a 1-year program divided into three phases. Phase one treatment required two 90-minute group sessions, 1 hour of individual counseling, and attendance at two, 12 Step self-help meetings each week. Participants came to court every week and showed proof on a card provided by the treatment provider of attendance at 12 Step meetings. The counselors assigned to the participants filled out a simple, 1-page form indicating progress for the week. This report was provided to the court the day before the scheduled hearing and placed in the file by the court clerk.

Prior to each drug court session, the treatment providers met with the judge and probation officer to discuss every participant and appropriate responses to deviations from treatment. Prosecutors and defense attorneys were invited to attend, but the district attorney and public defender chose not to, considering supervision of the participants to be the province of the court and probation. Each participant was called individually before the court to discuss progress, to make changes to the treatment program, and to receive a reward for good behavior or a sanction for undesirable behavior. The counselors performed drug testing as they felt necessary.

Participants were given the option of voluntarily leaving the program and accepting the punishment that would have been imposed had they initially decided not to participate. They were not punished with greater terms of incarceration because they attempted to go through treatment.

Initially, phase one lasted a minimum of 2 months. Advancement to phase two required at least 30 days' abstinence from drug abuse and substantial compliance with all treatment requirements. The only change between phase one and phase two was a 2-week interval between court appearances.

In phase three individual counseling sessions were reduced to every other week, with monthly court appearances. If the participants had been clean and sober for at least 180 days at the end of the 7 months of phase three, they graduated out of the drug court. They remained on probation but were encouraged to apply for early termination of probation.

Few offenders were terminated involuntarily, as the goal of the program was to keep the participants engaged in treatment as long as they were making progress. This was a subjective decision that was made by the judge after input from the treatment program and the probation officer. More frequently, participants voluntarily asked to be sent to jail or prison because they were unwilling or unable to continue to pay the cost of treatment or to abide by the strict requirements. About one fourth of those beginning the drug court were terminated without successful graduation.

Subsequent Refinements

The drug court proved immediately effective in reducing drug use and motivating participants toward accepting and embracing recovery. Experience also quickly revealed that many changes were necessary to improve outcomes. Because the treatment was based on the classic 12 Step model, mandatory attendance was increased to five meetings per week until a sponsor was obtained and then reduced to four meetings per week for the duration of the program. More emphasis was placed on completion of the 12 Step process and knowledge of the meaning of each step. Phase one was increased to 13 weeks, phase two remained at 13 weeks, and phase three was reduced to 26 weeks.

Additional treatment providers approached the court, wanting to be involved. Initially, all were accepted until it became apparent that some programs were substandard, so standards were adopted for all participating programs. Programs must now have certified treatment counselors, and, although most programs are certified by the state, some faith-based programs participate that have chosen not to be certified and regulated by the state. The court and probation department monitor those programs closely.

Inconsistencies in urinary testing were a concern. Different programs tested at different frequencies. There were also allegations that some counselors were not observing the collection of samples. Different laboratories and testing methodologies were used, and their reports followed varying formats that were hard to decipher in court. Varying cut-off levels between laboratories meant that participants were treated unequally after using drugs. To overcome this disparity, a protocol was developed and a solicitation was made for proposals from testing companies. One company was selected, and all participants were sent to a central testing location.

Each participant was assigned to a testing group based on the phase of treatment. Every morning every participant is expected to call the testing agency between 7:00 and 9:00 am and listen to a recorded message indicating which groups are to be tested that day. The short message lasts less than 30 seconds, so it requires only a very brief call. When a participant's group number was announced, he or she would go into the office and leave a urine sample before 5:00 pm that same day. The expectation is that they will begin the day focused on what is required for recovery.

There was a learning curve in the program regarding urinary drug testing. Participants tried various scams to avoid giving a positive drug test. There was an initial reluctance on the part of the court to have confidence in drug test results, thinking there might be another reason for a positive result. These hurdles were overcome by using a drug testing company that had a recovering addict on its staff who knew every trick in the book. A protocol was developed to minimize substitution or adulteration of a specimen. The second problem, lack of confidence in the results, was overcome by experience and consultation with a physician knowledgeable in the interpretation of drug-testing results.

Originally, various sanctions were imposed for missed tests, and up to 10% of participants failed to test on designated days. A wide range of excuses were given for missing tests, from death of relatives to malfunctioning vehicles. Because testing was such a critical part of drug court supervision, the sanction of incarceration was finally imposed for missing each test and compliance increased dramatically. It was explained to the participants that a positive test was seen as a clinical issue that indicated the need for increased treatment. Failure to test was treated as a behavioral issue, because it prevented the treatment provider from knowing whether or not the participant was responding to treatment. At present, less than 1% of participants fail to test as scheduled. The drug court judge has joked openly that sending people to jail for missing tests has tremendously improved the health of the participants' relatives and vehicles.

The philosophy of the drug court now is that behavioral issues are treated with punishment, whereas failure to maintain abstinence and drug use are considered treatment issues. Sanctions are intended to encourage compliance rather than to punish participants. A standard sanction list was adopted as a minimum response to deviations from treatment. These minimum sanctions are the general rule, with agreed upward departures imposed for aggravated violations.

Most clients responded more favorably to rewards than to sanctions, and the court adopted the goal of having participants feel better about themselves when they left the program than when they entered. Verbal accolades were freely given and small steps recognized. The courtroom audience was encouraged to applaud for milestones of sobriety, such as 30, 60, 90, or 180 days. As a humorous interlude, one participant was presented with a toy beach ball upon moving from phase one to phase two. Everyone laughed, but when the next participant was advanced, he asked, "Where's my beach ball?" It became the standard procedure to award participants small "trinkets" for milestones, most of which were obtained without cost. Court personnel donate miniature bottles of shampoo or lotion and bars of soap from hotel stays, and these are presented to recognize periods of sobriety. Pens, pencils, key chains, and similar useful items that are picked up on vacation trips are given freely to recognize improvement.

As the success of the program became apparent, other donations were received and used as rewards. A nonprofit foundation was created with a board of local community leaders that support the concept of recovery rather than incarceration. Although donations are not actively solicited, the foundation has received over $10,000 in donations. A business owner who employs a participant in a key position donated $500 to purchase key rings with a drug court logo and the message, "Recovery is a process that lasts a lifetime." The key rings are awarded to participants moving into phase two. The drug testing company donated mugs with a drug court logo to be presented to participants moving into phase three. Rotary clubs donated T-shirts with a logo to those graduating from the program. Some graduates donated to the foundation, giving between $5 and $100 dollars for each year of sobriety.

A significant number of the initial graduates experienced relapse, and counselors indicated that many felt a sense of abandonment when involvement in the program ended suddenly. To remedy this, a 6-month aftercare phase was added. The additional 6 months of involvement reduced relapse rates and allowed a more attenuated severance from the drug court and a cushioned release rather than an abrupt drop.

As a further reward to the graduates, an annual graduation ceremony has been held. Prominent figures in recovery have been keynote speakers, including musicians David Crosby, Joe Walsh, and Dallas Taylor and actors Larry Hagman, Art Linkletter, Mackenzie Phillips, and Todd Bridges. Up to 3,000 people attend the annual graduations, which are emotional events for participants, family members, and interested members of the community. Dignitaries, including law enforcement officials, prosecutors, legislators, city council members, and mayors, routinely attend and shake hands with the graduates.

The initial goal was to accept no more than 50 people into the program and then evaluate success. Because the positive effect was so immediately apparent, the population quickly rose above 50. Because participants pay their own cost of treatment, each additional participant adds only a small incremental burden on the system, principally in court time needed to review their cases. Larger populations increase the efficiency of the program because of economies of scale. For example, larger numbers help keep the cost of testing low, as fixed costs for the testing agency are spread among more clients. The treatment providers are able to add more counselors as needed to accommodate larger client bases. By early 2004, over 500 people were participating in the program.

The approach in Tulare County has been that if the drug court is to have a significant impact on the drug problem, as many people as possible should be directed into treatment. A system was developed whereby prosecutors, using agreed upon criteria, screened every offender and completed a form indicating whether the offender was eligible to participate in the program. If eligible, the program was offered at the first pretrial conference, encouraging an early settlement of the case and avoiding additional court hearings.

The concept that people can and will pay for the cost of their addiction treatment has flourished and enabled hundreds of people every year to avoid jail, embrace recovery, and return to a normal lifestyle. After 10 years, no evidence has come forth that any participant has committed theft, drug sales, or prostitution to pay for treatment.

The response of law enforcement was at first hostile. As graduation ceremonies, statistical studies, and word of mouth demonstrated the value of drug courts, many police officers and sheriff's deputies came to respect the program. Ironically, most senior law enforcement officers were open minded, freely admitting that nothing had worked before so why not try something different. Junior officers who worked the streets were angry at discovering that people they had worked hard to incarcerate were back on the streets and in some "do gooder" program. Over time, junior officers came to recognize the value of drug court, especially after participants sought them out to thank them for arresting them. Eventually, law enforcement officers were enlisted in a community effort to help the participants by giving them positive messages when they were encountered. Many officers came to appreciate their arrests of drug offenders as a therapeutic intervention.

Results

Anecdotal evidence indicated that the drug court was a huge success. To verify this, the Tulare County courts commissioned a statistical study of the first 3 years of operation. Every drug offender considered for placement in the drug court was tracked from the entrance interview to the close of the study period. Studied subjects were divided into four groups for research purposes, depending on their involvement in the program: (1) those who were considered for the drug court but found unsuitable, (2) those who were found suitable and offered the drug court but declined to participate, (3) those who began participating in the drug court but either left voluntarily to do custody time or were terminated involuntarily, and (4) those who successfully graduated from the drug court (24).

Five percent of the graduates were convicted of new drug charges during the course of the 3-year study period as compared with nearly 41% of those who were rejected for admission into the drug court and 27% of those who were found suitable but declined. In interpreting these figures, it is important to note that those who graduated were at liberty the entire 3-year period (except for some short-term incarcerations as sanctions). Those who were rejected or who declined spent all or a large part of the 3-year period in custody, where they were much less likely to be arrested for new drug charges (Table 1.1). Validating the probation officers' skill in sorting out violent offenders, only one person selected for drug court was convicted of a violent crime, and five of those rejected were convicted of violent crimes.

Because no funds are available to do a follow-up study, there is no current information about outcomes after 10 years of operation. It is the sense of the drug court team that the successful trend has continued but that recidivism of the graduates has probably increased to between 20% and 30%, which is consistent with other studies of programs around the

TABLE 1.1. Percentages of criminal recidivism after 3 years, Tulare County, California (N = 459).

Outcome	Rejected	Declined	Terminated	Graduated
Nondrug conviction	22.2	20.0	16.5	2.8
Drug conviction	40.7	27.0	21.5	5.0
County jail time	37.8	32.4	24.7	3.5
State prison time	19.8	9.5	8.2	1.4
Driver's license suspended	84.7	67.6	61.9	6.4

Source: Lessenger et al. (25).

nation. The stark difference between a 30% recidivism rate for drug court graduates after 10 years and a 70% to 80% recidivism rate for incarcerated offenders after 2 years demonstrates the need for more drug courts.

References

1. Jonnes J. Hep-Cats, Narcs, and Pipe Dreams: A History of America's Romance With Illegal Drugs. New York: Scribner; 1996.
2. White WL. Slaying the Dragon: A History of Addiction Treatment and Recovery in America. Bloomington, IL: Chestnut Health System/Lighthouse Institute; 1998.
3. Inaba DS, Cohen WE. Uppers, Downers, and All Arounders: Physical and Mental Effects of Psychoactive Drugs. Ashland, OR: CNS Publications; 1997.
4. Kalivas PW, Duffy P, DuMars LA, Skinner C. Behavioral and neurochemical effects of acute and daily cocaine administration in rats. J Pharmacol Exp Ther 1088;245(2):485–492.
5. U.S. Department of Justice: Recidivism of prisoners released in 1983. Washington, DC: Office of Justice Programs, Bureau of Justice Statistics, U.S. Department of Justice; 1989.
6. Hora PF, Schma WG, Rosenthal JTA. Therapeutic jurisprudence and the drug treatment movement: revolutionizing the criminal justice system's response to drug abuse and crime in America. Notre Dame Law Rev 1999;74(2):439–537.
7. Lynch T. War no more. National Review February 5, 2001.
8. Buckley WF. The war on drugs is lost. National Review February 12, 1996.
9. Association of the Bar of the City of New York, Special Committee on Drugs and Law. A Wiser Course: Ending Drug Prohibition. New York: Association of the Bar of the City of New York; 1994.
10. Caher J. Federal judge blasts mandatory minimal sentences. New York Law Journal January 20, 2006.
11. Becker FS, Murphy KM, Grossman M. The Economic Theory of Illegal Goods: The Case of Drugs. NBER working paper no. 10976. Cambridge, MA: National Bureau of Economic Research; 2004.
12. U.S. Department of Justice. Drug and Crime Facts, 1994. Washington, DC: Bureau of Justice Statistics, U.S. Department of Justice; 2004.
13. Huddleston CW, Freeman-Wilson K, Marlow DB, Roussel A. Painting the Current Picture: A National Report Card on Drug Courts and Other

Problem-Solving Programs in the United States. Alexandria, VA: National Drug Court Institute; 2005.
14. Mumola CJ. Substance Abuse and Treatment, State and Federal Prisoners, 1997. Washington, DC: Bureau of Justice Statistics, U.S. Department of Justice; 1999.
15. Belenko S. Research on drug courts: a critical review. Natl Drug Court Rev 1998;1(1):1–42.
16. Belenko S. Research on drug courts: a critical review. New York: The National Center on Addiction and Substance Abuse, Columbia University; 2001.
17. The California Department of Alcohol and Drug Programs, The Judicial Council of California, Administrative Office of the Courts. Drug Court Partnership Act of 1998, Chapter 1007, Statues of 1998, Final Report. Sacramento, CA: California Department of Alcohol and Drug Programs; 2002.
18. National Institute of Drug Abuse. Principles of Drug Addiction Treatment: A Research-Based Guide. Washington, DC: National Institute of Drug Abuse; 1999
19. Dearing RL, Stuewig J, Tangney JP. The secret message of shame. Addict Behav 2005;30(7):1392–1404.
20. Leshner AI. The Essence of Drug Addiction. Washington, DC: National Institute of Drug Abuse; 2005.
21. Substance Abuse and Mental Health Services Administration. Services Outcomes Research Survey. Washington, DC: U.S. Department of Health and Human Services; 2004.
22. Tucker-Ladd CE. Psychological Self-Help. Cleveland, OH: Mental Health Net, 2000.
23. National Highway Traffic Safety Administration. Traffic Safety Facts, 2004 Data. Washington, DC: National Center for Statistics and Analysis, National Highway Traffic Safety Administration, August 2005.
24. Bureau of the United States Census. 2000 United States Census. Washington, DC: Government Printing Office, 2002.
25. Lessenger JE, Lessenger LH, Lessenger EW. An outcome analysis of drug court in Tulare County, California. Visalia, CA: Tulare County Superior Court, 2000.

2
The Disease of Addiction

S. Alex Stalcup

Addiction is a disease of the pleasure-producing chemistry of the brain. Drugs of abuse share the ability to activate the chemical pathways in the brain. When active, they yield feelings of well-being, pleasure, and euphoria. By overstimulating the pleasure system, the drugs cause neuron-adaptive changes that damage the normal experience of pleasure (1).

Pleasure is a developmentally ancient sensation that is essential to survival. Virtually all organisms possess pleasure chemistry, located in the same midbrain region and activated by the same stimuli. Pleasure serves to reinforce behaviors that benefit the individual and the species. Natural reinforcers, naturally occurring stimuli that activate pleasure chemistry, include food, sex, and social contact.

The term *reinforcer* refers to stimuli that lead the organism to want to repeat the stimulus. There are two types of reinforcers, positive and negative. A positive reinforcer leads to repeated behavior because the stimuli feel good. A negative reinforcer leads to repeated behavior because a negative stimulation is diminished. Positive and negative reinforcements play large roles in the development of addictive disease and influence the behavior of people with addiction (2).

The pleasure pathways of the brain are activated during states of enjoyment, interest, motivation, and reward. Disease of the pleasure chemistry causes loss of pleasure from food, sex, and social contact and interferes with other reward-influenced behaviors. The individual loses enjoyment, interest, and motivation and finds the experience of life unrewarding.

Neuroadaptation

The initiating step in the development of addiction is neuroadaptation. Dopamine is the principal neurotransmitter associated with sensations of pleasure. Repetitive bouts of intoxication lead to high concentrations of dopamine in the reward and pleasure centers of the brain. In keeping with the body's overall need for homeostasis or balance, overstimulation forces a compensatory response in the brain through neuroadaptation (3).

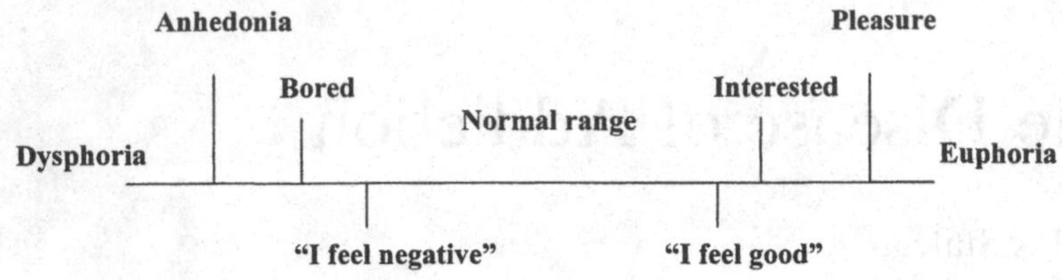

FIGURE 2.1. Pleasure scale.

Neuroadaptation is the process by which the brain adapts to the high concentrations of neurotransmitters released by drugs. Conversely, without the drug and under unstimulated conditions, there is a profound interference in the ability to experience pleasure. The pleasure centers, having adapted to drug-induced elevations in neurotransmitters, become unresponsive to the lower levels of neurotransmitters seen in natural reinforcers. Hence, the individual with a neuroadapted brain experiences dramatic shifts in mental state when drugs are absent, and sobriety is experienced as boring and unrewarding. Instead of pleasure and euphoria (maximum pleasure stimulation), the drug abuser experiences anhedonia (the loss of ability to experience pleasure) and dysphoria (a horrifically negative sensation that is the opposite of euphoria) (Figure 2.1).

The mechanisms of neuroadaptation involve multiple layers of physiologic function: receptor numbers and function change, the systems within the cell that mediate receptor function change, and, with prolonged drug use, adaptive changes extend into the cell nucleus to influence which genes are active and which genes are inactive (switched off). Once established, neuroadaptive changes persist for months to years, and the changes resurface upon reexposure to drug overstimulation even years after drug use is discontinued (4).

At the clinical level, the development of neuroadaptation is heralded by the appearance of *tolerance*, the need to escalate the dose to achieve the same effect as was previously achieved at a lower dose. Not only does a person with tolerance need to use increasing doses to get high, but the experience of sobriety is abnormal as well; sobriety becomes pleasureless. An early sign of brain neuroadaptive changes is a loss of pleasure in activities that previously were deemed rewarding. Moreover, whenever a drug user begins to develop tolerance, a degree of *withdrawal* upon cessation of drug use is experienced. In general, users feel as low as they had been high.

Physical Dependence and Drug-Specific Effects

Neuroadaptation of reward pathways is central to all addictions, whether to drugs or to the behavioral addictions involving sex, food, gambling, shopping, and, in some instances, exercise. However, in addition to marked changes in pleasure chemistry, neuroadaptive changes occur in other brain neurochemical systems influenced by drugs. This is termed *physical dependence*.

These drug-specific effects can produce florid pathology that contributes to progression in addictive disease and interferes with attempts at sobriety. For example, in addition to its pleasurable effect, alcohol also activates two of the brain's natural calming systems, gamma-aminobutyric acid and serotonin. Once neuroadapted because of repetitive overstimulation, the calming systems become impaired, and anxiety, panic, and depression result. Opiate drugs can be extraordinarily pleasurable in abused doses, but when overstimulation causes neuroadaptation, the body's natural opiate system, the endorphins, becomes impaired. Consequently, when sober, opiate addicts are quite pain-sensitive, anxious, and stressed, and they suffer interference with sleep and mood. These changes are superimposed on the core deficits in the dopamine pleasure system. Many addicts find these combined effects intolerable, especially when the discomfort persists for months after discontinuing drug use.

The term *physical dependence* is applied when drug use is discontinued in a tolerant individual and changes in other body functions occur, such as changes in blood pressure, pulse, gastrointestinal function, pain, sweating, and tremor. *Drug withdrawal* is the exact mirror image of the drug's effects: if the drug lowers blood pressure, it is increased during withdrawal.

Detoxification is the use of medications to treat distressing and, in some cases, life-threatening withdrawal symptoms. If detoxification services are not available, the addict is trapped in a relapse spiral caused by the inability to tolerate the inevitable withdrawal symptoms. For example, a severely affected alcoholic may relapse when afflicted with insomnia, anxiety, tremors, and vomiting that persists for days to weeks after discontinuing alcohol use.

As a result of these brain changes, brain pathophysiology appears, including hedonic dysregulation with dysphoria, persistent boredom, and drug hunger (craving). There also appears to be hypofrontality leading to decreased recall of adverse consequences, impaired impulse control, impaired reasoning, and a problem of overvaluing reward and undervaluing risk. Together, these entities underlie the progression of addiction and the propensity for the addict to relapse once sober.

Hedonic dysregulation refers to the injury that drugs cause to the pleasure and reward system in the brain. The tolerant drug user's ability to experience pleasure is impaired. Hence, addiction can be viewed as a disease of pleasure, fun, having a good time, enjoyment, interest, and motivation. Daily life for the newly sober addict is boring and empty. The symptoms caused by hedonic dysregulation may persist for months and, in the case of high-potency drugs such as methamphetamine, cocaine, and heroin, possibly for several years after initiating abstinence.

It has long been appreciated that an addicted person will persist in drug use even in the face of danger and will provide illogical answers to justify the risks taken. New brain neuroimaging research indicates that this is not willful misbehavior. Rather, it reflects a more pernicious aspect of addictive disease, hypofrontality.

The forebrain, the foremost portions of the brain, serves the highest developed brain functions, the executive functions of the brain. These include the appreciation of risk and the ability to weigh consequences and modify behavior accordingly. A critical element in normal executive brain function is the contribution made by dopamine in projection of the pleasure system to the prefrontal cortex. As a consequence of neuroadaptation, dopamine function in this essential brain activity is underactive (5).

In the desert of pleasure that is the addicted brain, activities that are dangerous are mistakenly judged to be worthwhile. By analogy, most individuals would avoid drinking obviously contaminated water. However, if one were lost in the desert and suffering from extreme thirst, the brain would judge contaminated water as worth the risk. In the addicted brain, natural warning systems fail to activate, and a falsely high value is assigned to drug use. The addict fails to appreciate the harm of use and overvalues the "high," at risk of self-harm. Bad decision making is not bad behavior or a character defect but is part of a disease process and the direct consequence of low dopamine activity in the decision-making part of the brain. In the individual with a lengthy history of addiction, the chronic lack of stimulation to the dopamine reward system in the forebrain leads to actual loss of volume in this critical brain region (6).

The development of the disease of addiction begins with *intoxication*, the overstimulation of the brain reward pathways, which is positively reinforcing. With repeated bouts of intoxication, the neuroadaptive response begins, both in the reward chemistry and in the other drug-specific neural pathways such as the calming or excitatory systems of the brain. Soon the user becomes tolerant to the levels of drug use that previously gave pleasure. At this point, the dosage must be escalated to maintain the drug effect, and the user begins to note changes in interest level when sober. Symptoms of physical dependence also occur at this time, and the user begins to suffer symptoms of insomnia, anxiety, appetite disturbance, pain, and muscle spasm. At this point, using drugs not only makes the user high but also relieves the discomfort of the withdrawal symptoms, a negative reinforcement. Over time, the user gets less and less enjoyment from the drug but continues use in an increasingly desperate attempt to avoid being sober (7).

Definition of Addiction

Although addicts use drugs frequently, the presence of addictive disease is not defined by drug use. Rather, the central issue in the disease is control. As addiction develops, the addict experiences diminished ability to control his or her use. This loss of control is reflected in loss of ability to stop use once started, to not use when it is inappropriate, to moderate use when necessary, and to remain abstinent when intending to do so. Use of drugs by an addict is not a choice but is compulsive and part of a disease process. Phrases such as "She chose drugs over her children" are incorrectly applied to use by an addict. It is more accurate to say, "She lost control and used, even knowing she could lose her children."

Many persons drink in an uncontrolled fashion from time to time, but this does not indicate addiction *per se*. In addition to loss of control, a second defining characteristic of addiction is continued use despite adverse consequences. Despite some awareness of the potential for harm, the addict continues to use. This concept underlies the staging of addictive disease: the more severe and numerous the adverse consequences faced by an addict, the more advanced the disease process.

The daily symptom of the disease of addiction is craving. *Craving* is broadly defined as the desire to use. Craving is one major effect of the changes that occur in the brain's reward circuitry as a result of repeated overstimulation. These changes manifest as boredom, restlessness, irritability, and distractibility and may occur without conscious awareness of the desire to use. These negative, uncomfortable sensations are identical to hunger for food or to sexual desire. Higher levels of craving produce feelings of anger, anxiety, frustration, a feeling of entitlement, depression, and mood swings. Neuroimaging studies of the brain in the craving state document a characteristic pattern of physiologic changes (8).

The brain machinery of hunger is activated during craving, and an addict suffers from a sense of desperate hunger. Intense levels of craving produce elevations in blood pressure, pulse, sweating, and dysphoria. Ultimately, craving induces an intense preoccupation with getting and using the drug. Craving that is too intense, too severe, or too uncomfortable results in loss of control over behavior and relapse to drug use.

Possibly the most dangerous symptom of addiction is the phenomenon previously termed *denial*. Heretofore, refusal to acknowledge out-of-control use was taken to mean denial. Such unwillingness to accept the diagnosis is more properly called *treatment resistance*, which often reflects the addict's previous experience with painful withdrawal or the appearance of distressing symptoms of boredom, anxiety, and depression, making continued pursuit of sobriety untenable. The modern definition of denial includes the concept of *hypofrontality*. As a critical component of the disease process, the lowered effectiveness of the brain's executive functions facilitates craving and relapse to drug use. In the face of craving, the addict is temporarily blinded to the risks of use even though those risks may include incarceration or death.

Risk of Addiction

A critical question arises as to why some people become addicted and others do not. Current research suggests that eventual development of addiction occurs when an individual's risk factors for addiction overwhelm that individual's protective factors. Indeed, the science of risk has progressed such that now it is clear that almost everyone who will eventually become addicted can be identified in childhood before ever trying a drug. Addiction is a pediatric disease, meaning that if risk factors are unaddressed and resilience is not promoted, addiction is more likely to result (9,10).

Three major risk factors predispose an individual to the disease of addiction: genetics, childhood trauma, and mental illness, including learning disabilities. In addition, the circumstances of first use and the properties of the drug or drugs used are predictive of further use. Finally, the presence of an enabling system that protects the user from the consequences of his use is predictive of further use. Although this set of factors, known inclusively as the *bio-psycho-social model*, does not directly cause addictive disease, the presence of one or more of these factors in an individual's history increases the likelihood that the individual will use alcohol and drugs in a manner that results in loss of control over behavior (11).

In assessing a person who presents with addiction, application of this model yields invaluable information explaining the development of the disease. It is clear that risk factors for addiction persist during the course of the disease and, in turn, represent potential obstacles to achieving sobriety. The factors that got them addicted will return in a more severe form when the individual attempts to get sober.

Decades of research indicate that the single most prevalent risk factor for addiction is genetic inheritance. Approximately 70% of addicts have a family history of addiction within two generations (parents and grandparents). Utilizing new genomic analytic tools, scientists have identified 51 chromosomal regions that are associated with increased risk of addiction (12). Not surprisingly, the most potent of these genes code for subtle differences in the brain pleasure system, predominantly having to do with dopamine receptor number and function. Prominent among these genetic discoveries is reward deficiency syndrome, associated with differences in the genes that code for dopamine receptor number. Individuals with this common gene variant have 20% to 30% fewer dopamine (reward) receptors and can be described as being born bored (13).

Those with these gene differences appear clinically to have attention deficit hyperactivity disorder, which is known from separate kinds of research studies to be a powerful risk factor for acquiring addictive disease. Without intervention, more than three fourths of children with attention deficit hyperactivity disorder will develop addiction. However, properly managed, the risk of attention deficit hyperactivity disorder yielding addiction falls to 24% (14).

Both childhood sexual abuse and mental health disorders are robust risk factors for addiction. Survivors of multigenerational domestic violence and verbal, physical, and sexual abuse are at high risk of experiencing a set of symptoms known collectively as *posttraumatic stress disorder*. Like other victims of prolonged trauma, the abused child, particularly when subjected to sexual abuse, learns dissociative behaviors that serve as a defense mechanism against the trauma. Through dissociative experiences, voluntary thought suppression, and denial, the child is able to survive the immediacy of the trauma. Many drugs mimic this dissociative state. Other child victims are given alcohol and other drugs as part of the abuse pattern. Recognition of the alarming prevalence of sexual abuse in addicts, both male and female, has been slow to develop. Approximately one in four women and one in six men have had an unwanted sexual contact prior to age 13 years (15).

Without intervention, many abused persons will develop late-stage addictive disease. Any seasoned addiction professional will readily confirm the wide prevalence of childhood sexual abuse among addicts and attest to the remarkable confounding effect it has on treatment outcomes. Only very recently have specific intervention tools been produced that address this widespread hidden cause of addiction (16,17).

Combat experience in the military may similarly result in posttraumatic stress disorder symptoms that increase the risk of addiction. For men, combat experience is a more potent risk factor than childhood sexual abuse. Other psychiatric diagnoses commonly known to co-occur with addictive disease are major depression and anxiety disorders. The obvious role of mental health disorders in producing addiction stems from the common observation that mental illness symptoms are painful and drugs effectively reduce that pain. When mental illness and addictive disease co-occur, the symptoms of each disease exacerbate the other. Not only does mental illness predispose the individual to a more severe presentation of addictive disease, but the person with untreated mental illness develops addiction at a younger age, progresses more rapidly, and does less well in treatment, unless the co-occurring mental illness is effectively treated along with the addiction.

In understanding why some people become addicts and others do not, it is important to include the concept of resilience, behaviors that afford a measure of protection from addiction. Many of these resilience factors operate by providing regular hedonic stimulus and protection from boredom.

In addition to risk and resilience, the bio-psycho-social model suggests that the properties of the drug itself and the circumstances in which the drug is first used, separately and in combination with risk, increase the likelihood of addiction. Some drugs are more addictive (likely to lead to loss of control) than others. Some drugs release very high levels of dopamine and, in turn, engender a rapid and pronounced neuroadaptive response. High-potency drugs, such as methamphetamine, cocaine, and heroin, lead to the more rapid acquisition of tolerance, forcing the user to escalate the dosage to maintain the euphoric drug effect, and using an inadequate dosage causes withdrawal symptoms (Table 2.1).

TABLE 2.1. Addiction: risk and resilience.

Risk	Resilience
Inherited predisposition (genetics)	No family history of addiction
Childhood trauma or abuse	Good mental health
Unwanted sexual involvement before age 13 years	Academic competence
Mental illness: depression, anxiety, personality disorder	Positive relationship with an adult
Attention deficit disorder	Family eats dinner together 5 days/week
Learning disabilities/school failure	Peer group participation (clubs)
Subjected to teasing, bullying	Participation in sports
Acne and/or obesity	Participation in music, drama, or dance
Other than heterosexual orientation	Involvement in faith-based activities
Social rejection	Taking care of pets
Early sexual involvement	Volunteer activities
Onset of drug use before age 16 years	Environment disapproves of drug use
Enabling environment	Immediate, appropriately scaled consequences for alcohol/drug use
Ignorance	Early intervention for alcohol/drug use

Source: From Najavits et al. (17), with kind permission of Springer Science and Business Media.

The route of administration also affects the drug-using experience. For example, use of methamphetamine by nasal insufflation (snorting) leads very slowly to physical dependence because the amount of drug entering the body is less and the speed of administration is relatively slow. Intravenous use of methamphetamine leads to physical dependence within 6 to 8 weeks because the route of administration is faster and more efficient. Intravenous use, like inhalation (smoking), produces an immediate, intense euphoria called a *rush* that prompts the user to try to recapture the euphoric feeling with subsequent use. Similarly, drugs used in a high-potency fashion, such as smoking and injecting, concentrate the high, leading to more rapid and extensive neuroadaptation. For example, cocaine when snorted is certainly addicting. However, when cocaine is smoked as crack, the high is dramatically higher, the comedown much lower, and the risk of severe addiction is enhanced.

There are times in a novice drug user's life when exposure to drugs is far more likely to lead to addiction. An independent risk factor for addiction is the age at onset of use. Early onset use, before the age of 16 years, leads to a disproportionately high percentage of users who will progress to addiction: the developing brain is critically sensitive to the neuroadaptive changes induced by drugs (18). Tragically, many youngsters begin drug experimentation before they fully appreciate the damage that their use is doing to the brain's reward system.

Drugs famously relieve distress. If initial drug exposures occur during stressful times in an individual's development, the perceived benefit of the drug use extends beyond getting high to relieving stress. It is thus more likely that the person will want to repeat the drug experience when similarly stressed. Adolescence, with its attendant social and academic pressures, is a particularly dangerous time to initiate drug use, primarily because the drug will work entirely too well in helping the teen to manage stresses.

Enabling is defined as behavior that protects the user from the consequences of use and therefore exacerbates the symptoms of the disease. The addict who lives in the drug subculture where selling and using drugs is a major part of life is often protected from some of the consequences of use by the addicts in his friendship circle. Parents, charged with preventing substance use in their offspring, may tacitly encourage and enable the use of substances by neglect or by failing to intervene when a youth begins to experiment with alcohol and other drugs (19). Other children are raised in environments where mental illness is self-medicated with alcohol or other drugs. Other types of enabling behavior include providing money to the addict to replace that spent on drugs or making excuses for an addict's performance failures at work or school. Often, identifying what enables the disease creates an opportunity to disable it, such as protecting an addict from exposure to unbudgeted money.

Conclusions

Once deemed a moral and character weakness, addiction is now understood to be a disease of neurochemical pathways in the brain that render sobriety intolerable. Drug use by an addict is not volitional but is part of a disease process characterized by loss of control (compulsion). Built into the disease is continued use despite adverse consequences. The disease is staged not on the basis of how often or in what quantities drugs are consumed but rather on the number and severity of adverse consequences that an addict sustains while continuing to use. Late-stage addicts will continue to use despite immediate risk of loss of freedom through incarceration, loss of the custody of their children, and even loss of their lives. Once established, the brain changes of addiction can persist for years after initiation of abstinence and even once resolved will return immediately on return to use.

Modern treatment of addiction is based on limiting exposure to environmental cues, effectively treating withdrawal symptoms, treating mental illness concurrently with addiction, and providing increased support around periods of life stress that activate the craving process. It is a national shame that despite the devastation in the lives of addicts, their families, and their communities, major shortfalls remain in the provision of services. Major barriers persist in availability of safe housing, detoxification services, and mental health services for addicts. It is inhumane to demand sobriety of addicted persons while failing to ease their pain. Drug courts offer hope of implementing integrated service models while supporting motivation through rational combinations of reward and sanctions.

References

1. Kosten TR. Neurobiology of abused drugs. J Nerv Ment Dis 1990;178:217–227.
2. Volkow ND, Fowler JS, Wang GJ. The addicted human brain: insights from imaging studies. J Clin Invest 2003;111:1444–1451.
3. Miller NS, Dackis CA, Gold MS. The relationship of addiction, tolerance, and dependence to alcohol and drugs: a neurochemical approach. J Subst Abuse Treat 1987;4:197–207.
4. Koob GF, LeMoal M. Plasticity of reward neurocircuitry and the "dark side" of drug addiction. Nat Neurosci 2005;8:1442–1444.
5. Koob GF. The neurobiology of addiction: a neuroadaptational view relevant for diagnosis. Addiction 2006;101:23–30.
6. Liu X, Matochik JA, Cadet JL, London ED. Smaller volume of prefrontal lobe in polysubstance abusers: a magnetic resonance imaging study. Neuropsychopharmacology 1999;18(4):243–252.
7. Miller NS, Kipnis SS, eds. Detoxification and Substance Abuse Treatment. Center for Substance Abuse Treatment. DHHS Publication No. 06-4131. Rockville, MD: Substance Abuse and Mental Health Services Administration; 2006.
8. Childress AR, Mozley PD, McElgin W, Fitzgerald J, Reivich M, O'Brien CP. Limbic activation during cue-induced cocaine craving. Am J Psychiatry 1999;156:11–18.
9. Kessler D, Natanblut S, Wilkenfeld J, Lorraine C, Mayl S, Bernstein I, Thompson L. Nicotine addiction: a pediatric disease. J Pediatr 1997;130:518–524.
10. Hingson RW, Heeren T, Winter MR. Age at drinking onset and alcohol dependence. Arch Pediatr Adol Med 2006;160:739–746.
11. Engel G. The need for a new medical model: a challenge for biomedicine. Science 1977;196:129–136.
12. Johnson C, Drgon T, Liu QR, Walther D, Edenberg H, Rice J, Foroud R, Uhl GR. Pooled association genome scanning for alcohol dependence using 104,268 SNPs: validation and use to identify alcoholism vulnerability loci in unrelated individuals from the collaborative study on the genetics of alcoholism. Am J Med Genet B Neuropsychiatric Genet 2006;141:844–853.
13. Blum K, Cull JG, Braverman ER, Comings DE. Reward deficiency syndrome. Am Scientist 1996;84:132–145.
14. Biederman J, Wilens R, Mick E, Spencer T, Faraone S. Pharmacotherapy of attention-deficit/hyperactivity disorder reduces risk for substance use disorder. Pediatrics 1999;104:20–24.
15. Finkelhor D, Hotaling G, Lewis IA, Smith C. Sexual abuse in a national survey of adult men and women: prevalence, characteristics, and risk factors. Child Abuse Neglect 1990;14:19–28.
16. Rohsenow DJ, Corbett R, Devine D. Molested as children: a hidden contribution to substance abuse? J Subst Abuse Treat 1988;5:13–18.

17. Najavits LM, Weiss RD, Shaw SR, Muenz LR. Seeking safety: outcome of a new cognitive-behavioral psychotherapy for women with posttraumatic stress disorder and substance dependence. J Trauma Stress 1998;11:437–456.
18. Weinberger DR, Elvevag B, Giedd JN. The adolescent brain: a work in progress. Washington, DC: The National Campaign to Prevent Teen Pregnancy; 2005.
19. National Survey of American Attitudes on Substance Abuse XI: Teens and Parents. New York: National Center on Addiction and Substance Abuse (CASA) at Columbia University; 2006:1–73.

3
The Biologic Basis of Drug and Alcohol Addiction

Olga A. Katz, Nikita B. Katz, and Steven Mandel

Many practitioners and researchers in the field have come to view drug addiction as a disease of the brain that is caused by both genetic and environmental factors and that may respond to pharmacologic and psychological therapies. The phenomenon of drug addiction is, however, far broader than the combination of genetics and neuropsychopharmacology. There are numerous social and political dimensions that add to the complexity of addiction that must also be considered.

The traditional view is that drug use is motivated by hedonism, the search for pleasure that follows the use of many drugs (heroin, cocaine) but not always or for all drugs (phencyclidine). For proponents of this theory, dependency develops through positive reinforcement: people take drugs to try to repeat a pleasant experience. This theory was formulated in the mid-1980s on the basis of self-stimulation experiments conducted in the 1950s on rats and other animals.

Research has shown that not all drug users are seeking the hedonistic, euphoric high. The view that drug addiction is a form of self-medication and that drug abusers choose a given substance according to their particular needs and the particular effect they are seeking is too limited to explain all the varieties of drug-associated habits and behaviors (1).

A fashionable approach is a variation on the hedonistic theory that benefits from the observation that dopaminergic neurons in the brain start secreting more of this neurotransmitter when the presence of a potentially rewarding agent (drug or food) is detected, before any actual consumption begins. Often, the dopaminergic surge is not diminished by the fact that the potentially rewarding agent is inaccessible. The conclusion is that drug-seeking behavior is a separate part of drug habituation and addiction and should be disassociated from the hedonistic satisfaction that drugs provide. This theory emphasizes the desire component of drug addiction and deemphasizes pleasure.

Berridge and Robinson (2) suggested a salience-based theory that a state of hyperexcitability (sensitization) of the mesolimbic dopaminergic system of the brain might be the source of the cravings for the drug, especially if the drug directly influences dopamine levels in the brain (cocaine) or directly modulates the dopaminergic activity (heroin). According to this theory, the dopaminergic system attributes a value, or salience, to stimuli associated with its activation, thus making them attractive or desirable incentives. Over time the salience itself becomes an incentive, creating a vicious circle of distortion of reality perception that is commonly observed in patients suffering from severe, complex addictions characterized by compulsions, denial, and splitting of reality. Thus, the values assigned to physical reality and values assigned to the social sphere of an addict are in a state of flux and may be continually warped by both the presence and absence of the dopamine-inducing drug (2).

A variation of this view is the idea that individual attitudes toward drugs and the likelihood of development of addiction fundamentally depend on the baseline activity of the dopaminergic neurons in the brain, mostly determined by genetic predisposition and early development of the brain, including growth and development in utero. If a person with genetically determined low activity of dopaminergic neurons is exposed to a drug of abuse (cocaine), the hyperactivated dopaminergic system will produce the feeling of satisfaction. As excessive dopamine is deactivated by the brain, the person will slide into a dissatisfaction that may be counteracted by repeated intake of the drug, thus predisposing the person to experience a craving for the drug whenever the dopaminergic system is functioning below or at the genetically normal level.

Tolerance and Sensitization

To continue getting the same sensation, for instance, euphoria, drug abusers often have to resort to increasing the dosage of the drug to achieve an effect that is comparable, if not equal, to their expectations. This well-known phenomenon is attributed to development of drug tolerance, or habituation (3).

Tolerance represents an adaptation at the cellular level. The brain's neurons may modify the number or sensitivity of their receptors to adapt to the increased dosage, much like a concert-goer reaches for ear plugs when the sound becomes too loud, or the neurotransmitter-deactivating systems of the brain may become more active. The drug-dependent person will have to go beyond the usual dosage, establishing a new threshold that has to be crossed to achieve the desired sensation. This moving threshold phenomenon often leads to constant increasing of the dosage, usually slowly at first and more rapidly later.

A different example of the tolerance-building mechanism is the development of drug-deactivating systems outside of the brain. For example, a habitual consumer of alcohol will have a higher amount of liver enzymes that convert alcohol into less harmful and nonaddictive chemicals.

Tolerance is not a necessary component of addiction, as many drug addicts do not report substantial tolerance. Neither is tolerance a sufficient condition; in many drug abusers dependence or addiction is manifest before significant tolerance sets in. Some substances that do not have any measurable mind-altering or psychoactive properties, such as hypertension or antiepileptic medications, are also subject to development of tolerance. There are certain psychoactive drugs, such as amphetamines, for which no true tolerance effects are observed.

The term *sensitization* refers to an increase in the effect of a drug when it is used repeatedly. Sensitization is often viewed as the opposite of tolerance, although it is only an incomplete opposite, as it is most commonly limited to psychomotor effects and reward effects of the drug. This limitation suggests involvement of the primitive brain structures that control the subconscious processes.

Pathways of the Brain Affected by Drugs of Abuse

Studies of the brain circuits that use dopamine and the locations of the dopamine receptors in these circuits have identified eight major dopaminergic pathways in the brain. Three of these pathways are especially important in the concept of addiction. All three originate in the midbrain (4–6).

The first is the *mesolimbic pathway*, which is composed of a bundle of dopaminergic fibers associated with the reward circuit. This pathway originates in the ventral tegmental area and innervates several structures of the limbic system, including the other major component of the pleasure circuit, the nucleus accumbens. The mesolimbic pathway is important for generation of sensations of pleasure and associated memories, as well as for motivating pleasure-seeking and pain-avoiding behavior.

The *mesocortical pathway* also originates in the ventral tegmental area but projects to the prefrontal cortex and surrounding structures. Some evidence indicates that a malfunction in this pathway might be the cause of some of the more alarming symptoms of drug use and addiction, such as hallucinations and disordered thinking.

The third, *nigrostriatal*, pathway projects axons from the substantia nigra to the striatum (caudate nucleus and putamen), which is involved in motor control. Degeneration of the neurons in this pathway is associated with the trembling and muscular rigidity symptomatic of Parkinson's disease. There is little evidence that this pathway is engaged in generation of pleasure, although patients suffering from Parkinson's disease commonly suffer from anhedonia, the inability to enjoy normally pleasurable activities.

Three structures of the brain are especially important from the standpoint of neuroanatomy of addiction: the ventral tegmental area, the nucleus accumbens, and the prefrontal cortex, all of which play central roles in the reward circuit. Located in the midbrain at the top of the brain stem, the ventral tegmental area is one of the most primitive parts of the brain. The neurons of the ventral tegmental area synthesize dopamine, which is used to modulate the activity of the more sophisticated parts of the reward circuitry, such as the nucleus accumbens and prefrontal cortex, and also to activate secondary structures of the reward circuitry, such as the amygdala, ventral pallidum, and, indirectly, the mediodorsal thalamus. The neurons of the ventral tegmental area receive inhibitive input from the nucleus accumbens and ventral pallidum that is mediated by the neurotransmitter gamma-aminobutyric acid (GABA) and receive excitatory input from the amygdala and the prefrontal cortex that is mediated by the neurotransmitter glutamate. The ventral tegmental area neurons are also influenced by endorphins, natural analogs of opioid drugs such as heroin and morphine.

Dopamine's role in the reward pathway is well accepted but is now viewed as far removed from the simple maxim of dopamine as the pleasure neurotransmitter. It has been argued that dopamine is more associated with anticipatory desire and motivation (commonly described as wanting) as opposed to actual consummatory pleasure (liking). Another consideration is the fact that dopamine is released whenever unpleasant or aversive stimuli are encountered, so it motivates the pleasure of avoiding or removing the unpleasant stimuli. The exact role of dopamine in the drug-naïve brain remains to be elucidated. However, the role of dopamine in addiction is universally accepted as that of the pleasure, reward, or euphoria-generating neuromodulator.

The prefrontal cortex serves as the seat of planning, executive function, and motivation. Its involvement in the reward circuit usually manifests itself through specific, most often conscious, decisions. On the other hand, the amygdala, which imparts agreeable or disagreeable affective colorations to perceptions, and the pallidum and the thalamus, which serve as relays for the sensory input from the body and the outside world, are generally regarded as the subconscious components of the reward circuitry.

Although not directly affected by many drugs (with the notable exception of stimulants), the hippocampus, often regarded as the initiator of consolidation of factual and procedural memories, has the ability to preserve the agreeable memories associated with the drug intake and, by association, the details of the environment in which it is taken. These details become the triggers or cues. If a person is exposed to them, they may reawaken the desire to take the drug, contributing to the perpetuation of the drug habit.

Aversive, painful, and unpleasant stimuli, such as punishment or withdrawal of reward, either earned or anticipated, activate the brain's punishment circuit, the periventricular system, which leads to a number of changes in behavior, from fight-or-flight responses to coping behaviors. The specific response is based on input from the amygdala and the hippocampus that often combines specific aspects of both factual and emotional memories of the individual. The punishment circuitry includes various brain structures, such as the hypothalamus, the thalamus, and the grey substance of the midbrain. Main neurotransmitters associated with the punishment system are acetylcholine, serotonin, and GABA. The influence of GABA may diminish the feeling of displeasure and punishment and may explain the addictive properties of GABA boosters, such as benzodiazepines and barbiturates (7).

Although the reward and the punishment circuits are the two major systems of motivation in human beings, they are not simple enough to be described in the terms of simple dichotomies. The active versus passive participation in the changes that happen in the environment is determined by yet another, equally important circuit: the behavioral inhibition system. This circuitry includes, once again, the amygdala, the septohippocampal system, and the basal nuclei, such as the thalamus and the pallidum. It receives inputs from the prefrontal cortex and modifies and transmits them as outputs via the fibers of the locus coeruleus and the medial raphe nuclei. Most researchers identify serotonin as the key neurotransmitter of this system.

The behavioral inhibition system is engaged when pleasure is impossible to attain, when punishment overwhelms, and when neither fight nor flight is possible. Such a high-level decision is made by the processing of the future-planning scenarios by the highly sophisticated neural networks of the prefrontal cortex. As opposed to the reward and punishment that seem to originate in the more primitive parts of the brain, behavior inhibition, often in the forms of acceptance, avoidance, and alienation, is generated by more advanced brain structures that are more amenable to learning and social interaction structures of the brain. While this may lead to successful application of psychological therapy and sociolegal interventions, the activity of this pathway may also lead to social withdrawal, habitual distortion of reality, scheming, and insincerity that are common components of the psychological profile of a drug addict (Table 3.1).

Neurochemical Effects of Specific Drugs

Cocaine

Cocaine is a dopamine transporter blocker that competitively inhibits dopamine reuptake, leading to an increase of dopamine levels in the synaptic cleft up to 150%. Cocaine prevents dopamine and other chemically related neurotransmitters from being reabsorbed by the neurons that released them and thus increases their concentration in the synapses. As a result, the natural effect of neurotransmitters on the postsynaptic neurons is amplified, producing the euphoria from dopamine, feelings of confidence from increased levels of serotonin, and energy from increased levels of norepinephrine that are typically experienced by cocaine abusers.

TABLE 3.1. Neurologic pathways and drugs of abuse.

Pathway	Components	Some neurotransmitters involved	Examples of drugs of abuse that may influence the pathway (possibly via a specified neurotransmitter)	Some prescription medications that may modulate
Reward	Ventral tegmental area (output)	Dopamine	Amphetamines (directly), cocaine (directly), opioids (indirectly), cannabis (indirectly), PCP (indirectly)	Stimulants, antiparkinsonian medications
	Ventral tegmental area (input), nucleus accumbens, prefrontal cortex and limbic/basal structures	Glutamate and gamma-aminobutyric acid (GABA)	Benzodiazepines (GABA), barbiturates (GABA), opioids (GABA/glutamate ratio), PCP and ketamine (directly, glutamate)	Benzodiazepines, GABA antagonists (flumazenil/Anexate®), GABA (as dietary supplement); Glutamate modulators: acamprosate/Campral®, memantine/ Namenda®; opioid antagonists (naltrexone/Revia®, Vivitrol®)
Punishment	Periventricular structures	Acetylcholine, serotonin, and GABA	Benzodiazepines (GABA), barbiturates (GABA), nicotine (acetylcholine) alcohol (GABA), MDMA/ "ecstasy" (serotonin)	Benzodiazepines, GABA antagonists (flumazenil/Anexate®), 5-hydroxytriptamine (as dietary supplement), GABA (as dietary supplement), antiserotonergic drugs (cyproheptadine/Periactin®, hydroxyzine/Atarax®)
Behavioral Inhibition	Prefrontal cortex	Many, including glutamate and GABA	PCP (may cause disinhibition), benzodiazepines, barbiturates	Benzodiazepines, GABA antagonists (flumazenil/Anexate®); Glutamate modulators: acamprosate/Campral®, memantine/Namenda®; antiepileptic drugs (e.g., gabapentin/Neurontin®);
	Basal nuclei, limbic system	Serotonin and norepinephrine	LSD and psilocybin (serotonin), stimulants (norepinephrine), cannabis (indirectly)	antidepressants (e.g., fluoxetine/Prozac®, venlafaxine/Effexor®); Atomoxetine/Strattera®; dextromethorphan (over-the-counter cough remedies)

Note: GABA, gamma-aminobutyric acid; LSD, lysergic acid diethylamide; MDMA, 3,4-methylenedioxymethamphetamine; PCP, phencyclidine.
Source: Data are from Robinson and Berridge (3) and Berridge and Robinson (4).

In addition, the norepinephrine neurons project their axons into all the main structures of the forebrain, including structures responsible for abstract thought, survival strategies, and planning for the future. The powerful overall effect of cocaine can be readily understood as warping of reality and the perception of the past and the future. Dependence on cocaine is closely related to its effect on the neurons of the reward circuit and is rarely associated with physical withdrawal (3,4).

Opioids

In addition to being influenced by dopamine, the reward circuit is modulated by endogenous opioids, such as enkephalins, endorphins, and dynorphins. In the ventral tegmental area, endorphins act on mu receptors on the dendrites of GABA-ergic neurons. Normally, these GABA-ergic neurons inhibit the dopaminergic neurons that project from the ventral tegmental area, activating the reward pathways. However, the influence of endorphins suppresses the release of GABA, thus removing the GABA-ergic inhibition of the dopaminergic neurons. Consequently, the nucleus accumbens is more stimulated by the dopamine from the dopaminergic neurons of the ventral tegmental area, creating a lasting sensation of pleasure and euphoria and a positive reinforcement.

The natural antagonists of endorphins, dynorphins, bind to kappa receptors of the GABA-ergic neurons and cause the inhibition of the release of dopamine in the nucleus accumbens. The stimulation of the nucleus accumbens is thereby reduced, which creates an aversive effect and may block the pleasurable effects of drugs of abuse. The so-called crash may be caused by a sudden change in the environment and may precipitate depression. Overproduction of dynorphins may explain some of the painful and psychologically aversive features of physical withdrawal associated with abuse of opioids.

In the thalamus and throughout the brain's nociceptive (pain perception) pathways, endorphins bind to the neurons involved in controlling pain and hyperpolarize them, thus reducing the amount of neurotransmitters, such as serotonin, released and serving as analgesics. Endorphins also inhibit the effect of the norepinephrinergic neurons involved in vigilance, anxiety, and feelings of uneasiness.

Exogenous, natural, or synthetic opioids such as heroin, methadone, and morphine are structurally similar to endorphins and attach to the same mu receptors when they reach the brain. By attaching to the *mu* receptors, exogenous opioids reduce the amount of GABA released by the neurons of the reward pathway. Normally, GABA reduces the amount of dopamine released in the nucleus accumbens. By inhibiting this inhibitor, the opioids ultimately increase the amount of dopamine produced and the amount of pleasure felt.

Although the exact mechanisms of opioid withdrawal are complex and have not been elucidated completely, one view is that chronic consumption of opioids inhibits the production of another neuroactive substance, cyclic adenosine monophosphate, but this inhibition is offset by activating additional cyclic adenosine monophosphate production mechanisms in the brain. When no opioids are available, increased cyclic adenosine monophosphate production leads to neural hyperactivity and the sensation of craving the drug that is amplified by the physical pain and discomfort of dynorphin-mediated withdrawal (3,6).

Alcohol

Alcohol is rapidly absorbed into the bloodstream and within minutes is found in the brain, as it passes directly through the blood–brain barrier. It affects the brain's neurons in several ways. As a solvent, it alters neuronal membranes and also acts on the ion channels, enzymes, and receptors. Alcohol exhibits direct binding to the receptors for acetylcholine, serotonin, GABA, and the N-methyl-D-aspartate subtype of the glutamate receptor.

The sedating function of alcohol is primarily due to its effect on GABA-ergic neurons. The GABA reduces neural activity by allowing the negatively charged chloride ions to enter the postsynaptic neuron, which makes the neuron less excitable. This physiologic effect is amplified when alcohol binds to the GABA receptor, probably because it enables the ion channel to stay open longer and thus allows more chloride ions into the cell. This effect is accentuated because alcohol also reduces glutamate's excitatory effect on N-methyl-D-aspartate receptors.

In cases of chronic consumption of alcohol, the N-methyl-D-aspartate receptors gradually become hypersensitive to glutamate and desensitized to GABA-ergic influences. In alcohol withdrawal, patients may enter a state of excitation involving motor activation and possibly seizures. Alcohol also increases the release of dopamine by a process that is still poorly understood but appears to involve curtailing the activity of the enzyme that deactivates dopamine (3,7).

Nicotine

Nicotine imitates the action of the neurotransmitter acetylcholine and binds to a particular type of acetylcholine receptor, commonly known as the *nicotinic receptor*. The nicotinic receptor, when activated, allows sodium ions to enter the neuron, depolarizing the membrane and exciting the cell. Depolarization causes the channel to close; the nicotinic receptor becomes temporarily unresponsive to any natural stimulation with neurotransmitters. It is this state of desensitization that is artificially prolonged by continual exposure to nicotine.

Tobacco dependence and tolerance tend to develop very quickly, possibly because nicotinic receptors are present on the neurons of the ventral tegmental area. In smokers, repeated nicotine stimulation also increases the amount of dopamine released in the nucleus accumbens.

After several hours without nicotine, the nicotinic receptors become functional again, causing the cholinergic neurotransmission to be raised to an abnormally high level. This affects all the cholinergic pathways in the brain, presenting with the typical agitation and discomfort that leads smokers to seek another dose of nicotine.

Another substance in tobacco smoke, not yet clearly identified, inhibits monoamine oxidase B, an enzyme that breaks down dopamine after its reuptake. The result is a higher concentration of dopamine in the reward circuit, which also contributes to the smoker's dependence and is similar to the already mentioned mechanism of alcohol dependence (3,8).

Amphetamines

Much like cocaine, amphetamines increase the concentration of dopamine in the synaptic gap but by a different mechanism. Amphetamines are similar in structure to dopamine and so can enter the terminal button of the presynaptic neuron via its dopamine transporters as well as by diffusing through the neural membrane directly. When entering inside the presynaptic neuron, amphetamines force the dopamine molecules out of their storage vesicles and expel them into the synaptic gap by making the dopamine transporters work in reverse. This leads to a significant increase in self-reported pleasure, often described as an immense high (9).

Amphetamines also seem to act by several other mechanisms, such as reduction of the reuptake of dopamine and, in high concentrations, inhibition of monoamine oxidase, thus preserving the excess amounts of dopamine. They may also excite dopaminergic neurons indirectly, via their action on the excitatory function of glutamate, making the dopaminergic neurons more excitable (10–12).

Cannabis

The sensations of mild euphoria, relaxation, and amplified auditory and visual perceptions produced by smoking or ingesting cannabis (marijuana) are almost entirely due to the effect on the cannabinoid receptors throughout the brain (13). Endocannabinoids are produced in the body and are natural ligands of the cannabinoid receptors. The first endocannabinoid compound was identified as arachidonyl ethanolamine and named *anandamide*, a name derived from the Sanskrit word for bliss. Anandamide is derived from the essential fatty acid arachidonic acid. It has pharmacology similar to 9-delta-tetrahydrocannabinol, although its chemical structure is very different (14).

Anandamide binds to both the central (CB1) and peripheral (CB2) cannabinoid receptors. It is about half as potent as 9-delta-tetrahydrocannabinol, the active ingredient in marijuana. Another endocannabinoid, 2-arachidonyl glycerol, binds to both the CB1 and CB2 receptors and is much less active than anandamide.

Endocannabinoids are similar to the well-known monoamine neurotransmitters, such as dopamine; however, their chemistry and pharmacology are significantly different. Neurotransmitters are usually small water-soluble molecules that tend to diffuse rapidly, whereas cannabinoids are fat soluble and can be stored in the neuronal membranes for days and even weeks.

Endocannabinoids are often described as retrograde transmitters because they most commonly travel backward against the usual synaptic transmitter flow. They are released from the postsynaptic cell and act on the presynaptic cell, often causing reduction of the amount of conventional neurotransmitter released. This endocannabinoid-mediated system permits the postsynaptic cell to control its own incoming synaptic traffic. The ultimate effect on the endocannabinoid-releasing cell depends on the nature of the conventional transmitter that is being controlled. When the release of the inhibitory transmitter GABA is reduced, the net effect is an increase in the excitability of the endocannabinoid-releasing cell that may lead to increased release of dopamine from the ventral tegmental area and the nucleus accumbens.

Conversely, when release of the excitatory neurotransmitter glutamate is reduced, the net effect is a decrease in the excitability of the endocannabinoid-releasing cell. As a result, marijuana produces effects that may appear contradictory when compared with drugs of abuse that directly affect neurotransmitters. For example, although both marijuana and amphetamines can produce the feelings of well-being and euphoria, appetite is strongly suppressed by amphetamines, whereas marijuana leads to potent liberation of appetite, overeating, and, possibly, appetite pathology (12–14).

In chronic consumers of cannabis, the brain compensates for the overstimulation of the cannabinoid receptors by reducing their overall number and sensitivity to both endocannabinoids and the exogenous cannabinoids such as tetrahydrocannabinol. The loss of CB1 receptors in the brain's arteries reduces the flow of blood, and hence the supply of glucose and oxygen, to the brain. The main results are attention deficits, memory loss, and impaired learning ability. Signs of physical dependence may be induced in animal models by rapid withdrawal of tetrahydrocannabinol. In dogs, ptosis and dysphoric behaviors such as wet shuddering appear, although in humans cannabis withdrawal is rarely, if ever, observed (12–14).

Methylenedioxymethamphetamine

3,4-Methylenedioxymethamphetamine (MDMA), or ecstasy, is a synthetic drug. It acts simultaneously as a stimulant and a hallucinogen because of its molecular structure, which is similar to that of both amphetamines and lysergic acid diethylamide. A single dose of MDMA may induce a general sense of openness, empathy, energy, euphoria, and well-being. Tactile sensations are enhanced for some users, making general physical contact with others more pleasurable. However, contrary to popular mythology, MDMA does not have aphrodisiac properties. Like amphetamines and cocaine, ecstasy blocks the reuptake of certain neurotransmitters and also potentiates the effects of norepinephrine and dopamine. It is distinguished from other psychostimulants by its strong affinity for serotonin transporters. The initial effect of ecstasy is an increased release of serotonin by the serotonergic neurons. The individual may then experience increased energy, euphoria, and the suppression of inhibitions in relating to other people (15).

This high may last several hours and is almost always followed by a decrease in serotonin levels, which is aggravated by the MDMA-induced reduction of serotonin synthesis. This down can last much longer than the initial high and may lead to feelings of immense dysphoria and discomfort.

Like all psychoactive drugs that increase the release of dopamine into the reward circuit, MDMA (ecstasy) induces short- and long-term changes in the ventral tegmental area, nucleus accumbens, and, significantly, the prefrontal cortex, leading to changes in the executive and planning functions of the brain. Research shows that the long-term changes in the levels of dopamine production may predispose drug abusers to development of Parkinson's disease or parkinsonism later in life. Whether this is true of MDMA specifically remains an area of conjecture. In addition, animal studies have shown that chronic high doses of MDMA lead to selective destruction of the terminal buttons of the serotonergic neurons, thus potentially causing severe depression that may respond poorly to conventional antidepressants (15,16).

Benzodiazepines and Barbiturates

Benzodiazepines, such as diazepam (Valium®) and alprazolam (Xanax®), are antianxiety agents that can also have hypnotic and amnesia-inducing effects. Like alcohol, these drugs increase the efficiency of synaptic transmission of the neurotransmitter GABA by acting on its receptors.

A GABA receptor is actually a complex of subunits that, in addition to containing sites for binding GABA, contain sites for binding other molecules such as benzodiazepines that modulate GABA's activity. When benzodiazepines bind to a specific site on a GABA receptor, they do not stimulate it directly. Instead, they make it more efficient by increasing the frequency with which the chlorine channel opens when GABA binds to its own site on this receptor. The physiologic result is the hyperpolarization of the neuron, which makes it less excitable. Behaviorally, the result is sedation and reduction of anxiety, which may be actively sought by the person and may contribute to dependence. Benzodiazepines can cause a drug dependency even in what are considered therapeutic dosages in a short course of treatment (17).

Barbiturates are similar to benzodiazepines in their behavioral effects, in particular, sleep induction. However, these bind to another site on the GABA receptor, causing direct opening of the chloride channel and serving as GABA substitutes. Addiction to barbiturates may also develop after a relatively short course of treatment (18). Because of the additive effect on the GABA receptors, a combination of benzodiazepines or barbiturates with alcohol may strongly potentiate the toxic and addictive properties of these agents and may lead to catastrophic events, such as respiratory arrest (17,18).

Genetics of Alcohol and Drug Addiction

Genetic predisposition to alcohol and drug addiction and dependence is commonly misunderstood. Genetic information, encoded in the DNA, determines whether the fruit of a tree will be orange, covered with a rind, and contain d-limonene or will be green, covered with a skin, and contain malic acid. Genetic information, however, does not determine whether the specific exemplar of an orange or an apple will, in the course of its development, grow to its fullest possible extent or wither and fall off the tree. Of course, when it comes to human beings, the role of genetics is immense but so is the importance of lifestyle and choices made in the process of growth and adaptation.

Genetics is best studied in the case of predisposition to alcohol abuse, although significant overlaps with other types of drug abuse may coexist. Although there is good evidence for substantial heritability for alcoholism, individual differences in clinical presentation suggest variation in origins of vulnerability. Alcoholics vary in their drinking patterns, in the severity of their symptoms, and in behavioral, physical, and psychiatric consequences of their condition. Vulnerability may be caused by personality or psychiatric traits that predispose to alcohol-seeking behavior, differential response to the effects of alcohol, or differential predisposition to addiction (19).

Alcohol dependence is often comorbid with other psychiatric disorders, including drug abuse, major depression, anxiety disorders, bulimia nervosa, and antisocial personality disorder (19). Alcohol, cocaine, opioid, and nicotine dependency co-occur more often in certain racial and ethnic populations than would be expected from their representation in the nation's population as a whole. This phenomenon may be explained by assuming that there exists a certain general genetic predisposition to abuse of addictive substances as well as a specific predisposition to abuse of a particular substance (19,20).

Two large-scale studies evaluated the familial aggregation of alcohol and drug dependence. In both studies it was established that relatives of drug-disorder patients had a much greater rate of drug disorders, including abuse of opioids, cocaine, and cannabis, than did relatives of controls. However, this finding does not necessarily suggest that the genetic predisposition to alcoholism is due to the same genes as the genetic predisposition to other drug disorders. In fact, the traits seem to be fairly independent. The only truly strong evidence of a shared, as well as a specific, genetically determined addictive tendency is between alcohol and nicotine, an observation that is hardly new or surprising (21–24).

General Observations on Inheritable Factors

Following are several inheritable factors that may predispose to alcohol or drug abuse:

1. Low level of response to alcohol or drugs of abuse.
2. Inherited patterns of the electrical activity of the brain.
3. Neuropeptide Y: alcohol, anxiety, and satiety.
4. Mutations of the proteins associated with neurotransmitters.

Low Level of Response to Alcohol or Drugs of Abuse

The low level of response factor reflects the need for higher doses of alcohol to produce a discernible effect. The low level of response to alcohol might enhance the probability of heavy drinking, encourage the formation of peer groups with similar drinking habits, and lead to rapid acquisition of tolerance. Low levels of response were seen in about 40% of children of alcoholics evaluated in several well-designed studies. Native Americans were identified as a specific group presenting with low levels of response. Conversely, high levels of response and, consequently, lower alcoholism risks have been noted for Jews and some Asian populations (22–25). A candidate gene study reported on mutations in the gene that codes for a subunit of GABA receptor and in the gene that codes for the serotonin transporter protein, whereas a different study linked the low response to alcohol with narrow areas of chromosomes 1 and 21 (26–29).

Inherited Patterns of the Electrical Activity of the Brain

An overall, low-voltage electroencephalography (EEG) pattern, lower amounts of alpha rhythm, and scarcity of synchronized EEG waves appear to be fairly common in alcoholics but also characterize a variety of conditions including major depression, anxiety, and drug withdrawal. Children of alcoholics may exhibit lower amounts of alpha EEG activity and respond to alcohol by increases in alpha activity. Some children of alcoholics also demonstrate overall lower EEG voltage (29–32). Evidence supporting genetic influences in EEG patterns includes greater similarities in identical versus fraternal twins and a report of classic dominant and recessive (mendelian) inheritance for predisposition to have mostly slow alpha EEG activity (32,33).

Neuropeptide Y: Alcohol, Anxiety, and Satiety

Chronic alcohol abuse is associated with increased levels of neuropeptide Y in the hypothalamus as well as with the increase in responsiveness of the brain to the action of neuropeptide Y. In animal models, alcohol-habituated rats have been shown to exhibit a mutation on chromosome 4 in the area that encodes for neuropeptide Y to which about one third of the increased alcohol intake may be attributed.

In other experiments, rats bred to consume high levels of alcohol have increased neuropeptide Y activity in the amygdala (which may reflect a higher level of anxiety), along with decreased neuropeptide Y in the frontal cortex and hippocampus (possibly reflecting a lower level of satiety). Genetically engineered mice that do not produce neuropeptide Y are observed to drink more alcohol and to have a lower intensity of response, while mice engineered to have higher than normal levels of neuropeptide Y consume less alcohol and produce higher responses to alcohol. Studies of the role neuropeptide Y may play in human beings are under way, with the neuropeptide itself being evaluated as a potential treatment of alcohol addiction (34–36).

Mutations of the Proteins Associated with Neurotransmitters

Most direct evidence in this field comes from studies of genes that code for serotonin receptors. Mutations in these genes may lead to higher alcohol intake either directly or through antisocial behavior, clinical depression, schizophrenia, or generalized anxiety.

Specific findings are limited to animal models and include higher density of serotonin receptor type 1A, observed in alcohol-addicted rats. Genetically engineered mice in which the gene for serotonin receptor type 1B has been deactivated consume more alcohol than the wild-type mice. A decrease in sensitivity of serotonin receptor 2C is found in alcoholics. In addition, children of alcoholics have been found to have lower levels of serotonin in the synapses of serotonergic neurons that might relate to proneness to depression or, separately, proneness to low response to alcohol and thus a higher risk of alcoholism (37–39).

Specific Genetics of Alcohol Addiction

The only genes that are known to have a major impact on the development of alcoholism are those that code for proteins involved in metabolism of alcohol: alcohol dehydrogenase and aldehyde dehydrogenase. The enzyme alcohol dehydrogenase metabolizes alcohol (ethanol) to acetaldehyde, a toxic intermediate product, which is later converted to the much less toxic acetate by the enzyme aldehyde dehydrogenase. In both cases, one gene variant appears to be protective and the other variant presents with increased vulnerability to development of alcohol addiction.

Specifically, the ADH2-2 and ALDH2-2 genetic variants of alcohol dehydrogenase and aldehyde dehydrogenase, respectively, lead to the specific changes in alcohol metabolism that resemble the results of aversion therapy with disulfiram (Antabuse). In persons who have inherited these variants, an unpleasant reaction develops upon ingestion of even small amounts of ethanol, characterized by facial flushing, headache, hypotension, palpitations, tachycardia, nausea, and vomiting.

In one study, the frequency of the dominantly acting ALDH2-2 variant was found to be approximately 30% in Japanese and Chinese populations. The risk of alcoholism in those individuals is reduced about 4- to 10-fold. At the same time, the popular view that genetics determines the outcome is not supported by any serious scientific studies, including those of the alcohol metabolism variants. A well-designed study found that the frequencies of the ADH2 and ALDH2 variants were very similar in examined Korean and Taiwanese populations. However, the incidence of alcoholism was 2.9% in the Taiwanese subjects and 17.2% in Koreans, suggesting that environmental factors play a major, and possibly determining, role in the actual development of alcoholism and, by extension, drug abuse. Recent findings of interest include the observation that the ADH2-3 allele, a high-activity variant that increases the rate of ethanol metabolism, is identified in approximately 25% of African Americans. In another report, the presence of ADH2-3 in African-American mothers who drank during pregnancy was associated with a lower rate of alcohol-related birth defects and fetal alcohol syndrome (40–45).

References

1. Solomon RL, Corbit JD. An opponent-process theory of motivation: I. Temporal dynamics of affect. Psychol Rev 1974;81:119–145.
2. Berridge KC, Robinson TE. What is the role of dopamine in reward: hedonic impact, reward learning or incentive salience? Brain Res Rev 1998;28:309–369.
3. Robinson TE, Berridge KC. Addiction. Annu Rev Psychol 2003;54:25–53.
4. Berridge KC, Robinson TE. Parsing reward. Trends Neurosci 2003;26: 507–513.
5. Tobler PN, Fiorillo CD, Schultz W. Adaptive coding of reward value by dopamine neurons. Science 2005;307:1642–1645.
6. Kelley AE. Opioid modulation of taste hedonics within the ventral striatum. Physiol Behav 2002;76:365–377.
7. Alcohol, the brain, and behavior. Mechanisms of addiction. Alcohol Res Health 2000;24(1):12–15.

8. Brauer LH, Cramblett MJ, Paxton DA, Rose JE. Haloperidol reduces smoking of both nicotine-containing and denicotinized cigarettes. Psychopharmacology (Berl) 2001;159:31–37.
9. Hart CL. Methamphetamine self-administration by humans. Psychopharmacology (Berl) 2001;157:75–81.
10. Wachtel SR. The effects of acute haloperidol or risperidone on subjective responses to methamphetamine in healthy volunteers. Drug Alcohol Depend 2002;68:23–33.
11. Leyton M. Amphetamine-induced increases in extracellular dopamine, drug wanting, and novelty seeking: a PET/11C raclopride study in healthy men. Neuropsychopharmacology 2002;27:1027–1035.
12. Volkow ND. Nonhedonic food motivation in humans involves dopamine in the dorsal striatum and methylphenidate amplifies this effect. Synapse 1002;44:175–180.
13. Gruber AJ, Pope HG, Hudson JI, Yurgelun-Todd D. Attributes of long-term heavy cannabis users: a case–control study. Psychol Med 2003;33:1415–1422.
14. Hoffman AF, Riegel AC, Lupica CR. Functional localization of cannabinoid receptors and endogenous cannabinoid production in distinct neuron populations of the hippocampus. Eur J Neurosci 2003;18:524–534.
15. Meyer JS, Ali SF. Serotonergic effects of MDMA (ecstasy) in the developing brain. Ann NY Acad Sci 2002;965:373–380.
16. Meyer JS, Grande M, Johnson K, Ali SF. Neurotoxic effects of MDMA (ecstasy). Int J Dev Neurosci 2004;22:261–271.
17. O'Brien CP. Benzodiazepine use, abuse and dependence. J Clin Psychiatry 2005;66(Suppl 2):28–33.
18. Zawertailo LA, Busto UE, Kaplan HL, Greenblatt DJ, Sellers EM. Comparative abuse liability and pharmacological effects of meprobamate, triazolam, and butabarbital. J Clin Psychopharmacol 2003;23(3):269–280.
19. Schuckit MA, Smith TL. An 8-year follow-up of 450 sons of alcoholic and control subjects. Arch Gen Psychiatry 1996;53:202–210.
20. Goldman D, Bergen A. General and specific inheritance of substance abuse and alcoholism. Arch Gen Psychiatry 1998;55(11):964–965.
21. Bierut LJ, Dinwiddie SH, Begleiter H. Familial transmission of substance dependence: alcohol, marijuana, cocaine and habitual smoking. Arch Gen Psychiatry 1998;55:982–988.
22. Pollock VE. Meta-analysis of subjective sensitivity to alcohol in sons of alcoholics. Am J Psychiatry 1992;149:1534–1538.
23. Monteiro MG, Klein JL, Schuckit MA. High levels of sensitivity to alcohol in young adult Jewish men: a pilot study. J Stud Alcohol 1991;52:474–469.
24. Ehlers CL, Garcia-Andrade C, Wall TL. Electroencephalographic responses to alcohol challenge in Native American Mission Indians. Biol Psychiatry 1999;45:776–787.
25. Wall TL, Johnson ML, Horn SM. Evaluation of the self-rating form of the effects of alcohol in Asian Americans with aldehyde dehydrogenase polymorphisms. J Stud Alcohol 1999;60:784–789.
26. Schuckit MA, Mazzanti C, Smith TL. Selective genotyping for the role of 5-HT2A, 5-HT2C, and GABAA6 receptors and the serotonin transporter in the level of response to alcohol: a pilot study. Biol Psychiatry 1999;45:647–651.
27. Schuckit MA, Edenberg HJ, Kalmijn J. A genome-wide search for genes that relate to a low level of response to alcohol. Alcohol Clin Exp Res 2001;25:323–329.

28. Ehlers CL, Schuckit MA. Evaluation of EEG alpha activity in sons of alcoholics. Neuropsychopharmacology 1991;4:199–205.
29. Enoch MA, White KV, Harris CR. Association of low voltage alpha EEG with a subtype of alcohol use disorders. Alcohol Clin Exp Res 1999;23:1312–1319.
30. Pollock VE, Volavka J, Goodwin DW. The EEG after alcohol administration in men at risk for alcoholism. Arch Gen Psychiatry 1983;40:857–681.
31. Bauer LO, Hesselbrock VM. EEG, autonomic and subjective correlates of the risk for alcoholism. J Stud Alcohol 1993;54:577–589.
32. van Beijsterveldt CEM, Boomsma DI. Genetics of the human electroencephalogram (EEG) and event-related brain potentials (ERPs): a review. Hum Genet 1994;94:319–330.
33. O'Connor S, Sorbel J, Morzorati S. A twin study of genetic influences on the acute adaptation of the EEG to alcohol. Alcohol Clin Exp Res 1999;23:494–501.
34. Ehlers CL, Li T-K, Lumeng L. Neuropeptide Y (NPY) levels in ethanol-naive alcohol preferring and non-preferring rats and in Wistar rats following ethanol exposure. Alcohol Clin Exp Res 1998;22:1778–1782.
35. Hwang BH, Zhang J-K, Ehlers CL. Innate differences of neuropeptide Y (NPY) in hypothalamic nuclei and central nucleus of the amygdala between selectively bred rats with high and low alcohol preference. Alcohol Clin Exp Res 1999;23:1023–1030.
36. Thiele TE, Marsh DJ, Ste Marie L. Ethanol consumption and resistance are inversely related to neuropeptide Y levels. Nature 1998;396:366–369.
37. Wong DT, Reid LR, Li T-K. Greater abundance of serotonin1A receptor in some brain areas of alcohol-preferring (P) rats compared to nonpreferring (NP) rats. Pharmacol Biochem Behav 1993;46:173–177.
38. Crabbe JC, Phillips TJ, Feller DJ. Elevated alcohol consumption in null mutant mice lacking 5-HT1B serotonin receptors. Nat Genet 1996;14:98–101.
39. Ernouf D, Compagnon P, Lothion P. Platelet 3H 5-HT uptake in descendants from alcoholic patients: a potential risk factor for alcohol dependence. Life Sci 1993;52:989–995.
40. Kreek MJ. Cocaine, dopamine and the endogenous opioid system. J Addict Dis 1996;15(4):73–96.
41. Merikangas KR, Stolar M, Stevens DE. Familial transmission of substance use disorders. Arch Gen Psychiatry 1998;55:973–979.
42. Harada S, Agarwal DP, Goedde HW. Aldehyde dehydrogenase deficiency as cause of facial flushing reaction to alcohol in Japanese. Lancet 1982;2(8253):982–990.
43. Goldman D. Genetic transmission. In Galanter M, ed. Recent Developments in Alcoholism. Volume 11: Ten Years of Progress. New York: Plenum Press, 1993;14:231–248.
44. Thomasson HR, Beard JD, Li TK. ADH2 gene polymorphisms are determinants of alcohol pharmacokinetics. Alcohol Clin Exp Res 1995;19(6):1494–1499.
45. McCarver DG, Thomasson HR, Martier SS. Alcohol dehydrogenase-2-3 allele protects against alcohol-related birth defects among African Americans. J Pharmacol Exp Ther 1997;283(3):1095–1101.

4
The Sociologic Basis of Drug and Alcohol Addiction

Noosha Niv

The sociologic model of addiction emphasizes the impact of environment and social relations on the development of addictive disorders. Developmental theories assert that socialization occurs in the context of primary relationships. Hence, this chapter focuses on the roles of parents, siblings, spouses, and peers as etiologic factors in the development and maintenance of addiction. Environmental stressors, including childhood abuse and neglect, exposure to violence, and poverty, are also examined as risk factors for substance use disorders. Other environmental factors, such as lack of appropriate law enforcement and societal attitudes and messages about substance use, have also been implicated in addiction. However, a review of these greater causes is beyond the scope of this chapter.

Family Factors

Given the significant role that families play in the development and well-being of adolescents, the family is regarded as the primary psychosocial determinant of susceptibility to substance use disorders. Family risk factors and protective factors—and how the two interact—are reviewed, primarily in the context of adolescent substance use. Less attention is given to the influence of family on adult substance abusers.

Parental Substance Use

Residing in a household with alcohol- or drug-using parents increases the risk in adolescents for substance use, and having a family history of substance abuse increases the likelihood of abuse (1–4). Compared with their peers, children who live with parents who abuse substances are at greater risk for both alcohol (5) and drug (6–8) use. One study found that 72% of parents who abstained from alcohol use had adolescents who also abstained, whereas 82% of parents who drank had children who also used alcohol (9). Parental substance abuse has been shown to be a strong predictor of alcohol and drug problems later in life (10). In a study of alcohol-dependent women, 77% reported alcoholism in a parent (11). Similarly, in a study of substance-dependent parents, 83% reported that one of their own parents had a substance abuse disorder (12).

In addition to actual parental substance abuse, adolescents' perceptions of the frequency of parental use is also predictive of adolescent use (13). Permissive attitudes regarding substance use on the part of the parent increases the likelihood of adolescent use (14,15). The literature suggests that this association between parental and adolescent use may be stronger for girls than for boys (16–18).

The transmission of alcohol and drug use from parent to child can be explained by a genetic transmission model and by a family systems model (19). The genetic transmission model contends that a genetic vulnerability makes individuals susceptible to low substance tolerance, which increases the likelihood of addiction. The family systems model stresses the role of family dysfunction in the etiology of addiction. Others posit that genetics and environmental influences (including family environment) combine to determine susceptibility to addiction (20,21).

Focusing on the family systems model, there are two competing theories that describe the relationship between parental psychopathology, including substance use, and adolescent adjustment (22). The first, social learning theory, hypothesizes that there is a direct link between parental and adolescent substance use. Parents may model substance-using behaviors and even positively reinforce them by sending the message that substance use is acceptable behavior (23). Furthermore, parental drug use may increase availability of substances, and many adolescents report that their first drinking or substance-using experiences occurred in the home (24,25). Although the association between parent and adolescent use provides support for this theory, the strength of these correlations is modest, suggesting that modeling explanations do not sufficiently explain the connection.

The second theory, the stress-coping model, asserts that parental substance use increases the number and severity of life stressors a family must face, which in turn alters family processes and increases an adolescent's risk for substance use (23,26). It is also believed that substance-using parents do not teach their children adequate coping skills (27), further increasing the risk for substance use. Lacking sufficient coping mechanisms, adolescents may turn to substance abuse to deal with adverse family situations and related emotional distress.

The stress-coping model is supported by findings that children in substance-abusing households report greater levels of stress, social isolation, and socioeconomic disadvantages than do children in nonabusing homes (28). Exposure to negative life stressors is associated with increased substance use (29,30), as well as decreased family cohesiveness, which in turn can lead to adolescent substance use (31). Substance-abusing parents experience a number of stressors, such as economic difficulties, unemployment, marital conflict and divorce, social isolation, parent–child conflict, and a range of other factors related to adolescent substance use (32–37). Some of these key variables are reviewed.

Studies indicate that family processes are disrupted when a parent abuses alcohol and drugs. For example, it can change the family composition by leading to the temporary or permanent loss of a parent as a result of incarceration, child custody proceedings, or even substance-related death. Parental substance use is related to greater parent–child conflict and lower levels of parental support (38). Parenting skills are also impacted by substance use. Compared with nonabusing mothers, substance-abusing mothers are less responsive to their infants' needs, spend less time with their children, and show deficient parenting skills (39,40). These changes in family interactions all increase the risk for adolescent substance abuse.

Parental substance abuse and, in particular, alcohol abuse have been associated with domestic violence (41). Children report that the greatest problem they view as associated with their parents' substance abuse is violence in the home and the resulting fear they experience (42). They may also put themselves at risk for harm in an attempt to stop the violence. Children exposed to parental violence are more vulnerable to substance abuse problems (43).

There is a large quantity of data showing that parental substance abuse elevates the risk for child maltreatment, including neglect and abuse. Parents who abused drugs or alcohol were 4.2 times more likely to be neglectful of their children than were parents who did not abuse substances (44). Drug-seeking behaviors, drug consumption, and even treatment involvement may increase the risk for child neglect (40). Children's medical care, food, shelter, and hygiene are often neglected, and these children are also at risk for getting involved in drug distribution or prostitution by their parents for the obtainment of drugs (45).

Furthermore, parental substance abuse can put a child's health or safety at risk or create a neglect or abuse situation that requires outside intervention and, often, out-of-home placement (46). Nearly 70% of child protective services cases come from homes characterized by parental substance use, and substance-abusing parents are more likely to lose custody of their children than are nonabusing parents (47,48). In a study comparing children who tested positive for cocaine at birth with a control group, the risk for neglect and abuse was nearly eight times higher in the drug-exposed group than in the control group (49). By their first birthday, about 50% of the drug-exposed babies had been removed from their home, whereas no children from the control group had been removed.

Children born to substance-abusing parents are also at greater risk for becoming "boarder babies." These babies remain in the hospital longer than necessary because parents are unable or choose not to take responsibility for them. A study of 7,000 boarder babies found that 85% of them had been prenatally exposed to drugs, and 58% were subsequently placed in foster care (50).

Little work has been done to identify relationships between abuse of specific substances and types of child maltreatment. However, in a review of 190 juvenile court cases involving child maltreatment, parental alcohol abuse was associated with physical abuse of the child, and parental cocaine abuse was associated with sexual abuse (51). In less severe cases, parental substance use is associated with higher levels of physical punishment and a greater risk for injury and unintended intoxication (52–54). The impact of childhood neglect and abuse on subsequent risk for substance use disorders is potent and is discussed later in this chapter.

Children living with alcohol-dependent parents are at higher risk for depression, anxiety, negative affect, low self-esteem, and oppositional and conduct disorders (55–57) and have lower school achievement and greater cognitive deficits compared with controls (58,59). These difficulties result in a greater number of hospital admissions and longer lengths of stay for children of substance abusers. Inpatient admission rates and average lengths of stay of children of alcoholics are reported to be 25% to 30% greater than for children of nonalcoholics (60). Furthermore, of children under 12 years old who were hospitalized for mental health problems, 53% came from families in which at least one parent abused substances (61). This increased likelihood of psychopathology puts these children at higher risk for developing substance use disorders themselves.

Poverty and unstable living conditions are potential consequences of having substance-dependent parents with employment difficulties or lower occupational status (40). Economic deprivation for children may only increase if their parents are too impaired to pursue public assistance programs. Low socioeconomic status of the parents, in turn, has been associated with drug use (62).

Clearly, the effects of parental substance use have a large impact on subsequent adolescent use both directly and indirectly. Concern for their children and/or fear of losing custody are common treatment motivators for parents, particularly mothers. The paradox is that lack of adequate child care and fear of losing custody of their children remain substantial barriers to getting proper treatment (63).

Sibling Substance Use

A high percentage of substance-dependent adolescents report that their siblings are regular drug users as well (64). Studies find that older siblings in particular play an important role, as use by older siblings is associated with the younger sibling's substance use (65,66), as well as with stage of use (67). Adolescents who have older drug-abusing siblings also start using drugs at an earlier age (68). The influence of sibling substance use has been found to be stronger than parental influence on use (69) and may even be equal to or greater than peer influences (68,70).

An adolescent's relationship and identification with the older sibling also impacts drug use. For example, one study found that drug use was inversely related to sibling fighting (71). This finding that heavier drug users have less conflicted relationships with their siblings suggests that these siblings may share the same attitudes regarding drug use. Alternatively, heavy drug-using adolescents may be alienated from their family members and may not have a relationship with their siblings. Identification with a sibling is also a factor in adolescent drug use. The combination of identification with an older brother, the older brother's drug use, and perceived peer drug use appeared to prompt adolescent drug use in one study (67). Interestingly, this combination of risk factors seemed to affect younger brothers' drug use more than younger sisters' drug use.

This association between siblings' substance use may be due to shared family or peer environments. However, this relationship remains significant even after accounting for measures of shared environment, such as family structure, parental substance use, socioeconomic status, and neighborhood risk (66,72). Therefore, it appears that the relationship between siblings' substance use is not due to shared environmental factors alone. Alternatively, there are multiple pathways in which a sibling's substance use may directly impact a younger sibling's use. Siblings, especially older ones, can act as role models by reinforcing certain attitudes and behaviors. Older siblings may influence substance use by modeling this behavior, as predicted by social learning theory, or by increasing the availability of substances. Older siblings may affect substance use behaviors indirectly by sharing a deviant peer group with the younger sibling or by influencing the younger sibling's choice of peers (73).

Siblings do not necessarily have to use substances together to influence one another's use. Younger siblings' substance use is associated with their perceptions of their older siblings' attitudes toward use, and older siblings may influence adolescent substance use by communicating their attitudes about drugs and alcohol verbally and nonverbally (74). The attitudes of 10- to 12-year-olds became more liberal about drinking behaviors the more their older siblings found it acceptable (75). Furthermore, younger siblings were more likely to have used substances in the past year if they believed their older sibling would not disapprove of this use (68). Older siblings' attitudes and willingness regarding substance use remained predictive of younger siblings' substance use even after accounting for parent, peer, and sibling substance use (76). However, substance use was more likely if adolescents had an older sibling who held positive attitudes about substance use and resided in a risky neighborhood. These findings, which are consistent with those found with regard to the influence of parental attitudes on adolescent substance, show that substance use norms and attitudes can be transmitted within families.

Siblings' substance use and attitudes regarding substance use may also serve as a protective factor. For example, adolescents with siblings who did not use substances were less likely to use substances themselves (68) and more likely to abstain from higher levels of use (67). The influence of peers' substance use on younger siblings was also reduced if they had a sibling who did not use or did not support substance use (67,76).

Family Composition

Family structure has been found to play an important role in the onset of adolescent substance abuse. Some researchers have highlighted birth order as a factor, but the data are conflicting. For example, there are reports of firstborns using substances as a way of escaping the pressures to achieve and reports of lastborns using substances as a way to maintain their "baby of the family" status (24,77).

Better understood is the effect of family composition and parental absence on adolescent substance use. Children in nonintact families due to breakups, divorce, or death are at greater risk for lifetime use and for more advanced stages of use (78). Children residing with both parents are less likely to use drugs and alcohol than are those living in single-parent households (79). The relationship between family composition and substance use, however, may be dependent on the drug of abuse. For example, nonintact families have been associated with increases in alcohol and marijuana use but not with hallucinogen use (80). Regardless, these findings are troubling given the increase in single-parent families.

It has been suggested that the relationship between family composition and adolescent drug use may not be due to family structure per se but rather that family structure may reflect other changes in family processes (81). Differences in single- and two-parent families may be accounted for by a reduction in parental monitoring (82,83), a reduction in family resources (84), a decline in the quality of family relationships (81,85), and increases in other stressors affecting single-parent families.

The role of the extended family as a risk or protective factor in adolescent substance use is not yet understood. Most studies examining family composition categorize families based on the presence or absence of a father figure. However, living with extended family members is fairly common, particularly in minority populations. Although extended family members play an important role in the development of adolescents (86), their impact on the etiology of substance use is not yet clear.

Family Discipline

Several aspects of parenting style have been associated with adolescent substance use. Aspects of parenting that have received the most attention are parental monitoring, control, and discipline.

Higher levels of parental monitoring (i.e., knowing where and with whom a child spends time) protects adolescents from affiliation with substance-using peers (82,87), and less parental monitoring has been associated with a greater likelihood of alcohol and drug use, more frequent use, and earlier initiation of use (88,89).

Jurich and associates (25) described three basic types of parental discipline: (1) democratic, (2) laissez-faire, and (3) authoritarian. Democratic discipline emphasizes discussion of rules in advance, joint decision making, and attempts to compromise by both parent and child. Laissez-faire discipline allows children to set their own rules with little or no direction from parents. In contrast, authoritative parents set all the rules and expect full, unquestioned obedience. There has been little research examining democratic discipline. The little that has been done, however, indicates that adolescents receiving democratic discipline are less likely to use drugs than are those who receive other forms of discipline (90,91).

Findings regarding discipline style and adolescent substance use have been inconsistent, with a tendency for parents of substance users to use either laissez-faire or authoritarian discipline (25). Parents of adolescents who use drugs typically adopt a permissive attitude compared with parents of nonusers (90). Substance-using adolescents report having parents who do not care about their actions (92), a lack of parental direction (93), perceptions of parental overpermissiveness, and a lowering of family expectations (94). Conversely, authoritative discipline has also been associated with adolescent substance use. Parents of adolescent substance abusers have been described as controlling, intrusive, possessive, and overprotective (93,95), and drug-using adolescents are often subject to much parental pressure (92).

These inconsistent findings associating both permissive attitudes and excessive control to substance use suggest that the relationship is best described by a U-shaped model with adolescents most at risk when parental discipline and control is inadequate or extreme. The general assumption is that parental disciplinary styles variously cause or prevent adolescent substance use. Another interpretation is that parental discipline changes in reaction to adolescent substance use. In response to their child's substance use, parents may either "give up" and become too lax or become too controlling. This in turn may lead to greater use on the part of the adolescent, resulting in a cycle of poorer parenting and greater substance use. Regardless of the type of discipline used, families of a substance-abusing adolescent are more erratic in their disciplining style than are families of non–substance abusers (96). Within these families, rules are poorly defined and seldom held constant (97,98).

Parenting styles and type of discipline used may also be influenced by parents' feelings about parenting. Compared with parents of nonabusing adolescents, parents of substance-abusing adolescents view parenting as a job requiring suffering and sacrifice, report more child-rearing problems and a lack of confidence in parenting, and perceive their child's behavior as impossible to change (90,93).

Family Environment and Communication

Relationship to Adolescent Substance Abuse

The adolescent substance abuse literature reveals a strong association between family conflict and antisocial behavior, including substance use (71,99,100). Families who report substance use problems are often characterized by stressful family relationships, family conflict, and negative parent–child interactions (101–103). Adolescent drug abusers perceive their parents more negatively than non–drug abusers, are more likely to report a hostile and controlling family environment (93,95), find their families less enjoyable (92), and often suggest that weak family relationships have contributed to their drug problems (104). Similarly, parents of adolescents with substance use disorders report greater dissatisfaction with their children (105) and have lower attachment to their children (106).

There is evidence that the effect of family conflict may be gender dependent. For example, Wu and associates (107) reported that family conflict was associated with severity of drug use for boys but not girls. This is consistent with other data suggesting that boys may be more directly influenced by family environment than girls (108).

Parental support and warmth have also received considerable attention, and the negative association between perceived parental support and alcohol and drug use in adolescents is well established (71,109,110). Teenage drug users are less likely to report feeling close to family members (111), report a lack of parental love (95), and report receiving less praise and recognition from their parents (111,112) than are nonusers. Adolescents with high levels of family support have lower rates of alcohol problems and are less likely to start smoking (113,114). Parental support also reduces the effect of life stressors on adolescent substance use (115). These studies all suggest that supportive parental behaviors such as approving, companionship, praise, physical affection, encouraging, and assisting have the potential for reducing the risk of adolescent substance use.

There have been some contradictory findings regarding the relationship between family substance use and family bonding: the extent to which families join together in a meaningful and integrated unit. Most studies find that adolescent substance users report a lack of family cohesiveness (90,91), and family bonding has generally been negatively associated with frequency of substance use (116). A low degree of bonding makes adolescents more likely to have substance abuse disorders (117). There are, however, some reports that excessive bonding, or overinvolvement of family members, may increase the risk for substance use as well (118). It has been suggested that at high levels of bonding, adolescents become conflicted between their need for autonomy and the family's need for connectedness, resulting in substance use as a way of coping.

Poor family communication has also been implicated in adolescent drug use, whereas open communication between parents and adolescents reduces the risk for substance use (119). Adolescent substance users describe their communication with parents as closed and unclear (93) and are less able to discuss substance use with their parents than are nonusing adolescents (80). Drug-abusing adolescents report blocking communication with their parents because they feel misunderstood (120). A small proportion of drug-using adolescents and their family members believe the other to be honest about their thoughts and feelings (91). Interestingly, parents acknowledge these deficits in communication, and a significant number of them report their own inadequacy in conveying understanding, trust, and acceptance to their children (93).

Rigid patterns of communication have been observed in families of drug-abusing adolescents, which make decision making and conflict resolution more difficult (121,122). In contrast, family flexibility, or the family's ability to modify interactions to accommodate different situations (including developmental changes in the adolescent), has been found to reduce the adolescent risk for substance abuse (109).

There is also a high frequency of blaming among families of substance-abusing adolescents, and family communication is often hostile and conflict ridden compared with families of nonabusing adolescents (25,123). For example, Humes and Humphrey (123) showed that drug-dependent adolescent girls displayed the same ambivalence about autonomy and separation from family as did non–drug-abusing girls. However, their parents responded to this ambivalence with contradictory messages of support and condemnation. Compared with parents of nonabusing girls, they were both more affirming and understanding of their daughter's autonomy and expressed greater belittling and blaming. In contrast, parents of nonabusing girls fostered their daughters' efforts at autonomy without hostility or conflicting messages.

Relationship to Adult Substance Abuse

Few studies have examined the family environment of adult substance abusers, and most of the studies conducted have looked at either families of dual-diagnosis patients (persons with both a substance use disorder and severe mental illness) or at marital relationships. Studies indicate that families of adults with dual disorders are characterized by more greatly disturbed family affect and more family problems than are families of persons without a substance abuse disorder (124,125). Dual-diagnosis patients also report greater family dissatisfaction than do those without a substance use disorder (126). However, the impact of these family variables on the initiation or maintenance of substance use disorders remains unstudied.

More is known about substance-abusing adults in the context of marital relationships. Substance use has been related to significant marital distress and problems in a number of domains of marital functioning (127,128). Common relationship problems of these couples include relationship instability and dissatisfaction, as well as physical and verbal aggression (129). Communication is also generally impaired. Compared with non–substance abusing couples, those with a drug-abusing husband show deficits in joint problem solving (i.e., an inability to stay focused on a topic or generate solutions to address the identified problem) and exhibit abusive communication (e.g., yelling, name calling, cursing, and making verbally abusive or threatening comments) (130).

The relation between marital friction and substance use is complicated and reciprocal. Partner alcohol and drug use has been implicated as a cause of a number of marital difficulties, such as financial stress, conflict, and poor communication and problem solving. In turn, any relationship problems are associated with increased substance use and posttreatment relapse (131). Among alcoholics, lower marital satisfaction predicts worse treatment outcomes (132). Similarly, alcoholic patients with spouses who are overly critical and/or overly protective of them are at greater risk for relapse, have a shorter time to relapse, and drink more frequently (133). In contrast, perceived family support is associated with reduced alcohol-related hospitalization rates 1 year postdischarge (134).

To further complicate the issue, substance use may in some ways serve relationship needs. For couples in which both partners use drugs or alcohol, more frequent use and comparable frequency of use have been associated with greater marital adjustment (128,129), whereas discrepant use is associated with poorer marital functioning (135). Substance use may become an important shared recreational activity for partners who use together. In fact, the relationship between drug use and relationship satisfaction increases the more time partners spend using drugs together (129).

Substance use may also allow for increased expressions of affection and intimacy (136). For example, a partner may express affection through substance-related caretaking behaviors such as taking care of a partner suffering from a hangover. Behaviors such as this are often referred to as *enabling behaviors*. These are coping behaviors that family members engage in that can, intentionally or unintentionally, exacerbate substance use. Examples of enabling behaviors include caretaking, attempting to stabilize situations, and fear and avoidance responses.

Peer Factors

One of the strongest predictors of adolescent drug use is peer influence (137,138). A higher probability of use and increased levels of use have been associated with peer pressure to use, perceptions of peer substance use, and association with drug-using peers (139,140). Some have argued that family factors may influence the choice of peers in the early stages of drug use and that peer interactions influence both the initiation and maintenance of continued substance use (141). The process by which peers influence substance use is not well understood. However, it appears that friends model drug-using behaviors, share and shape attitudes about drug use, provide drugs, and provide the social context for such use (142).

The findings that adolescent drug users associate with friends who use drugs, engage in other delinquent behaviors, and are not achievement oriented have been replicated in both cross-sectional and longitudinal studies (143,144). This raises the question of the directionality of this relationship. While having friends who use drugs increases the risk for an adolescent to use drugs as well, does adolescent drug use lead to making friends who engage in drug-abusing behaviors? Findings that adolescents were similar in their drug use prior to their friendship (145) and that drug use facilitated adolescents' access to drug-using peers (146) suggest that this relationship holds true. In a longitudinal study of adolescent marijuana users, Brook and associates (147) found that marijuana use led to an increase in drug-using peers 5 years later. These findings suggest that there is a feedback effect in which adolescent drug use leads to an increase in deviant peers and furthers the risk for subsequent drug use.

Adolescents' own drug use is not the only predictor of associating with drug-using peers. Poor relationships with parents, including family conflict and maternal rejection, also increase the likelihood of affiliation with drug-using and deviant peers (148,149). In contrast, family involvement and parental monitoring have been identified as factors protective against the selection of substance-using peers that reduce the likelihood of problem behaviors within the context of a deviant peer group (82,87).

Family factors not only impact the choice of peers among adolescents but they can also serve as a protective factor by buffering the influence of deviant peers (81). Specifically, the quality of the mother–child relationship has been found to moderate the relation between peer influences and adolescent drug use; mother–child discord was associated with a strengthening of the relation between the child's peers' drug use and the child's drug use. On the other hand, strong mother–child relationships may reduce the impact of peer influences. In contrast, the quality of father–child relationships has not been shown to moderate the peer–adolescent drug use relationship (81). However, the presence of a father or stepfather in the home appears to weaken the relationship between peer pressure and drug use, perhaps because of increased parental monitoring.

Substance-abusing adults have smaller social networks than controls, and those with smaller networks have greater substance-related problems, psychosocial stressors, and depressive symptoms (134). In contrast, support from friends is associated with reduced alcohol-related hospitalizations (134). The protective function of peer support may depend, however, on whether those peers use substances as well. Having a social network that supports sobriety aids recovery, whereas a substance-using social network increases the risk for relapse (150,151). Unfortunately, substance-abusing patients often have interpersonal relationships with other substance users and participate in leisure activities that include substance use; involvement in such a subculture may increase the risk of relapse (152–154).

Exposure to Trauma and Neglect

Exposure to trauma increases an individual's risk for alcohol and drug problems. A review of over 300 clinical studies concluded that 40% to 70% of those suffering from posttraumatic stress disorder will also meet criteria for alcohol abuse and that alcohol abusers report three times as much trauma as nonabusers (155). The types of trauma that have received the most attention include sexual and physical abuse, childhood neglect, and exposure to violence.

The risk for alcohol and drug abuse disorders is increased for adolescents who have been physically or sexually assaulted or who have witnessed violence, including domestic violence and violence among peers (156,157). Compared with their nonvictimized peers, adolescents who had experienced either physical or sexual abuse/assault were twice as likely to report a substance use disorder in the past year (156). Childhood neglect is also associated with adverse substance abuse effects in early adulthood (158).

The relationship between childhood maltreatment, including sexual and physical abuse, and later substance use has been demonstrated in adult populations as well. Most of the work in this area has focused on women, perhaps because adolescent girls and adult women are at greater risk for experiencing physical and sexual assault than are boys and men. The association between childhood maltreatment and substance abuse problems in women has been established repeatedly (159,160). Studies of the general population report that adults abused during childhood are approximately twice as likely as those who are not abused to have serious substance abuse problems (161). Among women in substance abuse treatment, 65% to 90% report having experienced either sexual or physical abuse (162,163). Even more problematic is that 21% of women in one treatment-based study reported experiencing both sexual and physical abuse (162). Experiencing multiple traumas puts individuals at greater risk for substance use disorders, and the risk for substance abuse is doubled for women with histories of both physical and sexual abuse (164).

Being a victim of domestic violence has also been associated with substance abuse disorders. Miller and Downs (162) reported that approximately 50% of a treatment sample had been victims of domestic violence, and having a violent partner led to worse treatment outcomes for women (165,166).

Studies indicate that the occurrence of a traumatic event usually precedes drug and alcohol abuse (155). Use of alcohol and drugs may help in forgetting abuse memories and in numbing negative feelings associated with the trauma, leading many to frame substance abuse as an avoidance mechanism among trauma survivors (167). When individuals discontinue substance use, they may experience a resurgence of trauma responses, such as intrusive flashback, nightmares, and fear. The return of these symptoms can thus reinforce the desire for renewed substance abuse.

Conclusions

Returning to the bio-psycho-social concept of disease formation and applying it to the problem of substance abuse, including drug abuse, the social concept clearly has three components: (1) parenting and family inputs, (2) the neighborhood or community in which the individual grew up, and (3) peers in and out of school. Interventions in reducing substance abuse must be targeted at all three areas of influence in the growing child to prevent them from becoming involved in the drug-using culture and in drug abuse.

References

1. Barnes GM, Farrell MP, Cairns A. Parental socialization factors and adolescent drinking behaviors. J Marriage Fam 1986;48:27–36.
2. Dishion TJ, Patterson GR, Reid JR. Parent and peer factors associated with drug sampling in early adolescence: implications for treatment. In Rahdert RE, Grabowski J, eds. Adolescent Drug Abuse: Analyses of Treatment Research. Monograph Series 77. Washington, DC: National Institute on Drug Abuse Research; 1988.
3. Jacob T, Johnson SL. Family influences on alcohol and other substance use. In Ott PJ, Tarter RE, Ammerman RT, eds. Sourcebook on Substance Abuse. Boston: Allyn and Bacon; 1999:165–174.
4. McGue M. The behavioral genetics of alcoholism. Curr Direct Psychol Sci 1999;8:109–115.
5. Chassin L, Pillow F, Curran P, Molina BS, Barrera M. Relations of parental alcoholism to early adolescent substance use: a test of three mediating mechanisms. J Abnorm Psychol 1993;102:3–19.
6. Gross J, McCaul ME. A comparison of drug use and adjustment in urban adolescent children of substance abusers. Int J Addict 1990;25:495–511.
7. Johnson GM, Shontz FC, Locke TP. Relationships between adolescent drug use and parental drug behaviors. Adolescence 1989;19:295–299.
8. Weintraub SA. Children and adolescents at risk for substance abuse and psychopathology. Int J Addict 1990;25:481–494.
9. Kandel DB, Kessler RC, Margulies RZ. Antecedents of adolescent initiation into stages of drug use: a developmental analysis. J Youth Adolesc 1978;7: 13–40.
10. Stein JA, Leslie MB, Nyamathi A. Relative contributions of parent substance use and childhood maltreatment to chronic homelessness, depression, and substance abuse problems among homeless women: mediating roles of self-esteem and abuse in adulthood. Child Abuse Negl 2002;26:1011–1027.

11. National Institutes of Health. Drinking in the United States: Main Finding from the 1992 National Longitudinal Alcohol Epidemiologic Survey (NLAES). NIH Publication No. 99–3519. Bethesda, MD: National Institutes of Health; 1998.
12. Bays J. Substance abuse and child abuse: impact of addiction on the child. Pediatr Clin North Am 1990;37:881–904.
13. Anderson AR, Henry CS. Family system characteristics and parental behaviors as predictors of adolescent substance use. Adolescence 1994;29:405–420.
14. Halebsky MA. Adolescent alcohol and substance abuse: parent and peer effects. Adolescence 1987;22:961–967.
15. McDermott D. The relationship of parental drug use and parents' attitudes concerning adolescent drug use. Adolescence 1984;19:89–97.
16. Duncan TE, Duncan SC, Hopps H, Stoolmiller M. An analysis of the relationship between parent and adolescent marijuana use via generalized estimating equation methodology. Multivariate Behav Res 1995;30:317–339.
17. Green G, MacIntyre S, West P, Ecob R. Like parent like child: associations between drinking and smoking behaviors of parents and their children. Br J Addict 1991;86:745–758.
18. Hundleby JD, Mercer GW. Family and friends as social environments and their relationship to young adolescents' use of alcohol, tobacco, and marijuana. J Marriage Fam 1987;49:151–164.
19. Steinglass P, Bennett LA, Wolin SJ, Reiss D. The Alcoholic Family. New York: Basic Books; 1987.
20. Alterman AI, Tarter RE. The transmission of psychological vulnerability: implications for alcoholism etiology. J Nerv Ment Dis 1983;171:147–154.
21. Schuckit MA. A clinical model of genetic influences in alcohol dependence. J Stud Alcohol 1994;55(1):5–17.
22. Akers RL. Drugs, Alcohol, and Society: Social Structure, Process, and Policy. Belmont, CA: Wadsworth Press; 1992.
23. Seilhamer RA, Jacob T. Family factors and adjustment of children of alcoholics. In Windle M, Searles JS, eds. Children of Alcoholics: Critical Perspectives. New York: Guilford; 1990:168–186.
24. Barnes GM. Impact of the family on adolescent drinking patterns. In Collins RL, Leonard KE, Searles JS, eds. Alcohol and the Family: Research and Clinical Perspectives. New York: Guilford Press; 1990:137–161.
25. Jurich AP, Polson CJ, Jurich JA, Bates RA. Family factors in the lives of drug users and abusers. Adolescence 1985;20:143–159.
26. West MO, Prinz RJ. Parental alcoholism and childhood psychopathology. Psychol Bull 1987;102:204–218.
27. O'Leary DE, O'Leary MR, Donovan DM. Social skill acquisition and psychosocial development of alcoholics: a review. Addict Behav 1976;1(2):111–120.
28. Kumpfer KL, DeMarsh JP. Family environmental and genetic influences on children's future chemical dependency. In Ezekoye S, Kumpfer K, Bukoski W, eds. Childhood and Chemical Abuse: Prevention and Intervention. New York: Hayworth Press; 1986:49–91.
29. Bruns C, Geist CS. Stressful life events and drug use among adolescents. J Hum Stress 1984;10:135–139.
30. Newcomb MD, Harlow LL. Life events and substance use among adolescents: mediating effects of perceived loss of control and meaninglessness in life. J Pers Soc Psychol 1986;51:564–577.

31. Sue SS, Hoffman JP, Gerstein DR, Johnson RA. The effect of home environment on adolescent substance use and depressive symptoms. J Drug Issues 1997;27:851–875.
32. Clair D, Genest M. Variables associated with the adjustment of offspring of alcoholic fathers. J Stud Alcohol 1987;48(4):345–355.
33. Moos R, Billings A. Children of alcoholics during the recovery process: alcoholic and matched control families. Addict Behav 1982;7:155–163.
34. Reich W, Earls F, Powell J. A comparison of the home and social environments of children of alcoholic and non-alcoholic parents. Br J Addict 1988;83:831–839.
35. Roosa MW, Tien J, Groppenbacker N, Michaels M, Dumka L. Mothers' parenting behavior and child mental health in families with a problem drinking parent. J Marriage Fam 1993;55:107–118.
36. Velleman R, Orford J. The importance of family discord in explaining childhood problems in the children of problem drinkers. Addict Res 1993; 1:39–57.
37. Werner EE. Resilient offspring of alcoholics: a longitudinal study from birth to age 18. J Stud Alcohol 1986;47:34–40.
38. Jacob T, Krahn GL, Leonard K. Parent–child interactions in families with alcoholic fathers. J Consult Clin Psychol 1991;59:176–181.
39. Bauman PS, Dougherty FE. Drug addicted mothers' parenting and their children's development. Int J Addict 1983;18:291–302.
40. Kumpfer KL. Special populations: etiology with the prevention of vulnerability to chemical dependency in children of substance abusers. In Brown BS, Mills AR, eds. Youth at High Risk for Substance Abuse. Washington, DC: National Institute on Drug Abuse; 1987:206–233.
41. Fitch FJ, Papantonio A. Men who batter: some pertinent characteristics. J Nerv Ment Dis 1983;171:190–192.
42. ChildLine. Beyond the Limit: Children Who Live With Parental Alcohol Misuse. London: ChildLine; 1997.
43. Kilpatrick DG, Saunders BE, Smith DW. Youth Victimization: Prevalence and Implications. Publication No. NCJ 194972. Washington DC: U.S. Department of Justice, Office of Justice Programs; 2003.
44. National Center on Addiction and Substance Abuse at Columbia University. No Safe Haven: Children of Substance-Abusing Parents. New York, NY: National Center on Addiction and Substance Abuse at Columbia University; 1999.
45. Johnson BD, Williams T, Dei KA, Sanabria H. Drug abuse in the inner city: impact on hard-drug users and the community. In Tonry M, Wilson JQ, eds. Drugs and Crime, vol 13. Chicago: University of Chicago Press; 1990.
46. Kelly SJ. Parenting stress and child maltreatment in drug-exposed children. Child Abuse Negl 1992;16:317–328.
47. McCord J. A forty year perspective on effect of child abuse and neglect. Child Abuse Negl 1983;7(3):265–270.
48. Murphy MJ, Jellinek MS, Quinn D, Smith G, Poitrast FG, Goshko M. Substance abuse and serious child mistreatment: prevalence, risk, and outcome in a court sample. Child Abuse Negl 1991;15:197–211.
49. Kelley SJ, Walsh JH, Thompson K. Prenatal exposure to cocaine: birth outcomes, health problems and child neglect. Pediatr Nurs 1991;17:130–135.

50. Child Welfare League of America and National Association of Public Hospitals. Boarder Babies in Selected Hospital in the United States, Washington, DC: Child Welfare League of America and National Association of Public Hospitals; 1992.
51. Famularo R, Kinscherff R, Fenton T. Parental substance abuse and the nature of child maltreatment. Child Abuse Negl 1992;16:475–483.
52. Kolar AF, Brown BS, Haertzen CA, Michaelson MA. Children of substance abusers: the life experiences of children of opiate addicts in methadone maintenance. Am J Drug Alcohol Abuse 1994;20:159–171.
53. Bijur PE, Kurzon M, Overpeck MD, Scheidt PC. Parental alcohol use, problem drinking and children's injuries. JAMA 1992;267(23):3166–3177.
54. Young SL, Vosper HJ, Phillips SA. Cocaine: its effect on maternal and child health. Pharmacotherapy 1992;12:2–17.
55. Chassin L, Pitts SC, DeLucia C, Todd M. A longitudinal study of children of alcoholics: predicting young adult substance use disorders, anxiety, and depression. J Abnorm Psychol 1999;108:106–119.
56. Reich W, Earls F, Frankel O, Shayka JJ. Psychopathology in children of alcoholics. J Am Acad Child Adolesc Psychiatry 1993;32:995–1002.
57. Tarter RE, Hegedus AM, Goldstein G, et al. Adolescent songs of alcoholics: neuropsychological and personality characteristics. Alcohol Clin Exp Res 1984;8:216–222.
58. Bennett L, Wolin S, Reiss D. Cognitive, behavioral and emotional problems among school-age children of alcoholic parents. Am J Psychiatry 1988; 145(2):185–190.
59. Marcus AM. Academic achievement in elementary school children of alcoholic mothers. J Clin Psychol 1986;42(2):372–376.
60. Children of Alcoholics Foundation. In the Medical System: Hidden Problems, Hidden Costs. New York: Children of Alcoholics Foundation; 1990.
61. Rivinus TM, Levoy D, Matzko M, Seifer R. Hospitalized children of substance-abusing parents and physically and sexually abused children. J Am Acad Child Adolesc Psychiatry 1992;31:1019–1023.
62. Dohrenwend BP, Levav I, Shrout PE, Schwartz SN, Naveh G, Link BG, Skodol AE, Stueve A. Socioeconomic status and psychiatric disorders: the causation–selection issue. Science 1992;255:946–952.
63. Powis B, Gossop M, Bury C, Payne K, Griffiths P. Drug-using mothers: social, psychological and substance use problems of women opiate users with children. Drug Alcohol Rev 2000;19:171–180.
64. Craig SR, Brown BS. Comparison of youthful heroin users and nonusers from one urban community. Int J Addict 1975;10:53–64.
65. Gfroerer J. Correlation between drug use by teenagers and drug use by other family members. Am J Drug Alcohol Abuse 1987;13:95–108.
66. Griffin KW, Botvin GJ, Scheier LM, Nichols TR. Factors associated with regular marijuana use among high school students: a long-term follow-up study. Subst Use Misuse 2002;37:225–238.
67. Brook JS, Whiteman MG, Gordon AS, Brenden C. Older brother's influence on younger sibling's drug use. J Psychol 1983;114:83–90.
68. Needle R, McCubbin H, Wilson M, Reineck R, Lazar A, Mederer H. Interpersonal influences in adolescent drug use: the role of older siblings, parents and peers. Int J Addict 1986;21:739–766.

69. Brook JS, Brook DW, Whiteman M. Older sibling correlates of younger sibling drug use in the context of parent–child relations. Genet Social Gen Psychol Monogr 1999;125(4):451–468.
70. Brook JS, Whiteman M, Gordon AS, Brook DW. The role of older brothers in younger brothers' drug use viewed in the context of parent and peer influences. J Genet Psychol 1990;151(1):59–75.
71. Johnson V, Pandina RJ. Effects of the family environment of adolescent substance use, delinquency, and coping style. Am J Drug Alcohol Abuse 1991;17(1):71–88.
72. Fagan AA, Najman JM. Sibling influences on adolescent delinquent behavior: an Australian longitudinal study. J Adolesc 2003;26:546–558.
73. Conger RD, Reuter MA. Siblings, parents and peers: longitudinal study of social influences in adolescent risk for alcohol use and abuse. In Brody GH, ed. Sibling Relationships: Their Causes and Consequences. Norwood, NJ: ABlex; 1996:1–30.
74. Bullock BM, Dishion TJ. Sibling collusion and problem behavior in early adolescence: toward a process model for family mutuality. J Abnorm Child Psychol 2002;30:143–153.
75. Brody GH, Flor DL, Hollett-Wright N, McCoy JK. Children's development of alcohol use norms: contributions of parent and sibling norms, children's temperaments, and parent–child discussions. J Fam Psychol 1998;71:211–222.
76. Pomery EA, Gibbons FX, Gerrard M, Cleveland MJ, Wills TA, Brody GH. Families and risk: prospective analyses of familial social influences on adolescent substance use. J Fam Psychol 2005;19(4):560–570.
77. Keltner NL, McIntyre CW, Gee R. Birth order effects in second-generation alcoholics. J Stud Alcohol 1986;47(6):495–497.
78. Flewelling R, Bauman K. Family structure as a predictor of initial substance use and sexual intercourse in early adolescence. J Marriage Fam 1990;52:171–181.
79. Needle RH, Su SS, Doherty WJ. Divorce, remarriage and adolescent substance use: a prospective longitudinal study. J Marriage Fam 1990;52:157–169.
80. Tolone WL, Dermott D. Some correlates of drug use among high school youth in a Midwestern rural community. Int J Addict 1975;10:761–777.
81. Farrell AD, White KS. Peer influences and drug use among urban adolescents: family structure and parent–adolescent relationship as protective factors. J Consult Clin Psychol 1998;66:248–258.
82. Brown BB, Nounts N, Lamborn SD, Steinberg L. Parenting practices and peer group affiliation in adolescence. Child Dev 1993;64:467–482.
83. Patterson G, Stouthamer-Loeber M. The correlation of family management practices and delinquency. Child Dev 1984;55:1299–1307.
84. Gabel S. Behavioral problems in sons of incarcerated or otherwise absent fathers: the issue of separation. Fam Process 1992;31:303–314.
85. Amato P, Keith B. Parental divorce and the well-being of children: a meta-nalysis. Psychol Bull 1991;110:26–46.
86. Wilson MN. Child development in the context of the black extended family. Am Psychol 1989;44:380–385.
87. Cohen DA, Rickardson J, LaBree L. Parenting behaviors and the onset of smoking and alcohol use: a longitudinal study. Pediatrics 1994;94:368–375.

88. Chilcoat HD, Anthony JC. Impact of parent monitoring on initiation of drug use through late childhood. J Am Acad Child Adolesc Psychiatry 1996;8:153–157.
89. DiClemente RJ, Wingood FM, Crosby R, et al. Parental monitoring: association with adolescents' risk behaviors. Pediatrics 2001;107:1363–1368.
90. Blum RH. White middle-class families. In Henry WE, Sanford N, eds. Horatio Alger's Children. London: Jossey-Bass; 1972.
91. Cannon SR. Social Functioning Patterns of Families of Offspring Receiving Treatment for Drug Abuse. New York: Libra; 1976.
92. Tec N. Parent–child drug abuse: generational continuity or adolescent deviancy? Adolescence 1974;4:351–364.
93. Rees CD, Wilborn BL. Correlates of drug abuse in adolescents: a comparison of families of drug abusers with families of nondrug users. J Youth Adolesc 1983;12:55–63.
94. Brook JS, Lukoff IF, Whiteman M. Family socialization and adolescent personality and their association with adolescent use of marijuana. J Genet Psychol 1978;133:261–271.
95. Pandina RJ, Schuele JA. Psychosocial correlates of alcohol and drug use of adolescent students and adolescents in treatment. J Stud Alcohol 1983;44(6): 950–973.
96. Hartmann DA. A study of drug taking adolescents. Psychoanal Study Child 1969;24:384–398.
97. Sloboda SB. The children of alcoholics: a neglected problem. Hosp Commun Psychiatry 1974;25:605–606.
98. Reilly DM. Family factors in the etiology and treatment of youthful drug abusers. Fam Ther 1975;2:149–171.
99. Andrews JA, Hops H, Ary D, Tildesley E, Harris J. Parental influence on early adolescent substance use: specific and nonspecific effects. J Early Adolesc 1993;13:285–310.
100. Duncan TE, Duncan SC, Hops H. The effects of family cohesiveness and peer encouragement on the development of adolescent alcohol use: a cohort-sequential approach to the analysis of longitudinal data. J Stud Alcohol 1994;55(5):588–599.
101. Duncan TE, Alpert A, Duncan SC, Hops H. Multilevel covariance structure analysis of sibling substance use and intrafamily conflict. J Psychopathol Behav Assess 1996;18(4):347–368.
102. Hops H, Tildesley E, Lichtenstein E, Ary D, Sherman L. Parent–adolescent problem-solving interactions and drug use. Am J Drug Alcohol Abuse 1996; 16:239–258.
103. Kuperman S, Schlosser SS, Kramer JR, et al. Risk domains associated with an adolescent alcohol dependence diagnosis. Addiction 2001;96:629–636.
104. Svobodny LA. Biographical, self-concept, and educational factors among chemically dependent adolescents. Adolescence 1982;17:847–853.
105. Ammerman RT, Leober R, Kolko D, Balckson TC. Parental dissatisfaction with sons in substance abusing families: relationship to child and parent dysfunction. J Child Adolesc Subst Abuse 1994;3:23–37.
106. Brook JS, Tseng L, Cohen P. Toddler adjustment: impact of parents' drug use, personality and parent–child relations. J Genet Psychol 1996;157:281–295.

107. Wu NS, Lu Y, Sterling S, Weisner C. Family environment factors and substance abuse severity in an HMO adolescent treatment population. Clin Pediatr 2004;43:323–333.
108. Baer JS, Garmezy LB, McLaughlin RJ, et al. Stress, coping family conflict, and adolescent alcohol use. J Behav Med 1987;10;449–466.
109. Anderson AR, Henry CS. Family system characteristics and parental behaviors as predictors of adolescent substance use. Adolescence 1994;29:405–420.
110. Wills TA, Vaccaro D, McNamara G. The role of life events, family support, and competence in adolescent substance use: test of vulnerability and protective factors. Am J Comp Psychol 1992;20(3):349–374.
111. Coombs RH, Paulson MJ. Contrasting family patterns of adolescent drug users and nonusers. J Chem Depend Treat 1988;1(2):59–72.
112. Alexander BK, Dibb GS. Interpersonal perception in addict families. Fam Process 1977;16:17–28.
113. Barnes GM, Welte JW. Patterns and predictors of alcohol use among 7–12th grade students in New York state. J Stud Alcohol 1986;47:53–62.
114. Chassin L, Curran PJ, Hussong AM, Colder CR. The relation of parent alcoholism to adolescent substance use: a longitudinal follow-up study. J Abnorm Psychol 1996;105:76–80.
115. Wills TA, Cleary SD. How are social support effects mediated: a test for parental support and adolescent substance use. J Pers Soc Psychol 1996;71:937–952.
116. Bahr SJ, Marcos AC, Maughan SL. Family, educational and peer influences on the alcohol use of female and male adolescents. J Stud Alcohol 1995;56:457–469.
117. Volk RJ, Edwards DW, Lewis RA, Sprenkle DH. Family systems of adolescent substance abusers. Fam Relations 1989;38:266–272.
118. Levine BL. Adolescent substance abuse: toward an integration of family systems and individual adaptation theories. Am J Fam Ther 1985;13(2):3–16.
119. Peterson GW, Leigh GK. The family and social competence in adolescence. In Gullota T, Adams GR, Montemayor R, eds. Advances in Adolescent Development: Social Competence. Newbury Park, CA: Sage; 1990:97–138.
120. Hambur BA, Kraemer HC, Jahnke W. A hierarchy of drug use in adolescence: Behavioral and attitudinal correlates of substantial drug use. Am J Psychiatry 1975;132(11):1155–1163.
121. Bartle SE, Sabatelli RM. Family system dynamics, identity development, and adolescent alcohol use: Implications for family treatment. Fam Relations 1989;38:258–265.
122. Steier F, Stanton MD, Todd TC. Patterns of turn-taking and alliance formation in family communication. J Commun 1982;32:148–160.
123. Humes DL, Humphrey LL. A multimethod analysis of families with a polydrug-dependent or normal adolescent daughter. J Abnorm Psychol 1994;103(4):676–685.
124. Kashner TM, Rader LE, Rodell DE, Beck CM, Rodell LR, Muller K. Family characteristics, substance abuse, and hospitalization patterns of patients with schizophrenia. Hosp Community Psychiatry 1991;42:195–197.
125. Osher FC, Drake RE, Noordsy DL, Teague GB, Hurlbut SC, Biesanz JC, Beaudett MS. Correlates and outcomes of alcohol use disorder among rural outpatients with schizophrenia. J Clin Psychiatry 1994;55:109–113.

126. Dixon L, McNary S, Lehman A. Substance abuse and family relationships of persons with severe mental illness. Am J Psychiatry 1995;152:456–458.
127. Kosten TR, Jalali B, Steidl JH, Kleber HD. Relationship of marital structure and interactions to opiate abuse relapse. Am J Drug Abuse 1987;14: 387–399.
128. O'Farrell T, Birchler GR. Marital relationships of alcoholic, conflicted, and nonconflicted couples. J Marital Fam Ther 1987;13:259–274.
129. Fals-Stewart W, Birchler GR, O'Farrell TJ. Drug-abusing patients and their intimate partners: dyadic adjustment, relationship stability, and substance abuse. J Abnorm Psychol 1999;108:11–23.
130. Fals-Stewart W, Birchler GR. Marital interactions of drug-abusing patients and their partners: comparisons with distressed couples and relationship to drug-using behavior. Psychol Addict Behav 1998;12:28–38.
131. Maisto SA. Alcoholics' attributions of factors affecting their relapse to drinking and reasons for terminating relapse episodes. Addict Behav 1988;13(1):79–82.
132. Moos RH, Finney JW, Cronkite RC. Alcoholism Treatment: Context, Process, and Outcome. New York: Oxford University Press; 1990.
133. O'Farrell TJ, Hooley J, Fals-Stewart W, Cutter HS. Expressed emotion and relapse in alcoholic patients. J Consult Clin Psychol 1998;66:744–752.
134. Westermeyer J, Thuras P, Waaijer A. Size and complexity of social networks among substance abusers: childhood and current correlates. Am J Addict 2004; 13:372–380.
135. Roberts LJ, Leonard KE. An empirical typology of drinking partnerships and their relationship to marital functioning and drinking consequences. J Marriage Fam 1998;60:515–526.
136. Critchlow B. The powers of John Barleycorn: beliefs about the effects of alcohol on social behavior. Am Psychol 1986;41:751–764.
137. Ary DV, Tildesley E, Hops H, Andrews J. The influence of parent, sibling, and peer modeling and attitudes on adolescent use of alcohol. Int J Addict 1993;28:853–880.
138. Hawkins JD, Catalano RF, Miller JY. Risk and protective factors for alcohol and other drug problems in adolescence and early adulthood: implication for substance abuse prevention. Psychol Bull 1992;112:64–105.
139. Dishion TJ, Loeber R. Adolescent marijuana and alcohol use: the role of parents and peers revisited. Am J Drug Alcohol Abuse 1985;11:11–25.
140. Simons RL, Robertson JF. The impact of parenting factors, deviant peers, and coping style upon adolescent drug use. Fam Relations 1989;38:273–281.
141. Kandel DB, Yamaguchi K. Developmental patterns of the use of legal, illegal and medically prescribed psychotropic drugs from adolescence to young adulthood. NIDA Res Monogr 1985;56:193–235.
142. Oetting ER, Beauvais F. Peer cluster theory, socialization characteristics and adolescent drug use: A path analysis. J Counsel Psychol 1987;34(2):205–213.
143. Brook JS, Whiteman M, Gordon AS. Qualitative and quantitative aspects of adolescent drug use: the interplay of personality, family, and peer correlates. Psychol Rep 1982;51:1151–1163.
144. Hundlesby J, Mercer GW. Family and friends as social environments and their relationship to young adolescents' use of alcohol, tobacco, and marijuana. J Marriage Fam 1987;49:151–164.

145. Kandel DB. On processes of peer influences in adolescent drug use: a developmental perspective. Adv Alcohol Subst Abuse 1985;4:139–163.
146. Lamanna M. Marijuana: implications of use by young people. J Drug Educ 1981;11(4):281–310.
147. Brook JS, Balka EB, Whiteman M. The risks for late adolescence of early adolescent marijuana use. Am J Public Health 1999;89(10):1549–1554.
148. Bahr SJ, Marcos AC, Maughan SL. Family, educational and peer influences on the alcohol use of female and male adolescents. J Stud Alcohol 1995;56:457–469.
149. Patterson GR, DeBaryshe BD, Ramsey E. A developmental perspective on antisocial behavior. Am Psychol 1989;44:329–335.
150. Beatie MC, Longabaugh R. Interpersonal factors and post-treatment drinking and subjective well-being. Addiction 1997;92(11):1507–1521.
151. Hall SM, Havassy BE, Wasserman DA. Social support and relapse: commonalities among alcoholics, opiate users, and cigarette smokers. Addict Behav 1991;16:235–246.
152. Caroll KM, Rounsaville BJ, Keller DS. Relapse prevention strategies for the treatment of cocaine abusers. Am J Drug Alcohol Abuse 1991;17(3):249–265.
153. Marlatt GA, Gordon JR. Relapse Prevention: Maintenance Strategies in the Treatment of Addict Behavior. New York: Guilford Press; 1985.
154. Tucker JA, Vuchinich RE, Gladsjo JA. Environmental influences on relapse in substance use disorders. Int J Addict 1991;25:1017–1050.
155. Stewart SH. Alcohol abuse in individuals exposed to trauma: a critical review. Psychol Bull 1996;120:83–112.
156. Kilpatrick DG, Acierno R, Saunders B, Resnick HS, Best CL, Schnurr PP. Risk factors for adolescent substance abuse and dependence: data from a national sample. J Consult Clin Psychol 2000;68:19–30.
157. Simpson TL, Miller WR. Concomitance between childhood sexual and physical abuse and substance use problems: a review. Clin Psychol Rev 2002;22:27–77.
158. Kirisci L, Dunn MG, Mezzich AC, Tarter RE. Impact of parental substance use disorder and child neglect severity on substance use involvement in male offspring. Prev Sci 2001;2(4):241–255.
159. Bensley LS, Van Eenwyk J, Simmons KW. Self-reported childhood sexual and physical abuse and adult HIV-risk behaviors and heavy drinking. Am J Prev Med 2000;18:151–158.
160. Wilsnack SC, Vogeltanz ND, Klassen AD, Harris TR. Childhood sexual abuse and women's substance abuse: national survey findings. J Stud Alcohol 1997;58:264–271.
161. Wilsnack SC, Klassen AD, Schur BE, Wilsnack RW. Predicting onset and chronicity of women's problem drinking: a five-year longitudinal analysis. Am J Public Health 1991;81:305–318.
162. Miller BA, Downs WR. The impact of family violence on the use of alcohol by women. Alcohol Health Res World 1993;17(2):137–143.
163. Wechsberg WM, Craddock SG, Hubbard RL. How are women who enter substance abuse treatment different than men? A gender comparison from the Drug Abuse Treatment Outcome Study (DATOS). Drugs Soc 1998;13:97–115.

164. Najavits LM, Weiss RD, Shaw SR. The link between substance abuse and posttraumatic stress disorder in women: a research review. Am J Addict 1997;6:273–283.
165. Comfort M, Sockloff A, Loverro J, Kaltenbach K. Multiple predictors of substance-abusing women's treatment and life outcomes: a prospective longitudinal study. Addict Behav 2003;28:199–224.
166. Haver B. Female alcoholics: IV. The relationship between family violence and outcome 3–10 years after treatment. Acta Psychiatry Scand 1987;75:449–455.
167. Briere J, Runtz MA. Childhood sexual abuse: long-term sequelae and implications for psychological assessment. J Interpers Violence 1993;8:312–330.

5
The Physical Consequences of Drug and Alcohol Abuse

Hitoshi Nakaishi

This chapter discusses the physical consequences of substance abuse, including the representative drugs of alcohol, opioids, cannabis, toluene, cocaine, and lysergic acid diethylamide (LSD). Nicotine is briefly addressed as a legal drug that is not involved in the drug court process but has significant health effects, particularly when used with another drug.

Alcoholism

Alcoholism, also known as *alcohol dependence* or *alcohol abuse*, is a chronic, often progressive disease marked by consumption of alcoholic beverages at a level that interferes with physical or mental health; disrupts social, family, or occupational responsibilities; and can result in death. Heavy alcohol use can affect nearly every organ (1,2).

Alcohol Poisoning

Alcohol poisoning is the sometimes deadly result of drinking excessive amounts of alcohol (ethanol), typically through binge drinking. The effects of alcohol depend on the concentration of alcohol in the blood and on the rapidity with which it was consumed.

Signs and symptoms of alcohol poisoning include confusion, vomiting, seizures, slow or irregular breathing, pale skin, and unconsciousness. Alcohol is a stomach irritant and may cause vomiting. It also affects the central nervous system, causing a decrease in breathing, heart rate, and gag reflex and an increase in the risk of choking on vomit. The blood alcohol level continues to rise even after the person has passed out (3).

Alcohol Withdrawal Syndromes

Withdrawal develops because the brain has physically adapted to the presence of alcohol and cannot function adequately in the absence of the drug.

Unlike withdrawal from opioids, which can be unpleasant but rarely fatal, alcohol withdrawal can kill the patient through uncontrolled convulsions or hypertension. The pharmacologic management of alcohol withdrawal is based on the fact that alcohol, barbiturates, and benzodiazepines have similar effects on the brain and can be substituted for each other. Because benzodiazepines are the safest of the three, alcohol consumption is terminated and a long-acting benzodiazepine is substituted to block alcohol withdrawal syndrome. The benzodiazepine dosage is then tapered slowly over a period of days or weeks (4,5).

There are four clinical alcohol withdrawal syndromes caused by alcohol withdrawal: tremulousness, seizures, hallucinosis, and delirium tremens.

Tremulousness

Tremulousness (the shakes) is characterized by tremor, restlessness or agitation, sweating, elevated temperature, rapid heart rate, and high blood pressure.

Seizures

Seizures, typically acute generalized tonic-clonic or grand mal seizures, can occur in alcohol withdrawal in patients who have no history of seizure or any structural brain disease.

Hallucinations

Hallucinations, usually visual or tactile, occur within 2 hours of the cessation of alcohol in chronic alcoholics. The person is extremely suggestive and may hallucinate about the appearance of elephants, beautiful women or men, or space ships when the observer suggests one is present in the room.

Delirium Tremens

Delirium tremens includes features of tremulosis and hallucinations and is accompanied by stupor and lack of contact with one's surroundings (delirium). It can be severe and is often fatal.

Brain Damage

Alcohol affects the central nervous system, acting as a sedative, resulting in a dose-dependent decrease of activity, anxiety, tension, and inhibitions. Even a few drinks can result in behavioral changes, a slowing in motor performance, and a decrease in the ability to think clearly. Concentration and judgment become impaired. In sufficient amounts, alcohol impairs speech and muscle coordination and produces sleep. Prolonged, excessive alcohol intake can result in nerve damage and severe memory loss, the

Wernicke-Korsakoff syndrome. With continued heavy drinking, and in the absence of vitamin supplementation, this injury may produce irreversible cognitive impairment. Chronic, heavy use of alcohol can produce psychotic symptoms in some individuals, either during acute intoxication or during the process of withdrawal (6,7).

Gastrointestinal Problems

Irritation of the gastrointestinal tract can occur with erosion of the lining of the esophagus and stomach, causing nausea, vomiting, and, possibly, bleeding. Vitamins are not absorbed properly, particularly folic acid and thiamine, which can lead to nutritional deficiencies and further nerve damage (8,9).

Liver Disorders

Alcohol is especially harmful to the liver. In the United States, approximately 1% of the population has alcoholic liver disease. Alcoholism and alcoholic liver disease are higher in minorities. Women are also more susceptible to the adverse effects of alcohol than men, developing alcoholic hepatitis in a shorter time frame and from smaller amounts. The effect of hormones on the metabolism of alcohol may play an important role in this phenomenon (10).

Excessive alcohol ingestion over many years leads to alcoholic hepatitis. Not only does alcohol destroy liver cells, but it also destroys their ability to regenerate, resulting in widespread liver cell damage and destruction. Signs and symptoms may include loss of appetite, nausea, vomiting, abdominal pain and tenderness, fever, jaundice (yellowing of the skin and eyes), and mental confusion. Over years of drinking, hepatitis may lead to cirrhosis, the irreversible and progressive destruction and fibrous degeneration of the liver. The destruction of the normal architecture and the loss of liver cells prevent the liver from functioning normally and playing an important part in digesting food, metabolizing drugs, and synthesizing proteins, including those that help the blood to clot. The rate of cirrhosis in a country is directly related to the average alcohol consumption (10). Half of all cases of cirrhosis are due to alcohol excess. Only 30% of patients with cirrhosis will survive 5 years after diagnosis, and the outlook is worse if the patient continues to drink. In the early stages, there may be no symptoms at all. As the disease progresses, symptoms similar to those of hepatitis may develop (11).

In the later stages, the liver struggles to perform all of its functions, and the following symptoms may be present: jaundice, nail clubbing, darkening of the skin, fluid retention (edema and/or ascites), abnormal blood vessels (a spider nevus, a red face, easy bruising), and enlargement of breasts in men. A cirrhotic liver leads to portal hypertension and the complication of bleeding esophageal varices with massive, life-threatening gastrointestinal hemorrhage. The blood may bypass the liver, which is responsible for removing toxic substances from the blood, so that these substances pass to the brain where they may result in alteration in brain function, causing confusion, drowsiness, and, finally, coma (hepatic encephalopathy). Furthermore, micronodular cirrhosis may lead to hepatocellular carcinoma (12,13).

Alcoholic Pancreatitis

There are two stages of alcoholic pancreatitis: acute and chronic. Acute pancreatitis consists of a sudden inflammation of the pancreas that can vary from mild to life threatening. However, the pancreas usually returns to normal function after the condition resolves.

When patients suffer repeated attacks of acute pancreatitis, the pancreas gradually becomes scarred, leading to chronic pancreatitis, an ongoing or recurring inflammation. Chronic pancreatitis always causes permanent damage to the pancreas. Over time, it is more difficult for the damaged pancreas to produce normal digestive enzymes and hormones.

Long-term alcohol abuse remains a leading cause of both acute and chronic pancreatitis in industrialized nations. Alcohol causes digestive enzymes to be released sooner than normal. It also increases the permeability of the small pancreatic ducts, which allows digestive juices to leak into and damage healthy tissue. Excessive alcohol intake leads to the formation of protein plugs, precursors to small stones that block parts of the pancreatic duct. Women with acute pancreatitis are more likely to have gallstones as the cause, while six times as many men as women suffer from acute pancreatitis due to alcoholism. As pancreatitis progresses, continuing to use alcohol greatly increases the risk of complications and death.

The symptoms of pancreatitis begin as a gradual or sudden severe abdominal pain. Pain usually begins in the upper abdomen and penetrates to the back. Breathing may become shallow because deep breathing causes more pain. This pain continues for hours or even days, or, in cases of chronic pancreatitis, the pain may last years and is likely to get worse if the patient ingests alcohol. Bending forward or curling into a fetal position may provide temporary relief. Other symptoms include nausea, vomiting, fever, abdominal swelling, rapid pulse, high or low blood pressure, feelings of faintness, and jaundice. In severe cases, dehydration and low blood pressure, internal bleeding, and shock may occur. It is thought that enzymes normally secreted by the pancreas in an inactive form become activated inside the pancreas and start to digest the pancreatic tissue (autodigestion) and cause swelling, hemorrhage, and damage to the blood vessels (14,15).

The symptoms of chronic pancreatitis are similar to those of acute pancreatitis. However, ongoing damage to enzyme-producing tissue in chronic pancreatitis leads to malabsorption of nutrients, especially fats. It causes frequent, malodorous stools, resulting from poor digestion and malabsorption of nutrients, particularly fats (steatorrhea). As the disease progresses, damage to or destruction of insulin-producing cells often leads to diabetes. Unusual, long-term inflammation of the pancreas increases the risk of pancreatic cancer. In severe cases, called *necrotizing pancreatitis*, the pancreatic tissue begins to die, producing a reddish-purple or greenish-brown area between the ribs and the hip bone (Turner's sign). In addition, the area around the navel may be purple (Cullen's sign). Both conditions are caused by the pancreas bleeding into the abdomen.

Other serious complications of chronic pancreatitis include kidney failure, adult respiratory distress syndrome, heart failure due to shock, blood clots, pancreatic abscess, and pancreatic pseudocyst. Pancreatic pseudocyst occurs as a result of the collection of pancreatic fluid, pancreatic tissue debris, blood cells, enzymes, and fluid leaked from the circulatory system within the pancreas or in an obstructed duct. Pseudocysts can abscess and rupture. Necrosis may be followed by a systemic inflammation response syndrome (SIRS) (16,17).

To diagnose pancreatitis, a complete medical examination is necessary. Diagnostic tests include blood and urine studies for elevated levels of the pancreatic enzymes amylase and lipase, white blood cell count, liver enzymes, and bilirubin. An elevated blood sugar level (hyperglycemia) and low levels of calcium in the blood (hypocalcemia) are highly suggestive; radiographs of the abdomen and chest, ultrasound examinations of the pancreas and gallbladder, and computed tomography scan of the pancreas may reveal obstruction, stones, or cysts. In severe cases, endoscopic retrograde cholangiopancreatography may be carried out, looking at the pancreas through an endoscope inserted into the patient's mouth and down to the pancreas. An endoscope is fitted with a tiny fiberoptic camera that gives the physician a detailed view of the pancreas. During the procedure, the physician can remove a biopsy specimen from the pancreas and remove obstructed stones. A stool sample may be needed to test for excess fats (18).

Cardiovascular Disorders

Excessive drinking can lead to high blood pressure and damage the heart muscle (cardiomyopathy). These conditions can cause increased risk of heart failure or stroke.

Alcoholic Hypertension

Systemic hypertension has been firmly established as a risk factor for cardiovascular diseases leading to stroke, heart attack, kidney failure, and congestive heart failure. Alcohol abuse is now recognized as an important contributor to elevated blood pressure.

Alcohol elevates blood pressure independently of the influences of age, body weight, or cigarette smoking. On the other hand, in some epidemiologic studies, light, occasional drinkers had lower blood pressures than did abstainers. Although the quantity of alcohol required to produce this pattern differed somewhat among studies, one or two drinks per day were generally sufficient to elevate blood pressure.

The relationship between blood pressure and alcohol use may not be as strong in blacks (a group in which hypertension is particularly prevalent) as in whites. There may also be an increased sensitivity to the blood pressure–elevating effects of alcohol in persons older than 50 years of age, which may be attenuated somewhat in women by the use of supplemental estrogens. Although alcohol influences both systolic and diastolic pressures, its effect on systolic pressure appears to be greater. Men are more sensitive to the hypertensive effects of alcohol than are women.

Overall, the blood pressure–elevating effects of alcohol seem to be relatively small compared with the independent effects of age and the proportion of body fat. Nevertheless, alcohol use is associated with an increased prevalence of hypertension, and heavy drinking has been shown to increase the risk of developing hypertension. Stroke, especially hemorrhagic events, occurs three to four times more frequently in moderate to heavy drinkers than in abstainers (19,20).

Alcoholic Cardiomyopathy

Alcohol is the most frequent identifiable cause of symptomatic heart muscle disease. It is pathologically indistinguishable from other dilated cardiomyopathies, so the diagnosis depends on a history of excessive alcohol consumption and the absence of any other known cause. Heart muscle abnormalities are believed to occur in most chronic alcoholics. Some researchers suggest that at least one half of all cases of dilated cardiomyopathy are caused by alcohol (21). Long-term damage to the heart muscle in drinkers is related to both the frequency and the duration of alcohol consumption. The estimated total lifetime dose of alcohol correlated inversely with the ejection fraction and directly with the left ventricular muscle mass (22).

A disproportionate number of both symptomatic and preclinical cases occur in men, even when results are adjusted for sex differences in alcohol consumption (23). The presence of alcohol has been shown to interfere with various aspects of the transport and binding of calcium, to depress cellular energy production, and to impair protein synthesis. Alcohol is also known to alter the function of the sarcoplasmic reticulum, contributing to the development of alcoholic heart muscle disease (22).

The symptoms of alcoholic heart muscle disease may appear suddenly or may develop gradually over the course of a few months. The development of symptoms reflects the progression of congestive heart failure in the patient. Shortness of breath and early fatigue during exercise are the predominant early complaints. As heart failure worsens, attacks of breathlessness become more frequent and may waken the patient from sleep; these attacks often can be relieved by sitting upright. Weakness and fatigue eventually may become chronic, presumably as a result of reduced cardiac output. In severe cases, sluggish blood flow may lead to signs and symptoms of oxygen deprivation in critical organs. There may also be liver enlargement accompanied by accumulation of fluid in the abdomen.

For patients whose disease progresses to congestive heart failure, the prognosis is poor. A person with congestive heart failure severe enough to require hospitalization has a 50% chance of dying within 1 year, usually from such complications as arrhythmias, blood clots in the brain or lung, or pneumonia. A common and potentially fatal complication of heart muscle disease is the development of blood clots (emboli). Emboli can be fatal when they occlude blood vessels in vital organs such as the lungs or brain. Left ventricular failure is frequently accompanied by various of the arrhythmias responsible for the sudden deaths of alcoholics (24–26).

Cancer

Considerable evidence suggests a connection between heavy alcohol consumption and increased risk for cancer, with an estimated 2% to 4% of all cancer cases thought to be caused either directly or indirectly by alcohol (27). A strong association exists between alcohol use and cancers of the esophagus, pharynx, and mouth, whereas a more controversial association links alcohol with liver, breast, and colorectal cancers.

An estimated 75% of esophageal cancers in the United States are attributable to chronic, excessive alcohol consumption. Nearly 50% of cancers of the mouth, pharynx, and larynx are associated with heavy drinking. The combination of alcohol and smoking increases the risk even more dramatically (28).

Alcohol may affect cancer development at the genetic level by affecting oncogenes at the initiation and promotion stages. It has been suggested that acetaldehyde, a product of alcohol metabolism, impairs the cell's natural ability to repair its DNA, resulting in a greater likelihood that mutations causing cancer initiation will occur. It has recently been suggested that alcohol exposure may result in overexpression of certain oncogenes in human cells, thereby triggering cancer promotion.

Although there is no evidence that alcohol itself is a carcinogen, alcohol may act as a co-carcinogen by enhancing the carcinogenic effects of other chemicals. The risk for mouth, tracheal, and esophageal cancer is 35 times greater for people who both smoke and drink than for people who neither smoke nor drink, implying a co-carcinogenic interaction between alcohol and tobacco-related carcinogens (29).

Chronic alcohol abuse may result in abnormalities in the way the body processes nutrients and subsequently promotes certain types of cancer. Reduced levels of iron, zinc, vitamin E, and some of the B vitamins, common in heavy drinkers, have been experimentally associated with some cancers (30,31). Alcoholism has been associated with suppression of the human immune system. Immune suppression makes chronic alcohol abusers more susceptible to various infectious diseases and, theoretically, to cancer (31).

Nutritional Deficiencies

Many alcoholics are malnourished either because they ingest too little of essential nutrients such as carbohydrates, proteins, and vitamins or because alcohol and its metabolism prevent the body from properly absorbing and/or digesting the nutrients. As a result, alcoholics frequently experience deficiencies in proteins and vitamins, particularly vitamin A, which may contribute to liver disease and other serious alcohol-related disorders. Furthermore, alcohol breakdown in the liver, both by the enzyme alcohol dehydrogenase and by an enzyme system called the *microsomal ethanol-oxidizing system*, generates toxic products such as acetaldehyde and highly reactive and potentially damaging, oxygen-containing molecules. These products can interfere with the normal metabolism of other nutrients, particularly lipids, and contribute to liver cell damage.

Alcoholic beverages primarily consist of water, ethanol, and variable amounts of sugars, while their content of other nutrients is negligible. The carbohydrate content varies greatly among beverage types. Pure alcohol provides approximately 7.1 kcal/g of energy compared with 4 kcal/g for carbohydrates. Under certain conditions, however, alcohol-derived calories when consumed in substantial amounts can have less biologic value than carbohydrate-derived calories. This suggests that some of the energy contained in alcohol is not available to the body for producing or maintaining body mass.

Many alcoholics do not consume a balanced diet, and excessive alcohol consumption may interfere with the alcoholics' ability to absorb and use the nutrients they do consume, leading to primary and secondary malnutrition. Primary malnutrition occurs when alcohol replaces other nutrients in the diet, resulting in overall reduced nutrient intake. Secondary malnutrition occurs when the drinker consumes adequate nutrients but alcohol interferes with the absorption of those nutrients from the intestine so that they are not available to the body.

The most severe malnutrition, which is accompanied by a significant reduction in muscle mass, generally is found in those alcoholics who are hospitalized for medical complications of alcoholism. This pattern applies to patients with and without liver disease. People who drink heavily but do not require hospitalization for alcohol-related medical problems, in contrast, often are not malnourished or show less severe malnutrition. In these people, drinking, especially when accompanied by a high-fat diet and lack of physical activity, may lead to obesity. This relationship between heavy drinking and obesity has been observed particularly in women.

In drinkers who consume more than 30% of their total calories in the form of alcohol, not only carbohydrate intake but also protein and fat intake decrease significantly. Consumption of vitamin A, vitamin C, and thiamine (vitamin B_1) by these drinkers also may fall below the recommended daily allowances. Malnutrition, regardless of its causes, can lead to liver damage and impaired liver function.

Alcoholic liver disease typically develops in several sequential and partially overlapping stages. The first stage, fatty liver, is characterized by fat accumulation in the liver, sometimes associated with inflammation, and is called *steatohepatitis* or *alcoholic hepatitis* when severe. At this stage, liver cells may begin to die and scar tissue may form, leading to the next stage of liver disease, fibrosis. Excessive scar tissue formation eventually destroys the normal liver structure, resulting in cirrhosis, the most severe type of liver disease (32,33).

Sexual Dysfunction

Alcohol abuse can cause erectile dysfunction in men. This is said to be due to a combination of the effects of alcohol and cirrhosis. Alcohol is a stimulant in its early phase, leading to disinhibition. This phase is rapidly followed by its depressant phase, whereby alcohol impedes erectile function. Excess drinking brings about both vascular problems and nervous system problems via atherosclerosis, diabetes, and hypertension. In women, it can interrupt menstruation (34,35).

Smoking and Nicotine

Nicotine is a legal drug, not targeted by the drug court program. Many people in recovery turn to nicotine and smoking to fill their time and reduce their craving. However, it must be recognized that smoking tobacco is associated with an increased overall morbidity and mortality. Smoking remains the primary cause of preventable death in both developing and developed countries.

Among smokers aged 35 to 69 years, smoking accounts for a threefold increase in the death rate, and approximately half of all regular smokers who begin smoking during adolescence will experience fatal diseases precipitated by smoking. Smokers have more acute and chronic illnesses than those who never smoke, more bed disability days, and miss more school and work days. Of all cancer deaths in the United States, 30% could be prevented if cigarette smoking was eliminated.

Tobacco smoke contains various substances, some of which are irritants, oxidants, free radicals, and carcinogens. These substances have a direct and profound effect on the human body and are the direct cause of the diseases associated with smoke, including cardiovascular disease, cancer, and pulmonary disease (36,37).

Nicotine and Nicotine Withdrawal

Nicotine is a drug found naturally in tobacco. It is highly addictive, at least as addictive as heroin and cocaine. Over time, the body becomes physically and psychologically dependent on nicotine. When smoke is inhaled, nicotine is carried deep into the lungs, where it is absorbed quickly into the bloodstream and carried throughout the body. Nicotine affects many parts of the body, including the cardiovascular, hormonal, metabolic, and central nervous systems. Nicotine can be detected in breast milk and in cervix mucous secretions of smokers. During pregnancy, nicotine freely crosses the placenta and has been found in amniotic fluid and in the umbilical cord blood of newborn infants (38).

When smokers try to cut back or quit smoking, the absence of nicotine leads to physical and psychological withdrawal symptoms. The symptoms can include depression, feelings of frustration and anger, irritability, insomnia, difficulty concentrating, restlessness, headache, tiredness, and increased appetite. If a person has smoked regularly for just a few weeks, withdrawal symptoms will occur. Symptoms usually start within a few hours of the last cigarette and peak about 2 to 3 days later. Withdrawal symptoms can last for a few days to several weeks (39,40).

Cardiovascular Disease

Cardiovascular disease is the leading cause of death in developed countries, and smoking is considered one of the eight major risk factors in its development. Coronary artery disease, cerebrovascular disease, abdominal aortic aneurysm, and peripheral vascular disease are all caused by smoking. The degree of this risk is proportional to the amount of cigarette smoking (41).

Cancer

There is irrefutable evidence linking cigarette smoking and cancer of various sites in the body. The urine of cigarette smokers is strongly mutagenic in bacterial test systems. There are at least 43 carcinogens described in cigarette smoke, including polyaromatic hydrocarbons, heterocyclic hydrocarbons, N-nitrosamines, aromatic amines, aldehydes, volatile carcinogens, inorganic compounds, and radioactive elements. Organs with direct contact with smoke (lung, oral cavity, and esophagus) are at the greatest risk of developing cancer. However, as the substances delivered in cigarette smoke are absorbed and spread through the human body, smoking causes cancer at various distant sites. For instance, cigarette smoking is a risk factor for the development of cervical cancer.

The irritant and inflammatory effect of tobacco smoke leads to increased cell turnover and interferes with the normal barrier and clearance mechanism of the lungs, potentiating the carcinogenicity of cigarette smoking. Tobacco-initiated DNA damage can be accentuated by exposure to other toxic agents, such as asbestos and alcohol (42–44). Heavy alcohol consumption increases the risk of laryngeal cancer in a smoker by approximately 75% (45).

Pulmonary Disease

Studies have indicated that smoking is the primary risk factor for accelerated decline in respiratory function. Smokers of all ages are more likely to report pulmonary symptoms such as chronic cough, phlegm production, wheezing, and shortness of breath.

Chronic obstructive pulmonary disorder refers to a group of conditions that cause shortness of breath and are associated with obstruction of air flow within the lung. These conditions are chronic bronchitis, bronchiectasis, asthma, and emphysema. Smoking is the single most important risk factor in the development of chronic obstructive pulmonary disease, contributing to 81.5% of all chronic obstructive pulmonary disease deaths. Studies have found that smoking is associated with an increased rate of acute respiratory infection. Furthermore, mortality from influenza and pneumonia is increased, and this increase is directly proportional to the number of cigarettes smoked (46).

Pregnancy and Infant Health

Smoking is associated with multiple complications in pregnancy. Studies have confirmed that smoking increases the rate of low-birth-weight babies, premature babies, spontaneous abortions, stillbirths, neonatal death, abruptio placentae, placenta previa, bleeding during pregnancy, prolonged rupture of membranes, and impaired development of the infant. This can be attributed to several factors such as the vasoconstriction of placenta blood flow by nicotine, elevated fetal carboxyhemoglobin and catecholamine levels, and fetal tissue hypoxia, reduced delivery of nutrients to the fetus, and increased heart rate and blood pressure (47).

Other Smoking Risks

Smoking is associated with the development, delayed healing, and recurrence of peptic ulcer, as well as resistance to treatment (48). Smoking is also a risk factor for osteoporosis and bone fractures (49).

Opioids

Acute Effects

Some of the opioids share an acute intoxicating effect with alcohol and cannabis, although the sedative effect is more pronounced with opioids. Acute administration of heroin causes euphoria in many users, although other opioids such as methadone do not have this effect in tolerant individuals. The extent of euphoria is also affected by the route of administration. Some naive users report unpleasant feelings with opiate use, specifically nausea and dysphoria. All opioids are central nervous system depressants and as such can reduce the level of consciousness and cause sleep (50).

High doses of most opioids can lead to suppression of breathing rate and blood pressure and can cause respiratory arrest by suppressing the function of the medulla oblongata. The risk of overdose is worsened by use in combination with alcohol or other drugs and by variations in the potencies of opiates obtained illegally. Opioids cause some suppression of hormone levels. The opiates have been associated with miscarriage, fetal death, and low birth weight.

Chronic Effects

The specific health effects of opioid use largely depend on the route of administration. Local tissue and organ damage may result from the adulterants in injection drugs obtained on the street. Injecting heroin or morphine can lead to trauma, inflammation, and infection at the site of administration. Liver damage in opiate addicts may be caused by viral hepatitis contracted through needle sharing or from chronic alcohol abuse. Serious infection such as endocarditis is also reported. Intravenous drug use is a major concern for the transmission of other communicable diseases such as human immunodeficiency virus (HIV). Chronic use of noninjected opioids appears to carry little risk of adverse health effects other than a modest effect on endocrine activity, some suppression of the immune system, and chronic constipation.

Physical dependence on opiates has been recognized for centuries. Opiate withdrawal is associated with considerable discomfort but is rarely life threatening. The withdrawal syndrome is generally less dangerous than rapid withdrawal from sedative-hypnotics or from alcohol, although it may be life threatening in neonates. Despite the low risk, avoidance of withdrawal appears to be a powerful motive for continued use of opiates among heavy users.

Chronic opioid users may experience instability of mood, anorexia, lethargy, and depression related to acute drug effects. Opioids have not been linked to chronic psychiatric disorders, but street addicts have a shortened life expectancy and more frequently experience social and emotional problems. This is in part due to their exposure to infection, violence, and poor living conditions rather than to their drug use (51).

Cannabis and Marijuana

Marijuana is a mixture of dried, shredded leaves, stems, seeds, and flowers of the hemp plant. Cannabis refers to marijuana and other drugs made from that plant. Other forms, less common in the United States, are hashish and hashish oil. Marijuana is the most commonly used illicit drug, and at least one third of Americans have used this drug sometime in their lives. Marijuana is usually smoked as a cigarette (called a *joint*) or in a pipe or bong.

Health risks of cannabis use exist, most particularly when it is used daily over a period of years or decades. Considerable uncertainty remains about whether these effects are attributable to cannabis use alone and about the quantitative relationship between frequency, quantity, and duration of cannabis use and the risk of experiencing these effects. Using analogies with the known effects of alcohol and tobacco, the most probable health risks of chronic heavy cannabis use over a period of years are the development of a dependence syndrome and increased risk of being involved in motor vehicle accidents, developing chronic bronchitis or respiratory cancers, giving birth to low-birth-weight babies when used during pregnancy, and, perhaps, developing schizophrenia in vulnerable individuals. Many of these risks are shared with alcohol and tobacco, which is not surprising given that cannabis is an intoxicant like alcohol and is typically smoked like tobacco.

With existing patterns of use, cannabis poses a much less serious public health problem than is currently posed by alcohol and tobacco in Western societies. This is no cause for complacency, however, as the public health significance of alcohol and tobacco is major, and the public health significance of cannabis could increase if the prevalence of its heavy daily use were to approach that of heavy alcohol use among young adults or the prevalence of daily cigarette smoking among adults. Marijuana use may cause frequent respiratory infections, impaired memory and learning, increased heart rate, anxiety, panic attacks, tolerance, and physical dependence. Use of marijuana during the first month of breast-feeding can impair infant motor development.

Chronic smokers may have many of the same respiratory problems as tobacco smokers, including daily cough and phlegm, chronic bronchitis symptoms, and frequent chest colds. Chronic abuse can also lead to abnormal functioning of lung tissues. A study of college students has shown that skills related to attention, memory, and learning are impaired among people who use marijuana heavily, even after discontinuing its use for at least 24 hours (52,53).

Methamphetamine

Amphetamine, dextroamphetamine, methamphetamine, and their various salts are collectively referred to as *amphetamines*. Methamphetamine is the most commonly abused. During 2000, 4% of the U.S. population reported trying methamphetamine at least once in their lifetime. Methamphetamine comes in many forms and can be smoked, snorted, orally ingested, or injected. The drug alters moods in different ways, depending on how it is taken. Effects of usage include addiction, psychotic behavior, and brain damage.

Health Hazards

Methamphetamine releases high levels of the neurotransmitter dopamine, which stimulates brain cells, enhancing mood and body movement. It also appears to have a neurotoxic effect, damaging brain cells that contain dopamine and serotonin, another neurotransmitter. Over time, methamphetamine appears to cause reduced levels of dopamine, which can result in symptoms like those of Parkinson's disease.

The central nervous system actions that result from taking even small amounts of methamphetamine include increased wakefulness, increased physical activity, decreased appetite, increased respiration, hyperthermia, and euphoria. Other central nervous system effects include irritability, insomnia, confusion, tremors, convulsions, anxiety, paranoia, and aggressiveness. Hyperthermia and convulsions can result in death.

Methamphetamine stimulates the sympathetic nervous system, causing increased heart rate and blood pressure, and can cause irreversible damage to blood vessels in the brain (strokes). Other effects of methamphetamine on the sympathetic nervous system include respiratory problems, irregular heartbeat, and extreme anorexia. Its use can result in cardiovascular collapse and death (54).

Short-Term Effects

Methamphetamine is taken orally or intranasally (snorting the powder), by intravenous injection, and by smoking. Immediately after smoking or intravenous injection, the methamphetamine user experiences an intense sensation, called a *rush* or *flash*, that lasts only a few minutes and is described as extremely pleasurable. Oral or intranasal use produces euphoria—a high, but not a rush. Users may become addicted quickly and use it with increasing frequency and in increasing doses.

As with similar stimulants, methamphetamine most often is used in a binge and crash pattern. Because tolerance occurs within minutes, meaning that the pleasurable effects disappear even before the drug concentration in the blood falls significantly, users try to maintain the high by binging on the drug. A single high dose of the drug has been shown to damage nerve terminals in the dopamine-containing regions of the brain. High doses can elevate body temperature to dangerous, sometimes lethal, levels, as well as cause convulsions (55).

Long-Term Effects

Long-term methamphetamine abuse results in many damaging effects, including addiction. Addiction is a chronic, relapsing disease, characterized by compulsive drug seeking and drug use that is accompanied by functional and molecular changes in the brain. In addition to being addicted to methamphetamine, chronic methamphetamine abusers exhibit symptoms including violent behavior, anxiety, confusion, and insomnia. They also can display a number of psychotic features, including paranoia, auditory hallucinations, mood disturbances, and delusions (e.g., the sensation of insects creeping on the skin, which is called *formication*). The paranoia can result in homicidal as well as suicidal thoughts.

With chronic use, tolerance for methamphetamine can develop. In an effort to intensify the desired effects, users may take higher doses of the drug, take it more frequently, or change their method of drug intake. In some cases, abusers forgo food and sleep while indulging in a form of binging known as a *run*, injecting as much as 1 g of the drug every 2 to 3 hours over several days until the user runs out of the drug or is too disorganized to continue.

Although there are no physical manifestations of a withdrawal syndrome when methamphetamine use is stopped, there are several symptoms that occur when a chronic user stops taking the drug. These include depression, anxiety, fatigue, paranoia, aggression, and an intense craving for the drug.

In scientific studies examining the consequences of long-term methamphetamine exposure in animals, concern has arisen over its toxic effects on the brain. Researchers have reported that as much as 50% of the dopamine-producing cells in the brain can be damaged after prolonged exposure to relatively low levels of methamphetamine. Damage to the brain caused by methamphetamine use is similar to Alzheimer's disease, stroke, and epilepsy (56). Researchers also have found that serotonin-containing nerve cells may be damaged even more extensively. However, the relation of such toxicity with the psychosis seen in some long-term methamphetamine abusers still remains unclear (57).

Risk of Contracting Human Immunodeficiency Virus and Hepatitides B and C

Increased HIV, hepatitis B, and hepatitis C transmissions are likely consequences of increased methamphetamine abuse, particularly in individuals who inject the drug and share injection equipment. Infection with HIV and other infectious diseases is spread primarily through the shared reuse of contaminated syringes, needles, and/or other instruments. In nearly one third of Americans infected with HIV, injection drug use is thought to be a risk factor, making drug abuse the fastest growing vector for the spread of HIV in the nation.

Methamphetamine and related psychomotor stimulants are recognized to increase the libido in users in contrast to opiates, which actually decrease the libido. However, long-term methamphetamine use may be associated with decreased sexual functioning, at least in men. Additionally, methamphetamine seems to be associated with rougher sex, which may lead to bleeding and abrasions. The combination of injection and sexual risks may result in HIV becoming a greater problem among methamphetamine abusers than among opiate and other drug abusers, something that already seems to be occurring in California (58).

Toluene

Solvent abuse is a relatively common form of substance abuse. The representative organic solvent is toluene. Chronic toluene abuse can lead to muscle weakness, gastrointestinal disturbances, neuropsychiatric problems, peripheral neuropathy, and renal tubular acidosis. It is estimated that 3% to 4% of teenagers and young adults abuse solvents on a regular basis. Toluene readily crosses the placenta, although the magnitude of risk for an individual pregnancy remains unknown (59).

Cocaine

Cocaine is a powerful central nervous system stimulant. It is a chemical derived from the leaf of the *Erythroxylon* coca bush, which grows primarily in Central and South America. Cocaine was initially used in patent medicines and tonics to treat a wide variety of symptoms. It was later used as a local anesthetic for minor surgery, but this role today is limited as synthetic anesthetics are more widely used. Cocaine has no other medicinal application. Its low cost, easy availability, and false reputation as a nonaddictive drug has led to widespread use among young people, where 9% of those aged 20 to 24 years who were asked in 1998 said they had taken it.

Abuse

Cocaine is generally sold on the street as cocaine hydrochloride, a fine, white crystalline powder, soluble in water, known by slang names such as *coke*, *C*, or *Charlie*. Cocaine in powder form is usually sniffed, or snorted, up the nose through a rolled-up bank note or similar type of tube. To experience cocaine's effects more rapidly and to heighten their intensity, some users inject the drug directly into their veins.

Pure cocaine is a chemical base. Free base or crack takes the shape of relatively large crystals. It is not soluble in water and therefore must be smoked in order to be taken. Crack is absorbed into the body much faster than when cocaine powder is snorted, and it takes effect very quickly. It is also highly addictive (60).

Health Effects

Cocaine, like most drugs, acts on neurotransmitters in the brain. Cocaine interferes with the normal action of at least two neurotransmitters, serotonin and dopamine. When cocaine is taken in any form, brain activity increases together with sympathetic functions (heart rate, breathing rate, blood pressure, and body temperature). Physical symptoms of cocaine use may include chest pain, nausea, blurred vision, fever, and muscle spasms.

Cocaine produces feelings of mental well-being and exhilaration. A user may feel energetic, talkative, and mentally alert—especially to sensations of sight, sound, and touch. At the same time cocaine inhibits appetite and the desire for sleep. In some respects the effect of cocaine is grossly similar to that of amphetamines and, like those drugs, cocaine use can produce anxiety or panic attacks. The aftereffects of cocaine can include tiredness and depression. Excessive doses can sometimes cause death from heart failure (60).

Short-Term Effects

When cocaine is snorted, its euphoric effects appear soon after it is taken, peak in about 15 to 30 minutes, and disappear completely within one half to 2 hours. The short-lasting high encourages users to repeat the dose in order to maintain the effect. It is common for cocaine users to take cocaine again after about half an hour. Many repeated dosages taken over a short period can lead to extreme states of agitation, anxiety, or paranoia. The compulsion to repeat cocaine use is even more evident when the drug is taken as crack. The effects of crack cocaine occur and peak immediately after the drug is smoked and begin to fade shortly afterward. Crack users commonly repeat the dosage at short intervals in an attempt to maintain the high.

When large amounts of cocaine are taken (several hundred milligrams or more) the high is intensified up to a point, but such doses can also lead to bizarre, erratic, and violent behavior. These users may experience severe tremors, vertigo, muscle twitches, and paranoia (61).

Long-Term Effects

If cocaine is taken over a period of time, the euphoric high is gradually replaced by restlessness, extreme excitability, insomnia, paranoia, and, eventually, hallucinations and delusions. These conditions are very similar to amphetamine psychosis and paranoid schizophrenia, although they disappear in most cases after cocaine use is ended.

Many of the physical effects of heavy continuous use are essentially the same as those of short-term use, but the heavy user may also suffer from mood swings, loss of interest in sex, weight loss, and insomnia (62).

At present there is no evidence to suggest tolerance to cocaine's stimulant effect occurs. Users may keep taking the original amount over extended periods and still experience the same euphoric effects. However, some users do increase their dosage in an attempt to intensify and prolong the effects.

Dependency

At present, it is unclear if physical dependence on cocaine hydrochloride can occur. However, when some regular heavy users stop taking the drug, they experience a powerful negative reaction, which may indicate physical dependence. Crack cocaine does produce a strong physical dependency. With regular heavy use, increasingly unpleasant symptoms occur. Euphoria is replaced by restlessness, overexcitability, and nausea. With continued use this can lead to paranoid psychosis. Regular users may appear chronically nervous, excitable, and paranoid. Confusion as a result of exhaustion, due to lack of sleep, is common.

Among heavy cocaine users, an intense psychological dependence can occur; they suffer severe depression when the supply of cocaine runs out that lifts only when they take it again. Experiments with animals have suggested that cocaine is perhaps the most powerful drug of all in producing psychological dependence. When not taking cocaine, many regular users complain of sleep and eating disorders, depression, and anxiety, and the mental craving for the drug often compels them to take it again (63).

Health Consequences

Death from a cocaine overdose can occur from convulsions, heart failure, or the depression of vital brain centers that control breathing. Chronic cocaine snorting often causes sinus stuffiness, runny nose, and eczema and commonly damages the nasal membranes and the structure separating the nostrils. Severe respiratory tract irritation has been noted in some heavy users of crack cocaine.

Users who inject the drug risk not only overdosing but also getting infections from nonsterile needles and hepatitis or acquired immunodeficiency syndrome from needles shared with others. The risk of using cocaine to mental health is high. As mentioned earlier, regular use can lead to anxiety, paranoia, and psychosis, which can sometimes produce permanent mental health problems (61–63).

Lysergic Acid Diethylamide

Lysergic acid diethylamide is the most potent hallucinogen ever known. An oral dose of as little 25 μg of LSD is capable of producing vivid hallucinations. Lysergic acid diethylamide became popular in the 1960s together with an antiestablishment movement by youth. Lysergic acid diethylamide use has varied over the years, but it still remains a significant drug of abuse. In 1999, over 12% of high school seniors and college students reported that they had used LSD at least once in their lifetime. Because of its structural similarity to a chemical present in the brain and its similarity in effects to certain aspects of psychosis, LSD was used as a research tool to study mental illness. The average effective oral dose is from 20 to 80 μg, with the effects of higher doses lasting for 10 to 12 hours.

Physical reactions include dilated pupils, lowered body temperature, nausea, goose bumps, profuse perspiration, increased blood sugar, and rapid heart rate. During the first hour after ingestion, the user may experience visual changes with extreme changes in mood. In the hallucinatory state, the user may suffer impaired depth and time perception, accompanied by distorted perception of the size and shape of objects, movements, color, sound, touch, and the user's own body image. During this period, the users' ability to perceive objects through the senses is distorted: they may describe hearing colors and seeing sounds. The ability to make sensible judgments and to see common dangers is impaired, making the user susceptible to personal injury. After an LSD trip, the user may suffer acute anxiety or depression for a variable period of time. Flashbacks have been reported days or even months after taking the last dose.

References

1. Ringold S, Lynm C, Glass RM. Alcohol abuse and alcoholism. JAMA 2006; 295(17):2100.
2. Nagel M, Ferbert A. Diseases due to alcoholism. Fortschr Neurol Psychiatry 2005;73(8):470–482.
3. Al-Sanouri I, Dikin M, Soubani AO. Critical care aspects of alcohol abuse. South Med J 2005;98(3):372–381.
4. Ebell MH. Benzodiazepines for alcohol withdrawal. Am Fam Physician 2006; 73(7):1191.
5. Petignat PA. The management of the alcohol withdrawal syndrome in the intensive care unit. Rev Med Suisse 2005;1(45):2905–2911.
6. Harper C, Matsumoto I. Ethanol and brain damage. Curr Opin Pharmacol 2005; 5(1):73–78.
7. Yamamoto M, Ukai W, Tateno M, Saito T. Possible alterations in brain neural network by ethanol. Nihon Arukoru Yakubutsu Igakkai Zasshi 2004;39(1): 51–60.
8. Schenker S, Bay MK. Medical problems associated with alcoholism. Adv Intern Med 1998;43:27–78.

9. Hislop WS, Heading RC. Caledonian Society of Gastroenterology. Impact of alcohol related disease and inpatient workload of gastroenterologists in Scotland. Scott Med J 2004;49(2):57–60.
10. Wakim-Fleming J, Mullen KD. Long-term management of alcoholic liver disease. Clin Liver Dis 2005;9(1):135–149.
11. Crews FT, Bechara R, Brown LA, Guidot DM, Mandrekar P, Oak S, Qin L, Szabo G, Wheeler M, Zou J. Cytokines and alcohol. Alcohol Clin Exp Res 2006;30(4):720–730.
12. D'Amico G, Garcia-Tsao G, Pagliaro L. Natural history and prognostic indicators of survival in cirrhosis: a systematic review of 118 studies. J Hepatol 2006;44(1):217–231.
13. Motola-Kuba D, Zamora-Valdes D, Uribe M, Mendez-Sanchez N. Hepatocellular carcinoma: an overview. Ann Hepatol 2006;5(1):16–24.
14. Kloppel G. Acute pancreatitis. Semin Diagn Pathol 2004;21(4):221–226.
15. Gullo L, Migliori M, Brunetti MA, Manca M. Alcoholic pancreatitis: new insights into an old disease. Curr Gastroenterol Rep 2005;7(2):96–100.
16. Kloppel G. Chronic pancreatitis of alcoholic and nonalcoholic origin. Semin Diagn Pathol 2004;21(4):227–236.
17. Go VL, Gukovskaya A, Pandol SJ. Alcohol and pancreatic cancer. Alcohol 2005;35(3):205–211.
18. Kingsnorth A, O'Reilly D. Acute pancreatitis. BMJ 2006;332(7549):1072–1076.
19. Hendriks HF, van Tol A, Alcohol. In von Eckardstein A, ed. Atherosclerosis: Diet and Drugs. New York: Springer; 2005;339–361.
20. Tykarski A. Resistant hypertension. Blood Press Suppl 2005;2:42–45.
21. Russo D, Purohit V, Foudin L, Salin M. Workshop on alcohol use and health disparities 2002: a call to arms. Alcohol 2004;32(1):37–43.
22. Zhang X, Li SY, Brown RA, Ren J. Ethanol and acetaldehyde in alcoholic cardiomyopathy: from bad to ugly en route to oxidative stress. Alcohol 2004; 32(3):175–186.
23. Fernandez-Sola J, Nicolas-Arfelis JM. Gender differences in alcoholic cardiomyopathy. J Gend Specif Med 2002;5(1):41–47.
24. Spies CD, Sander M, Stangl K, Fernandez-Sola J, Preedy VR, Rubin E, Andreasson S, Hanna EZ, Kox WJ. Effects of alcohol on the heart. Curr Opin Crit Care 2001;7(5):337–343.
25. Schoppet M, Maisch B. Alcohol and the heart. Herz 2001;26(5):345–352.
26. Fauchier L. Alcoholic cardiomyopathy and ventricular arrhythmias. Chest 2003;123(4):1320.
27. Rothman KJ. The proportion of cancer attributable to alcohol consumption. Prev Med 1980;9(2):174–179.
28. Boffetta P, Hashibe M. Alcohol and cancer. Lancet Oncol 2006;7(2):149–156.
29. Ferguson LR, Philpott M, Karunasinghe N. Dietary cancer and prevention using antimutagens. Toxicology 2004;198(1–3):147–159.
30. Crabb DW, Matsumoto M, Chang D, You M. Overview of the role of alcohol dehydrogenase and aldehyde dehydrogenase and their variants in the genesis of alcohol-related pathology. Proc Nutr Soc 2004;63(1):49–63.
31. Barshes NR, Goodpastor SE, Goss JA. Pharmacologic immunosuppression. Front Biosci 2004;9:411–420.

32. Leevy CM, Moroianu SA. Nutritional aspects of alcoholic liver disease. Clin Liver Dis 2005;9(1):67–81.
33. Lieber CS. Relationships between nutrition, alcohol use, and liver disease. Alcohol Res Health 2003;27(3):220–231.
34. Fabbri A, Caprio M, Aversa A. Pathology of erection. J Endocrinol Invest 2003; 26(3 Suppl):87–90.
35. Clayton AH. Sexual function and dysfunction in women. Psychiatr Clin North Am 2003;26(3):673–682.
36. Critchley JA, Capewell S. Mortality risk reduction associated with smoking cessation in patients with coronary heart disease: a systematic review. JAMA 2003;290(1):86–97.
37. Andrews JO, Tingen MS. The effect of smoking, smoking cessation, and passive smoke exposure on common laboratory values in clinical settings: a review of the evidence. Crit Care Nurs Clin North Am 2006;18(1):63–69.
38. Crooks PA, Dwoskin LP. Contribution of CNS nicotine metabolites to the neuropharmacological effects of nicotine and tobacco smoking. Biochem Pharmacol 1997;54(7):743–753.
39. Warner C, Shoaib M. How does bupropion work as a smoking cessation aid? Addict Biol 2005;10(3):219–231.
40. Brown RA, Lejuez CW, Kahler CW, Strong DR, Zvolensky MJ. Distress tolerance and early smoking lapse. Clin Psychol Rev 2005;25(6):713–733.
41. Ford CL, Zlabek JA. Nicotine replacement therapy and cardiovascular disease. Mayo Clin Proc 2005;80(5):652–656.
42. Lerman C, Patterson F, Berrettini W. Treating tobacco dependence: state of the science and new directions. J Clin Oncol 2005;23(2):311–323.
43. Westmaas JL, Brandon TH. Reducing risk in smokers. Curr Opin Pulm Med 2004;10(4):284–288.
44. Hecht SS. Tobacco carcinogens, their biomarkers and tobacco-induced cancer. Nat Rev Cancer 2003;3(10):733–744.
45. McCoy GD, Hecht SS, Wynder EL. The roles of tobacco, alcohol, and diet in the etiology of upper alimentary and respiratory tract cancers. Prev Med 1980; 9(5):622–629.
46. Bartal M. COPD and tobacco smoke. Monaldi Arch Chest Dis 2005;63(4):213–225.
47. Melvin C, Gaffney C. Treating nicotine use and dependence of pregnant and parenting smokers: an update. Nicotine Tobacco Res 2004;(6 Suppl 2):S107–S124.
48. Thomas GA, Rhodes J, Ingram JR. Mechanisms of disease: Nicotine—a review of its actions in the context of gastrointestinal disease. Nat Clin Pract Gastroenterol Hepatol 2005;2(11):536–544.
49. Templeton K. Secondary osteoporosis. J Am Acad Orthop Surg 2005;13(7):475–486.
50. Sporer KA. Acute heroin overdose. Ann Intern Med 1999;130(7):584–590.
51. Warner-Smith M, Darke S, Lynskey M, Hall W. Heroin overdose: causes and consequences. Addiction 2001;96(8):1113–1125.
52. Kalant H. Adverse effects of cannabis on health: an update of the literature since 1996. Prog Neuropsychopharmacol Biol Psychiatry 2004;28(5):849–863.
53. Castle DJ, Ames FR. Cannabis and the brain. Aust NZ J Psychiatry 1996; 30(2):179–183.

54. Centers for Disease Control and Prevention. Acute public health consequences of methamphetamine laboratories—16 states, January 2000–June 2004. MMWR Morbid Mortal Wkly Rep 2005;54(14):356–359.
55. Lundqvist T. Cognitive consequences of cannabis use: comparison with abuse of stimulants and heroin with regard to attention, memory and executive functions. Pharmacol Biochem Behav 2005;81(2):319–330.
56. Cho AK, Melega WP. Patterns of methamphetamine abuse and their consequences. J Addict Dis 2002;21(1):21–34.
57. Schuster CR, Fischman MW. Amphetamine toxicity: behavioral and neuropathological indexes. Fed Proc 1975;34(9):1845–1851.
58. Worth H, Rawstorne P. Crystallizing the HIV epidemic: methamphetamine, unsafe sex, and gay diseases of the will. Arch Sex Behav 2005;34(5):483–486.
59. Filley CM, Halliday W, Kleinschmidt-DeMasters BK. The effects of toluene on the central nervous system. J Neuropathol Exp Neurol 2004;63(1):1–12.
60. Nnadi CU, Mimiko OA, McCurtis HL, Cadet JL. Neuropsychiatric effects of cocaine use disorders. J Natl Med Assoc 2005;97(11):1504–1501.
61. Prakash A, Das G. Cocaine and the nervous system. Int J Clin Pharmacol Ther Toxicol 1993;31:575–590.
62. Majewska MD. Cocaine addiction as a neurological disorder: implications for treatment. NIDA Res Monogr 1996;163:1–26.
63. McClelland GT. The effects and management of crack cocaine dependence. Nurs Times 2005;101(29):26–27.

6 Drugs and Alcohol in Pregnancy and the Affected Children

Ira J. Chasnoff

Over the past three decades, the use of alcohol and illicit drugs during pregnancy has become a major public health concern. A number of studies have found poor pregnancy outcomes among women who used alcohol or illegal drugs during pregnancy (1–5), and effects on their newborns also have been documented (6–9). Recent publications have begun to track the long-term impact of prenatal alcohol or illicit drug exposure on the development and behavior of the exposed child (10–16).

In addition to public health problems, child welfare systems across the nation have found that substance use in the family has become a leading reason for children to be referred into out-of-home placement. In some states, up to 80% of children in custody are there because of substance abuse problems in the family (17,18). On a daily basis, courts are being called on to make decisions in the best interest of a child whose birth parents are unable or unwilling to address their substance abuse problems. This chapter examines the policy and practice issues related to identification of pregnant women at risk for alcohol and drug use and discusses what is known about the impacts of prenatal exposure to maternal substance abuse on a child's long-term physical and mental health and on behavioral and learning outcomes.

Early Identification of Pregnant Women at Risk for Substance Abuse

The harm done by substance abuse in pregnancy was documented by Aristotle, who noted the damage alcohol can cause in the unborn child. Etchings from the 1700s depicting the scourge of the gin epidemic in England portray children with facial features characteristic of fetal alcohol syndrome. However, despite this early recognition of the problems alcohol consumption during pregnancy can cause, little progress has been made in reducing the rate of alcohol or other drug use by pregnant women. In fact, physicians rarely ask a pregnant woman about her alcohol use, and fetal alcohol syndrome remains the most common cause of diagnosable mental retardation in the United States as well as one of the leading causes of behavioral problems in children (14).

Despite professed public and professional concern over the consequences of prenatal alcohol and drug exposure, the American College of Obstetricians and Gynecologists documented the low priority that obstetricians place on advising their patients about alcohol use during pregnancy (19). Although 97% of obstetricians declared that they asked their patients about alcohol use, 80% confirmed that they advise their patients that "a little alcohol" does not pose a threat to the pregnancy or the developing fetus. In addition, 4% of the obstetricians surveyed stated that eight drinks or more per week was a safe level of alcohol consumption for pregnant women. This of course is in direct contrast to a recent study that documented that any alcohol use in pregnancy places the child at more than three times increased risk for delinquent behavior (20).

Although the lack of an appreciation for alcohol's toxicity stands at the heart of the problem, legal, social, and attitudinal barriers often come together to restrain open communication between physician and patient. Most pregnant women state that they simply will not talk to primary care providers about their alcohol or drug use, the most common reason given being the fear of prosecution or loss of their baby to the child protection system (21).

There is good reason for this fear. When screening for alcohol or drug use is implemented in clinical practice, it often focuses on targeted populations rather than on the general population. Providers often state that they can tell who is an alcoholic or drug user by looking at the person. A 1990 study of substance use in pregnancy in Pinellas County, Florida (22), revealed that although the overall use of licit and illicit substances was approximately 15% in African-American women and in white women within the population, African-American women were 10 times more likely to have a urine toxicology performed or to have intensive evaluation for substance use than were white women. This study demonstrated that physicians' selection of pregnant women for toxicology testing was influenced by race and social class.

On a more positive note, recent work has focused on universal screening of pregnant women for the risk of alcohol or drug use. However, it is important that screening take place in the context of a much larger integrated system of screening, assessment, referral, and treatment. If there is no capability to educate the pregnant woman about the dangers of substance use, if there is no ability to link a pregnant woman who is drinking or using drugs to a treatment program, or if there is no treatment available, identifying the at-risk woman usually results in more punitive policies that disrupt families and drive women out of prenatal care, further complicating medical risk for the pregnancy and the baby.

A successful approach to community-based screening and early intervention can be found in data developed through the use of the 4Ps Plus© Screen for Substance Use in Pregnancy in prenatal care sites in eight California communities (23). The 4Ps Plus© was administered in the prenatal care provider's office at the first prenatal visit. Any woman who had a positive 4Ps Plus© screen (i.e., admitted use of any alcohol or any tobacco in the month before she knew she was pregnant) immediately underwent a structured clinical interview to further assess for substance use.

In response to the 4Ps Plus© screening instrument, 18% of the 26,249 women admitted to tobacco use in the month prior to knowledge of the pregnancy, 21% admitted to alcohol use, and 10% admitted to both alcohol and tobacco use in the month prior to knowledge of pregnancy. Eliminating duplicative counts, the rate of positive screens was 31%. On follow-up assessment at the doctor's office, 8% of the women continued to drink alcohol even though they knew they were pregnant, 5% were using marijuana, and 6% were using other illegal drugs such as cocaine, heroin, or methamphetamine. Overall, this means that 27% of the infants (over 7,000 babies in this sample alone) were exposed to alcohol or illicit drugs that affect the structure and function of the developing fetal brain.

Interesting patterns of substance use emerged when subsets of the data were evaluated. For example, among pregnant women in San Bernardino County, Caucasian women had consistently higher rates of substance use in pregnancy (46%) than African-American (36%) or Latina women (21%). In addition, it was found that although women on public aid and women with private insurance had similar rates of substance use before they knew they were pregnant, women on public aid had a significantly higher likelihood of stopping use once they found out they were pregnant than women with private insurance.

This type of screening relies on self-reporting. There are those who advocate for more direct markers of substance abuse, such as urine toxicologies. However, in a related study conducted at a clinic in Southern Illinois (23), clinical policies instruct physicians to obtain urine toxicologies on all pregnant women suspected of substance use based on clinical criteria. These criteria include no prenatal care or abruptio placentae, preterm labor, and intrauterine growth retardation for no apparent reason. Of the 1,435 pregnant women seen in the prenatal clinics, 651 (45%) had a urine toxicology ordered. Among these urine results, 2.6% were positive, giving a positive urine toxicology rate in the overall population of 1.2%. However, 37% of the women admitted to the use of alcohol or illicit drugs during pregnancy when administered the 4Ps Plus© screening with follow-up assessment. Thus, the verbal screening and assessment process uncovered a more than 30 times higher rate of alcohol or illicit drug use than did the use of clinically guided urine toxicologies (6).

From a prevention perspective, the high rate of alcohol use in the month before the woman knew she was pregnant is of concern, given the documented structural changes in the fetal brain that can be induced by early alcohol exposure. Thus, public education campaigns must focus on preconception as well as postconception health. Failing alcohol abstinence in early pregnancy, several studies have demonstrated that many of the maternal and child complications associated with the prenatal use of alcohol or illicit drugs are preventable with early identification of the pregnant substance-using woman and referral into treatment. Infants whose alcoholic mothers enter treatment and become alcohol free by the third trimester have been shown to have substantially improved outcome at birth (24). Studies of cocaine use in pregnancy have found that cessation of cocaine use by the third trimester significantly reduces the rate of low-birth-weight infants and prematurity (25). In addition, a recent study at Kaiser Permanente Medical Care Program documented the cost savings accrued when pregnant substance-using women are identified early in pregnancy and provided substance abuse interventions within the prenatal care setting (5).

A highly sensitive screening instrument moves us away from selecting high-risk women based on race and economic level and addresses the need to identify all women at risk. It identifies not only those pregnant women who are drinking heavily or whose drug use is at a high enough level to impair daily functioning but also identifies those women whose pregnancies are at risk from tobacco use as well as relatively small amounts of alcohol, marijuana, or other drugs. Specifically, women with a positive screen but whose assessment is negative can receive prevention materials and education regarding the impacts of even low levels of tobacco use, drinking, or illicit drug use during pregnancy. Educational input provided by the prenatal care provider significantly increases the woman's likelihood to make healthy decisions during pregnancy (26). In addition, interventions in the current pregnancy are likely to influence the woman's behavior in subsequent pregnancies, and successful intervention during pregnancy lessens the likelihood that the woman and her child will end up in the jurisdiction of the courts and the child welfare system.

Alcohol Effects

Fetal alcohol syndrome is the original name given to a cluster of physical and mental defects present from birth that is the direct result of a woman's drinking alcoholic beverages while pregnant (27). The prevalence of fetal alcohol syndrome is estimated to range from 0.2 to 2 cases per 1,000 live births, depending on ethnic, cultural, and regional factors (28). If one considers that there are approximately 4 million births per year in the United State, this means there are up to 6,000 children born each year with fetal alcohol syndrome.

Criteria for Diagnosis of Fetal Alcohol Syndrome

Individuals with fetal alcohol syndrome have findings in three categories (29): growth deficiencies, central nervous system involvement, and changes in shape and structure of the face.

Growth Deficiencies

In the United States, the average birth weight of babies born at full term (38 to 42 weeks' gestation) is 7 pounds 8 ounces, with a normal range down to 5 pounds 8 ounces. Babies born to mothers who use alcohol have an average birth weight of around 6 pounds and are more likely to weigh less than 5 pounds 8 ounces. As children with fetal alcohol syndrome grow older, they tend to continue to be small for their age, short, and underweight. To meet the guidelines for growth criteria, a child must have either reduced weight or reduced height at or below the 10th percentile on standard growth charts at birth or at any one point in time after birth (29).

Central Nervous System Involvement

Problems in the central nervous system can be manifest through structural, neurologic, or functional changes in the brain. Structurally, a small head circumference, at or below the 10th percentile, at birth or at any time after birth indicates poor brain growth. For example, the average head size of full-term infants is 35 cm, whereas the head size of a baby with fetal alcohol syndrome often is less than about 33 cm. Structural changes also can be found on specialized x-ray studies of the brain, which show changes in the shape and placement of different areas of the brain. Neurologic damage can show up in the child as seizures, wandering eye, problems in coordination, difficulty with motor control, or a number of other soft neurologic deficits. Functionally, fetal alcohol syndrome is recognized as the most common cause of diagnosable mental retardation, with an overall average IQ of about 68. However, the range of IQs for children with fetal alcohol syndrome is quite wide, as evidenced by children and adolescents with fetal alcohol syndrome in our program at Children's Research Triangle. We have found children with fetal alcohol syndrome who have IQs that range from the 20s to 135; the average IQ is about 72. Alcohol-exposed children, with or without the characteristic facial features or growth retardation, have consistently lower IQ scores than nonexposed children. Importantly, even alcohol-exposed children with a normal IQ demonstrate difficulty with behavioral regulation, impulsivity, social deficits, and poor judgment, causing difficulties in day-to-day management in the classroom and at home (29,30).

In fact, a wide range of other functional difficulties are much more common than mental retardation in children with fetal alcohol syndrome: learning disabilities, poor school performance, poor executive functioning (organization of tasks, understanding cause and effect, following several steps of directions), clumsiness, poor balance, and problems with writing or drawing, to name a few. Behaviorally, many of the children appear to have a short attention span, are impulsive, and are described as hyperactive (30).

The impact of prenatal alcohol exposure is not determined only by the dosage of alcohol to which the child was exposed. Many reports demonstrate that binge drinking, with high peak blood alcohol levels, is more dangerous than chronic drinking, and long-term studies have shown that even small doses of alcohol are damaging (16).

Prenatal alcohol exposure not only causes the child to have a small brain overall but also can stunt the growth of individual parts of the brain (31–35). This can be present regardless of the child's facial features. Problems with the growth and formation of different parts of the brain can result in a wide range of behavioral and learning deficits. The children have trouble moving information between different brain regions; they cannot keep information in mind in order to self-direct their behavior or think in the abstract. They may have trouble recording information in the brain and then have difficulty retrieving information they already learned. Therefore, the child learns his or her multiplication tables one day but forgets them the next. Other parts of the brain can be affected so that the child's ability to coordinate planned motor movements is impaired, resulting in impulsive movement and clumsiness. Reduction in the size of the cerebellum produces difficulties with balance and arousal and may be a source of sleep or problems. It is important to remember that such problems occur not only in children with the abnormal facial features associated with prenatal alcohol exposure but also in alcohol-exposed children who look normal (35).

Changes in Facial Features

Facial features (29) of children and adults with fetal alcohol syndrome are consistent with overall flattening of the middle portion of the face:

1. Epicanthal folds (extra skin folds coming down around the inner angle of the eye).
2. Short palpebral fissures (small eye openings).
3. A flattened, elongated philtrum (no groove or crease running from the bottom of the nose to the top of the lip).
4. A thin upper lip.
5. A small mouth with high arched palate (roof of the mouth).
6. Small teeth with poor enamel coating.
7. Low-set ears.

These features can vary in severity but usually persist over the life of the child. Most people will not recognize any differences when they see the child, but someone with experience in working with children prenatally exposed to alcohol will be able to detect the features.

Children with fetal alcohol syndrome also may have a variety of malformations of major organs, especially the heart, kidneys, eyes, and ears. Many children with fetal alcohol syndrome have vision problems; a good number of them have an eye that turns in or a lazy eye. In addition, children with fetal alcohol syndrome have a predisposition to ear infections and a high rate of hearing loss (eighth nerve deafness), so a thorough hearing examination is usually beneficial (30).

The mother's confirmed use of alcohol is not necessary to make a diagnosis of fetal alcohol syndrome if the child meets criteria in all three categories (growth, central nervous system functioning, and facial features) (29). However, physicians will note when the diagnosis is made without confirmation of the mother's drinking.

Terminology Related to Alcohol-Exposed Children

For the past 40 years, a child whose mother drank alcohol during pregnancy but who had only partial or no apparent expression of physical features of alcohol exposure was said to have *fetal alcohol effects*. These children may have had minimal to moderate facial changes or no changes at all but usually had some problems in intellectual, behavioral, or emotional development. These difficulties had a significant impact on learning and long-term development.

Over the past few years, research has demonstrated that children with so-called fetal alcohol effects have significant structural and functional changes in the brain, even though there is little, if any, overt physical manifestation of the alcohol exposure (31–35). Currently, preferred terminology for children who have been exposed to alcohol but do not meet criteria in all three diagnostic categories is *alcohol-related neurodevelopmental disorder* or *alcohol-related birth defects*. In April 2004, a group of U.S. agencies (36) developed a consensus definition of a new term, *fetal alcohol spectrum disorders,* as follows:

> An umbrella term describing the range of effects that can occur in an individual whose mother drank during pregnancy. These effects may include physical, mental, behavioral, and/or learning disabilities with possible lifelong implications.

It is important to understand that *fetal alcohol spectrum disorder* is not meant to serve as a diagnostic term but rather to be a unifying one to help us all appreciate the many ways in which prenatal alcohol exposure can manifest itself in the affected individual. Research is underway to determine the subtle differences in physical, neurologic, behavioral, and executive functioning status that exist among children who fall within the spectrum of alcohol exposure. In the meantime, diagnostic terminology in daily use focuses on *fetal alcohol syndrome* and *alcohol-related neurodevelopmental disorder*, both of which fall within the larger continuum of *fetal alcohol spectrum disorder*.

Brain Structure and Functioning in Alcohol-Exposed Children

The behavioral, emotional, and learning difficulties of children with fetal alcohol syndrome can best be understood as a deficit in processing information:

1. Input: recording information (bringing it into the brain).
2. Integration: organizing and bringing different forms of information.
3. Memory: storing the information in memory for later use.
4. Output: using the information to guide actions, behavior, emotions, language, and movement.

Different areas of the brain account for these successive steps in information processing. Unfortunately, depending on the timing of the mother's alcohol use and other factors, alcohol can damage formation and growth of any area of the brain, disrupting information processing and brain function at any step along the way.

Damage in the First Trimester

Damage from drinking in the first trimester mainly occurs in the midline structures of the brain responsible for information processing, the way we bring information into the brain and use it to manage our behaviors, emotions, and thinking. Visual information enters the brain through the back part of the brain, the occipital lobe. Touch, taste, and smell enter through the parietal lobe. Auditory information enters through the ear, and the eighth cranial nerve carries the information from the ear to the inner midline section of the brain. A primary job of the brain is to bring all these bits of sensory input together and to conduct the information to the front part of the brain where neurotransmitters regulate actions, behavior, emotion, and speech and language. In other words, the individual is able to use information from the environment to guide and respond appropriately to the environment.

Alcohol's damage to the midline structures of the brain, the limbic system, is what produces many of the functional difficulties we see in children exposed prenatally to alcohol (31–35). For example, the hippocampus connects sensory input to motor output. Damage to the hippocampus interferes with the child's using sensory information such as vision and connecting that information to a motor activity. This causes learning and memory problems: asking a child to take a note to the teacher often will result in her taking the note to school, but she cannot remember what to do with it when she gets there. Another example is when a child sees a truck coming but runs out in front of the truck anyway because she cannot connect that visual input, the visual image of the truck, to motor output, that is, stopping her running out in front of the truck.

Other alcohol-induced structural changes in the brain can occur in the corpus callosum, the section of the brain that permits the two major halves of the brain to share information. For example, alcohol use early in pregnancy can produce thinning of the corpus callosum at its posterior segment (31). This interrupts communication within the brain. If this communication is interrupted, as it is in alcohol-exposed children, then some types of information cannot reach consciousness. For example, a child can recite the rules for good behavior in the school lunchroom but cannot control or regulate his behavior in accordance with the rules. He then is described as disobedient or, worse, is misdiagnosed with oppositional defiant disorder and is placed on inappropriate medications.

Finally, the thalamus receives input from all over the body and sends it to the cerebral cortex, the area of the brain responsible for cognition and learning. The thalamus helps organize behavior related to survival such as fighting, feeding, and fleeing. This is why children with fetal alcohol syndrome often get a look of panic in their eyes when faced with a sudden change or threat or when they are overloaded with information (30). Parents describe the children as "not there." The child does not learn from experience. Parents describe the child as stubborn, but the connections between past instructions or experience and current behavior just do not exist (30).

Damage in the Third Trimester

Although formation of the brain begins in the earliest stages of gestation, the majority of growth of the brain occurs in the last trimester. In fact, the brain grows so rapidly during the last 3 months of pregnancy that it cannot fit inside the skull. Therefore, the outer shell of the brain, the cortex, begins to fold in upon itself as demonstrated in a normal magnetic resonance image of the brain. This folding effectively increases the surface area of the brain, and, in general, the greater the surface area of the brain, the greater the intellectual functioning.

When a woman uses alcohol during the last 3 months of pregnancy, the alcohol disrupts appropriate development of the brain, particularly the cortex. In addition to the small size of the brain (microcephaly), there are reduced folds in the cortex of the brain, and the surface of the brain is quite flat. This is a condition known as *lisencephaly* and is associated with profound mental retardation.

Marijuana Effects

Marijuana does not have a direct health effect on pregnancy or the fetus; there is no increased rate of preterm labor, growth retardation, or other such complications. However, a woman who uses marijuana is more likely to have also used other substances, including alcohol, tobacco, and other illegal drugs. More important, even though marijuana does not affect pregnancy outcome, it does have an impact on fetal brain development. Long-term studies document that children whose mothers used marijuana during pregnancy have a significantly higher rate of learning and behavioral problems, especially related to executive functioning (37).

Cocaine and Methamphetamine

Early research on the effects of prenatal methamphetamine exposure shows that the outcome of the infants is similar to that of cocaine-exposed children. This makes sense, because both cocaine and methamphetamine affect the way neurotransmitters such as serotonin, dopamine, and norepinephrine are stored in the brain. Thus, we discuss cocaine and methamphetamine use in pregnancy jointly. However, it should be noted that the world of methamphetamine abuse is replete with violence and pornography; this is at the heart of methamphetamine's impact on families, especially as related to the child welfare system.

Cocaine and methamphetamine each produces a high by increasing the availability of the neurotransmitters at the nerve endings and increasing the excitability of the nerves. The excess neurotransmitter can interfere with blood flow from the mother to the fetus, resulting in poor growth in the womb, and can cause contractions of the uterus, producing premature labor (30).

Chronic exposure to cocaine and methamphetamine can result in the downregulation of the neurotransmitter receptors, meaning that there is a decreased number of receptors left at the nerve endings (38). Positron emission tomography scans of adults with a long history of cocaine or methamphetamine use have shown an absence of functioning dopamine receptors in the prefrontal cerebral cortex (30). The prefrontal cortex is the area of the brain that controls impulsive and aggressive behavior. Animal studies have shown that prenatal exposure to cocaine alters the brain metabolism of neurotransmitters in the motor, limbic, and sensory systems, which results in difficulties regulating different types of responses. All of this information suggests that prenatal exposure to cocaine or methamphetamine has long-term effects on the function of the central nervous system in general and on behavioral regulation specifically (38).

Children who have been prenatally exposed to cocaine or methamphetamine may suffer a range of additional physical problems, often based on the interruption of adequate blood flow to developing organs. Use of either of these substances during pregnancy can result in limb reduction deformities in which the baby is born missing an arm, leg, or fingers. There are reports of babies prenatally exposed to cocaine missing a kidney or portions of the bowel because of infarction: death of the organ from inadequate blood supply and oxygen (25).

Brain defects also have been reported in babies whose mothers used cocaine or methamphetamine during pregnancy. Small areas of infarction, or strokes, in the brain can occur throughout fetal development, or the baby can have a large stroke if the mother uses cocaine or methamphetamine toward the end of pregnancy. Similarly, constriction of blood flow to the heart can cause the baby to have a heart attack while still in the womb (39).

Adding to these difficulties, prenatal exposure to cocaine or methamphetamine interferes with the infant's neurobehavior: the ability to interact with her environment, to respond to sound and visual stimulation, and to interact appropriately with her parents or other caretaker (25). Although physical difficulties occur in only about 25% to 30% of infants exposed prenatally to cocaine, neurobehavioral difficulties are far more common and are the basis of many of the more difficult challenges a parent may have in caring for the child.

Heroin and Other Opiates

Heroin, opium, and other opiates are used by pregnant women across the country in the form of illegal drugs (heroin) and the abuse of legal drugs (methadone, Vicodin®, OxyContin®). Each of these drugs is a narcotic that can result in the physical addiction of both the mother and the fetus. Infants born to opiate-addicted women frequently are low birth weight and have a high rate of prematurity. If the pregnant woman suddenly ceases her use of opiates, miscarriage, preterm labor, and significant fetal stress can result (40).

The newborn infant can be born addicted and can go through opiate withdrawal after birth. The most significant features of the neonatal abstinence syndrome are a high pitched cry, sweating, tremulousness, abrasions of the chin, knees, and elbows from rubbing on the bed sheets, vomiting, and diarrhea. In addition, the child can run a low-grade fever, the muscle tone is increased, and the reflexes are hyperactive. Seizures are not uncommon in severe withdrawal, and feeding can be so difficult that the child suffers failure to thrive (7,40,41).

Symptoms of neonatal withdrawal from opiates may be present at birth, but they usually do not appear until 3 to 4 days of life. Withdrawal depends on many factors; in some cases, symptoms may not appear until 10 to 14 days after birth. The withdrawal symptoms peak around 6 weeks of age and can persist for 4 to 6 months or longer (40,41).

When discussing opiate use during pregnancy, it is important to at least mention methadone treatment for narcotic addiction. It is not unusual to find a pregnant woman being treated with methadone, a synthetic narcotic that is used to treat people who are addicted to heroin, opium, or other narcotics. The advantage of methadone treatment is that it usually requires only one oral dose each day to suppress the desire to use heroin. The risk of infection from the human immunodeficiency virus that causes acquired immunodeficiency virus or from forms of hepatitis is reduced when the pregnant woman is on methadone rather than continuing to use heroin or other narcotics. However, it is important to be aware that infants whose mothers are on methadone during pregnancy can undergo the same difficulties as infants whose mothers continue to use heroin through the pregnancy (40,41).

Long-Term Impact of Prenatal Exposure to Alcohol and Illicit Drugs

In the past several years, research on the effects of prenatal alcohol and other drug exposure has begun to focus on the longer term implications of prenatal substance exposure. Drawing firm conclusions from many of these studies is difficult because of the challenge of distinguishing the purely biologic effects of the prenatal exposure from the ongoing environmental problems caused by living in a home with a substance-abusing parent. However, these studies still provide us with valuable insight into the potential issues to be faced in the older child who was prenatally exposed to drugs or alcohol.

Studies consistently report that prenatal exposure to cocaine and other drugs, with the exception of alcohol, has minimal direct influence on intellectual development in children (38,42). It is becoming increasingly clear that the single most important predictor of cognitive development, other than genetics, is the environment in which the child is raised. This reiterates the principle of infant mental health: all aspects of a child's development occur within the context of a positive, secure, parent–child relationship.

On the other hand, there is clear evidence that there is a biologic basis to the behavioral difficulties seen in prenatally exposed children as they grow older. The studies of alcohol exposure cited earlier support this hypothesis, as do the studies of children exposed to illicit substance (30–35,37,38,42). Difficulties in executive functioning appear to lie at the basis of many of the problems the children suffer long term, presenting as a behavioral pattern that often appears to be attention deficit hyperactivity disorder (30). However, there is more to the picture than classic attention deficit hyperactivity disorder. Table 6.1 provides an overview of the most common problems seen in children who have been prenatally exposed to alcohol or illegal drugs. In the larger picture, it is important to recognize that no one substance of abuse can be associated with any one particular problem, and studies of long-term effects are still going on. It also is impor-

TABLE 6.1. Behavioral patterns in children prenatally exposed to alcohol and illicit drugs.

Anxiety or depression
Social problems
Thought problems
Attention problems
Delinquent behavior
Aggressive behavior
Poor executive functioning

Source: Data from Bertrand et al. (29) and Chasnoff (30).

tant to remember that early deprivation and neglect can produce some of these same long-term behaviors in children.

Impact of Prenatal Alcohol and Drug Exposure on Children

The impact of prenatal alcohol and drug exposure extends over all aspects of a child's life. This point is illustrated in a recent study of 78 children, aged 6 to 12 years, conducted at the Children's Research Triangle. The children and their families underwent a comprehensive assessment across multiple domains of functioning. All the children had a diagnosis of fetal alcohol syndrome or alcohol-related neurodevelopmental disorder, all had been exposed to illicit substances in addition to alcohol, and all were currently in foster care or had been adopted through the Illinois Department of Children and Family Services.

Assessment results revealed that there were significant academic difficulties for a significant number of the children: 13% already had repeated at least one grade. Almost half of the children were requiring special education services as compared with 12% of the children in the Chicago Public Schools. Because of behavioral problems at school, 11% of the children had suffered an in-school suspension, 11% had received an out-of-school suspension, and 3% had been placed in a 10- to 45-day interim placement. In comparison, the overall suspension rate in the Chicago Public Schools is 4.6%. Two percent of the children in this study had been expelled from school, which is three times higher than the Chicago Public Schools' rates.

The average IQ of the children was 92, but a clear correlation between head size and IQ was found. Children with a head circumference below the 3rd percentile had an average IQ of 85, whereas children with a head circumference above the 3rd percentile had an average IQ of 97. Executive functioning problems were documented in significant numbers of the children, with children who had been diagnosed with fetal alcohol syndrome demonstrating significantly worse academic, memory, cognitive, and adaptive functioning compared with the children with alcohol-related neurodevelopmental disorder.

On psychological evaluation, it was found that 75% of the children met criteria for a diagnosis of a significant mental health disorder, including attention deficit hyperactivity disorder, posttraumatic stress disorder, attachment disorder, and depression. The incidence of the various disorders was similar for children with fetal alcohol syndrome as compared with children with alcohol-related neurodevelopmental disorder except that attention deficit hyperactivity disorder occurred significantly less frequently in the children with a diagnosis of fetal alcohol syndrome.

It is notable from this study that children who meet a diagnosis of fetal alcohol syndrome are different from children who are exposed but do not meet criteria in all three categories: growth, facial features, and neurodevelopmental functioning. This is important because it demonstrates that while children exposed to alcohol are at great risk for cognitive and neurocognitive functioning, children with alcohol-related neurodevelopmental disorder (those alcohol-exposed children who do not meet all criteria for fetal alcohol syndrome) present a different clinical picture from that of children with the full picture of fetal alcohol syndrome. The question thus arises as to how much of the neurodevelopmental difficulties seen in alcohol- and drug-exposed children are due to biologic damage induced by alcohol exposure and how much of the damage is due to environmental factors, especially those related to the foster care system. This point currently is being explored in a study of this same population of children. Preliminary results indicate that disabilities such as attention deficit hyperactivity disorder, processing problems, and mood disorders are related to the biologic impact of the alcohol and illicit drugs. However, it appears that the more severe mental health disorders of reactive attachment disorder, posttraumatic stress disorder, and disruptive behaviors with conduct disorder are most strongly related to the number of placements the child has endured within the child welfare system.

The bottom line is that all families, biologic, foster, and adoptive, who are raising children affected by prenatal exposure to maternal substances of abuse need support, education, and training as they deal with the multiple issues the children bring to their family. Most important, substance-exposed children must be identified early in order to receive the early intervention services they so sorely need. Unfortunately, there is no reliable screening process that can reliably identify children at risk from prenatal alcohol and drug exposure, but there are validated screening instruments that screen for risk across multiple domains of developmental, behavioral, and mental health functioning in young children. A universal screening and assessment process within the court system can help to ensure that all children at risk receive the support and services they need in order to reach their full potential.

References

1. Chasnoff IJ, Burns WJ, Schnoll SH, Burns KA. Cocaine use in pregnancy. N Engl J Med 1985;313:666–669.
2. Chasnoff IJ, Griffith DR, MacGregor S, Dirkes K, Burns KA. Temporal patterns of cocaine use in pregnancy. JAMA 1989;161:1741–1744.
3. MacGregor SN, Keith LG. Cocaine use during pregnancy, adverse perinatal outcome. Am J Obstet Gynecol 1987;157:686–690.
4. Shiono PH, Klebanoff MA. The impact of cocaine and marijuana use on low birth weight and preterm birth: a multicenter study. Am J Obstet Gynecol 1995; 172:19–27.
5. Armstrong MA, Osejo VG, Lieberman L, Carpenter, DM, Pantoja PM, Escobar GJ. Perinatal substance abuse intervention in obstetric clinics decreases adverse neonatal outcomes. J Perinatol 2003;23:3–9.

6. Eisen LN, Field TM, Bandstra ES, Roberts JP, Morrow C, Larson SK, Steele BM. Perinatal cocaine effects on neonatal stress behavior and performance on the Brazelton Scale. Pediatrics 1995;88:477–480.
7. Finnegan LP, Connaughton JF, Kron RE, Samuels SJ, Batra KK. Neonatal abstinence syndrome: assessment and management. In Harbison RD, ed. Perinatal Addiction. New York: Spectrum Publications; 1975:141–158.
8. Frank DA, Bauchner H, Parker S, Huber AM, Kyei-Aboagye K, Cabral H, Zuckerman B. Neonatal body proportionality and body composition after in-utero exposure to cocaine and marijuana. J Pediatr 1990;117:622–626.
9. Lester BM, Corwin MJ, Sepkoski C, Seifer R, Peucher M, McLaughlin S, Golum HL. Neurobehavioral syndromes in cocaine-exposed newborn infants. Child Dev 1991;62:694–705.
10. Azuma SD, Chasnoff IJ. Outcome of children prenatally exposed to cocaine and other drugs: a path analysis of three-year data. Pediatrics 1993;92:396–402.
11. Fried PA, Watkinson B. 36- and 48-month neurobehavioral follow-up of children prenatally exposed to marijuana, cigarettes, and alcohol. Dev Behav Pediatr 1990;11(2):49–58.
12. Hurt H, Brodsky NL, Betancourt L, Braitman LE, Malmud E, Giannetta J. Cocaine-exposed children: follow-up through 30 months. J Subst Abuse 1995; 7(3):267–280.
13. Mayes LC, Bornstein MH, Chawarska K, Granger RH. Information processing and developmental assessments in 3-month-old infants exposed prenatally to cocaine. Pediatrics 1995;95:539–545.
14. Streissguth AP, Sampson P, Barr H. Neurobehavioral dose–response effects of prenatal alcohol exposure in humans from infancy to adulthood. Ann NY Acad Sci 1989;562:145–158.
15. Wekselman K, Spiering K, Hetteberg C, Kenner C, Flandermeyer A. Fetal alcohol syndrome from infancy through childhood: a review of the literature. J Pediatr Nurs 1995;15:296–303.
16. Sood B, Delaney-Black V, Covington C. Prenatal alcohol exposure and childhood behavior at age 6 to 7 years: I. Dose–response effect. Pediatrics 2001; electronic 1–9, 2001.
17. Tatara T. U.S. Child Substitute Care Flow Data for FY 1993 and Trends in the State Child Care Substitute Populations. Washington DC: American Public Welfare Association; 1995.
18. Kilborn PT. Priority on safety is keeping more children in foster care. New York Times. April 29, 1997.
19. Rayburn WF, Bogenschutz MP. Pharmacotherapy for pregnant women with addictions. Am J Obstet Gynecol 2004;191:1885–1897.
20. Sood B, Delaney-Black V, Covington C. Prenatal alcohol exposure and childhood behavior at age 6 to 7 years: I. Dose–response effect. Pediatrics 2001;e34, 1–9.
21. Maliza B. Most Pregnant Women Don't Disclose Drug Use. New Orleans: Society for Maternal–Fetal Medicine; 2002.
22. Chasnoff IJ, Landress HJ, Barrett ME. The prevalence of drug or alcohol use during pregnancy and discrepancies in mandatory reporting in Pinellas County, Florida. N Engl J Med 1990;1202–1206.
23. Chasnoff IJ, McGourty RF, Bailey GW, Hutchins E, Lightfoot SO, Pawson LL, Fahey C, May B, Brodie P, McCulley L, Campbell J. The 4Ps Plus© Screen for

Substance Use in Pregnancy: clinical application and outcomes. J Perinatol 2005;25:368–374.
24. Larrson G. Prevention of fetal alcohol effects: an antenatal program for early detection of pregnancies at risk. Acta Obstet Gynecol. Scand 1983;62:171–178.
25. Chasnoff IJ, Griffith DR, MacGregor S, Dirkes K, Burns KA. Temporal patterns of cocaine use in pregnancy: perinatal outcome. JAMA 1989;261: 1741–1744.
26. U.S. Preventive Services Task Force Ratings: Strength of Recommendations and Quality of Evidence. Guide to Clinical Preventive Services, 3rd ed. Periodic Updates, 2000–2003. Rockville, MD: Agency for Healthcare Research and Quality; 2003.
27. Stratton K, Howe C, Battaglia F. Fetal Alcohol Syndrome: Diagnosis, Epidemiology, Prevention, and Treatment. Washington, DC: National Academy Press, Institute of Medicine; 1996.
28. National Institute on Alcohol Abuse and Alcoholism and Office of Research on Minority Health, National Institutes of Health. Rockville, MD: U.S. Department of Health and Human Services; 2000.
29. Bertrand J, Floyd RL, Weber MK, O'Connor M, Riley P, Johnson KA, Cohen DE, National Task Force on FAS/FAE. Fetal Alcohol Syndrome: Guidelines for Referral and Diagnosis. Atlanta, GA: Centers for Disease Control and Prevention; 2004.
30. Chasnoff IJ. The Nature of Nurture: Biology, Environment, and the Drug-Exposed Child. Chicago: NTI Publishing; 2001.
31. Riley EP, Mattson SS, Sowell ER, Jernigan TL, Sobel DF, Jones KL. Abnormalities of the corpus callosum in children prenatally exposed to alcohol. Alcohol Clin Exp Res 1995;19:1198–1202.
32. Mattson S, Riley EP, Sowell ER, Jernigan TL, Sobel DF, Jones KL. A decrease in the size of the basal ganglia in children with fetal alcohol syndrome. Alcohol Clin Exp Res 1996;20:1088–1093.
33. Swayze VW, Johnson VP, Hanson JW, Sato J, Giedd Y, Mosnik JN, Andreasen NC. Magnetic resonance imaging of brain anomalies in fetal alcohol syndrome. Pediatrics 1997;99:232–241.
34. Mattson SN, Riley EP, Gramling L, Delis DC, Jones KL. Neuropsychological comparison of alcohol-exposed children with or without physical features of fetal alcohol syndrome. Neuropsychology 1998;12:46–153.
35. Clark CM, Li DC, Conry J, Loock R. Structural and functional brain integrity of fetal alcohol syndrome in nonretarded cases. Pediatrics 2000;105:1096–2011.
36. Bertrand J, Floyd RL, Weber MK, O'Connor M, Riley P, Johnson KA, Cohen DE, National Task Force on FAS/FAE. Fetal Alcohol Syndrome: Guidelines for Referral and Diagnosis. Atlanta, GA: Centers for Disease Control and Prevention; 2004.
37. Fried PA, Smith AM. A literature review of the consequences of prenatal marihuana exposure: an emerging theme of a deficiency in aspects of executive function. Neurotoxicol Teratol 2001;23:1–11.
38. Chasnoff IJ, Anson A, Hatcher R, Stenson H, Iaukea K, Randolph L. Prenatal exposure to cocaine and other drugs: outcome at four to six years. In Harvey JA, Kosofsky BE, eds. Cocaine Effects on the Developing Brain. New York: New York Academy of Sciences, 1998;314–328.

39. Chasnoff IJ, Bussey M, Savich R, Stack CA. Perinatal cerebral infarction and maternal cocaine use. J Pediatr 1986;108:456–459.
40. Chasnoff IJ, Hatcher R, Burns WJ. Early growth patterns of methadone-addicted infants. Am J Dis Child 1980;134:1049–1051.
41. Chasnoff IJ, Burns WJ and Hatcher R. Polydrug- and methadone-addicted newborns: a continuum of impairment? Pediatrics 1982;70:210–212.
42. Hurt H, Giannetta J, Brodsky NL, et al. Are there neurologic correlates of in utero cocaine exposure at age six years? J Pediatr 2001;138:911–913.

7 The Social Consequences of Drug and Alcohol Abuse

Heather R. Hayes and Julie M. Queler

In this chapter, we discuss the social consequences of drug and alcohol abuse from the following viewpoints: legal, societal, family, domestic abuse, and women's issues. In addition, the Orchid treatment model is presented.

Of the total arrests for all crimes in the United States (14,004,327) in 2004, nearly 12.5% (1,745,712) were for drug abuse–related violations. In the period from 1995 to 2004, arrests for drug abuse violators of all ages increased by nearly 22%. In contrast to the overall increase, during the same period from 1994 to 2004, the number of drug abuse violations reported for persons under the age of 18 years was down 3.6%. Although this is not a large decrease, it does show an improvement among the younger generation. Drug abuse violations in persons over 18 years of age, however, increased by nearly 26%. If this is not controlled, the country stands to lose the progress made with our youth. The decline in drug abuse violations among persons under the age of 18 years may be credited to the increase in education and awareness in the learning environment. One may also speculate that the decrease may be credited to stiffer penalties imposed by the judicial system in response to rising drug abuse violations and drug-related crime (1).

Cost to Society

The effects of substance abuse reach beyond the walls of the penal system. Substance abuse also places an enormous financial strain on our economy. The overall cost of drug abuse to society in 1998 was almost $143.5 billion. This cost estimate was composed of three main components: health care, loss of production, and other miscellaneous costs, to be defined later (2).

Just as the number of drug arrests has risen in recent years, so has the cost of substance abuse to society. From 1992 to 1998, the overall cost of drug abuse rose by 5.9% annually, outpacing the growth of both the adult population and the consumer price index for the period. A National Office of Drug Control Policy report also estimated that the cost of substance abuse–related health care was $12.9 billion, comprising 9% of the overall cost of substance abuse to society. For the purposes of that report, health care was defined as services provided by community-based specialty treatment, federally provided specialty treatment, support (prevention, training, and research), and medical consequences of substance abuse, including crime victim–related costs (2).

The other miscellaneous costs to society were costs of goods and services lost to substance abuse-related crime, criminal justice system and other public costs, private costs (including private legal defense and property damage of crime victims), and social welfare. In 1998 alone, these miscellaneous costs to society totaled $32.1 billion, making up 22% of society's substance abuse–related costs (2).

The largest cost associated with substance abuse to society in 1998 was the loss of productivity, accounting for 69%, or $98.5 billion, of the total cost to society for substance abuse. The loss of productivity includes premature death of a substance user, substance abuse-related illness, institutionalization, production losses due to crime victims being unable to work, incarceration, and crime careers. These figures begin to demonstrate the scope of the substance abuse problem in the United States. Not only does it affect individual substance users and their families, but the ripples affect every facet of our society (2).

According to the Federal Bureau of Prisons, 53% of the nation's federal inmate population is incarcerated for drug offenses. This makes it the largest sector of the federal prison system, followed by weapons, explosives, and arson at 13.9% (3). If one were to assume that each of the 93,437 persons incarcerated in federal prisons for drug-related crimes represents one family unit, this alone is a staggering statistic. If you add the number of drug abusers and addicts at large and those incarcerated in local jails across the United States, each representing a family of their own, the number of affected families is enormous. This begins to illustrate the impact on the country's family structure.

Family Disruption

In today's environment of fast-paced social, economic, and technical change, the role of the family is constantly being altered. The changes and new roles that the family must assume to ensure the survival of its next generation places strain on the already stressed family unit. The family is a powerful force: a basic source of society's strength and stability and the institution that ensures generational continuity for the community and the culture. The family acts to protect its members, to sustain both the strong and the weak while nurturing the young and protecting its more vulnerable members. As the family strives to maintain stability and to preserve its moral influence, stress on the family is generated from outside and inside its structures: job stress, financial stress, and the emotional stress of keeping a family together in uncertain times. When substance abuse is introduced into a family unit, the emotional stress becomes enormous, and the financial stress greatly increases. An individual who abuses alcohol or other drugs can put a family under increased economic strain as a result of hospital bills from substance abuse-related injuries, fatalities, increased general health care costs, lost workdays, and the potential for job loss.

There are other factors to consider that affect the family and not just the individual substance abuser. The family incurs the direct cost of drug and alcohol abuse in the form of time, money, and in-kind contributions. The indirect costs may be even greater and may include lost career opportunities, social and physiological stress, and stress-related medical complications for other family members.

The time spent helping or caring for a substance-abusing family member has the potential to increase the time away from work and reduce family earnings. While many parents provide financial and other forms of support to ensure their adult children's success, parents of adult children with substance abuse problems spend significantly more time and financial resources in comparison to parents of non–substance-abusing children. The average family of an adult substance abuser with other psychiatric problems spends between \$8,489 and \$13,891 each year compared with parents of adult children without comparable problems, who spend \$3,547 to \$4,279. Families of substance abusers spend on the average 16% of the total family income on their adult children compared with 6% for families without substance-abusing adult children. The family of a substance abuser commits time as well as financial support to deal with the problem. Parents of an adult substance abuser spend on the average 21.2 hours over a 2-week period in care compared with 12.5 hours spent by parents of other families without comparable problems (4).

Drug and alcohol abuse creates a great strain on the family unit, as we have shown, but the greatest impact is on the younger members of the family. It is estimated that one in four children (23.8%, 17 million) in the United States live in a household in which one adult or a parent is a heavy drinker of alcohol or is a binge drinker. Additionally, more than 1 in 10 children (12.7%, 9.2 million) live in a household in which an adult or a parent uses illegal drugs (5). Substance abuse is not merely a disease of the individual but a disease that affects the entire family. The effects of substance abuse radiate through the family members and outside of the family, including school, work, and other social activities. Substance-abusing families tend to be less involved in social, religious, and cultural activities than families without substance-abusing members (6).

Families of substance abusers often experience self-imposed isolation because of embarrassment caused by the efforts of the abuser to conceal the substance abuse. In some cases, the family of a substance abuser is ostracized from the community due to community prejudice or rejection. As a result, many children suffer in silence, with their needs taking a backseat to the addiction or abuse in the family's efforts to maintain the secrecy or to deny the existence of the problem. This isolation reduces the family's chances of getting help and adds further strain to the family life (6).

In this environment, compounded with anxiety and stress, children may become more withdrawn and uncommunicative, increasing their susceptibility to isolation and loneliness. As a direct result of this isolation, children of substance abusers have fewer opportunities to interact with other children and therefore have fewer age-appropriate social skills than children not in an isolated environment. In the education environment, teachers' and peers' expectations of the abilities of children with substance-abusing parents can affect the child's academic progress and social relationships. Teachers of children whose parents are known to be substance abusers may have lower academic expectations for the children and may attribute poor academic achievement to the parents' drug abuse rather than work to unlock the child's full potential. These self-fulfilling prophecies are a common feature in education settings and can have long-lasting effects on children (7). Similar effects can be observed among a child's peers who know thc parents are substance abusers; they too may label the children as different and avoid contact with them or interact with them in ways that can be detrimental to their ability to do well in the education environment (8).

Anyone who has observed a family member struggle with substance abuse or addiction can attest to the pain and disruption in the family life. The most vulnerable children in our society are the children in families where substance abuse exists. In families with one or more substance abusers, children are more likely to experience physical or emotional neglect or sexual abuse than are children in families without substance abuse. When parents abuse drugs, the basic needs of the child become secondary to the addiction because of physical and mental impairments, use of limited financial resources for the addiction, time spent seeking out the drug, and time spent administering or consuming the drugs (8–12).

In families where one or both parents are substance abusers, the family is often faced with other problems such as mental illness, higher rates of unemployment, higher stress levels, and impaired family functioning, all of which can place the children at greater risk for abuse and neglect (13). Studies have shown that from one third to two thirds of reported child maltreatment cases in the United States involved substance abuse (14). According to the National Center on Child Abuse Prevention Research, 85% of the states reported that substance abuse was one of the two major problems exhibited by families in which abuse of children was suspected (15).

Children who are abused are at risk for having chronic problems stemming from the abuse, such as poor physical, mental, and emotional states in their adult lives. Studies have indicated that children from substance-abusing families are more likely to be removed from the home and placed in foster care than are other children. These children of substance-abusing homes typically remain in foster care for longer periods than abused children from non–substance-abusing households (16).

Chemical dependence does not explain violence and abuse, but it is a contributing factor. We know that alcohol and other drugs can act as disinhibitors, lowering the inhibitions that would normally keep a person from acting violently. Frustration tolerance may also be lowered by drug and alcohol abuse. A parent is more likely to strike out at a child while using drugs than when sober and faced with the same circumstances. Chemical consumption may also act to diminish or anesthetize any shame or guilt the perpetrator may experience in regard to the offense, especially after the offense has occurred. The absence of negative emotions or internal inhibitors further perpetuates the abuse by defending the abusers from their own internal processes and inhibiting the distinction between right and wrong. This may account for the fact that children abused by a substance abuser require more time in foster care and more social services. It is indeed an atrocity what these children suffer in their own homes at the hands of the ones they love. The cost is significantly greater for expenditures related to substance-abusing families in the child welfare system. It has been estimated that of the $24 billion the United States spends annually to address aspects of substance abuse, more than 20% ($5.3 billion) is spent on child welfare issues related to substance abuse (16).

Domestic Abuse

It is well documented in the United States that the leading cause of injury to adult women is domestic violence. Domestic violence is defined as any sort of physical, sexual, or emotional abuse perpetrated on another in a past or current intimate relationship. Domestic violence refers to abuse of spouses, children, and the elderly. Although the problem of domestic abuse is vastly underreported, it potentially affects 10% to 15% of the women in the United States (17). Researchers have illustrated that the behavior of domestic abusers closely resembles the behavior of substance abusers, including loss of control, maintenance of behaviors regardless of consequences, blaming others, denial, minimization, and cycles of escalation. Therefore, it is not surprising that domestic abuse and substance abuse often co-occur.

It has also been shown that both women and men tend to hold an intoxicated victim more responsible than the intoxicated perpetrator (18). The argument is that the "act" would not have occurred had the person been in a sober state of mind. It is possible to argue that "they deserved it or "they were asking for it," thus unvictimizing the true victim. Furthermore, in some subcultures of our society, chemically dependent or chemically intoxicated women are viewed as being more sexually available, which may explain the perpetrator's rationale that sexual aggression toward them is acceptable, although as a society we condemn the action (19).

Substance abuse has been shown to be a factor in 92% of reported domestic violence episodes, with the perpetrator or the victim using drugs or alcohol (20). Alcohol is frequently seen as a disinhibitor that facilitates or acts as the catalyst for violence in domestic abuse cases. Other illicit drugs such as cocaine, crack cocaine, and amphetamines are also frequently implicated in cases of domestic violence, because they reduce the user's impulse control and at the same time increases feelings of paranoia. In over 50% of reported domestic sexual assault cases, alcohol is a major contributor. Studies have determined that alcoholism rates are much higher among violent married men than among their nonviolent counterparts (21). Researchers have reported that alcoholism rates among domestic abusers range from 63% to 93% (22). When male alcoholics in treatment were surveyed, 20% to 33% indicated that they had assaulted their wives in the year prior to the survey. When the wives of these men were surveyed separately, they indicated that the incidence was much higher than reported by their spouses (23). The American Medical Association has reported that in cases of marital violence, 54% involved rape or another form of sexual abuse of the female spouse (24).

Substance abuse can trigger domestic violence in arguments over financial matters. Substance abusers may use money for household bills or even steal money from their spouses to support their habits and may react violently when confronted (25). In contrast, women may use alcohol and other drugs to cope with problems, such as to medicate the physical and emotional pain suffered in a violent relationship (26). Alcohol and drug abuse is two to three times higher in women who are abused by a male partner than are women not in abusive relationships. It has been suggested by Gilbert and associates (27) that the fear, anger, and humiliation associated with domestic violence toward women may serve as a trigger for substance abuse. These substances may function as a coping mechanism to buffer the long-term psychological stresses of domestic violence (28). Women in treatment for alcohol and other drug abuse report an elevated rate of violence by their male partners (29). Male partners of these women are twice as likely to abuse alcohol and four times as likely to use illicit drugs than are men not in an abusive relationship (30,31). Women who use psychoactive substances are at a higher risk of violence, as a result of their own drug abuse and that of their partners. The relationship between female substance abuse and increased violence has been reported in several studies (32–34).

Women's Issues

Over the years, women's roles have been redefined, providing them with more autonomy and more opportunity than ever before. Even as the tides of change have afforded women great advances in society, women are still anchored to traditional responsibilities and roles. Modern women are in a constant balancing act between their career and family. Even beyond the dual role modern women play, in boardroom by day and the family room by night, many women are alone as single parents. Many women begin to view the natural aging process through the tainted looking glass of society, and they too begin to see themselves as invisible and to undermine their own personal value (35,36).

In addition to the societal advances women have made for themselves, the tides of change have also brought about the equality of substance abuse and addiction. As young women's bodies begin to experience the hormonal changes brought on by puberty and natural growth, their risk of substance use rises. Young woman who mature faster than their peers are at an increased risk for negative outcomes, including substance use and abuse (37,38). Girls who attain sexual maturity earlier have an increased possibility of engaging in substance abuse earlier and in greater quantities than their peers who reach sexual maturity later (39,40).

The incidence of early puberty and substance use also share similar biologic mechanisms (41). One biologic explanation is that of increased testosterone. Higher testosterone levels in young girls have been shown to accelerate the onset of puberty and have also been linked to an increase in substance use and abuse (42,43). The link between increased testosterone levels and substance use may also explain the tendency for early-maturing girls to spend more time with older, more risk-taking peers (37,44) and to engage in substance abuse to cope with the physiologic and emotional stresses associated with their changing bodies (45,46).

A young woman's increased risk of substance abuse, however, does not pass with the diminishing pubertal hormone cascade. Research has shown that women are affected by substance abuse differently from their male counterparts. Women can become addicted faster, even though consuming smaller amounts. As women mature, their tolerance for substances decreases because of decreasing amounts of lean body mass (46,47). Metabolism also slows as women age; thus alcohol and other drugs remain in their systems longer and lower quantities are needed to achieve the same effect as when they were younger (48). For example, older adults consuming the same quantity of alcohol as younger adults have higher concentrations in the blood (49,50). These changes can be a shock to women, as what was considered safe to moderate consumption in their thirties and forties can become extremely dangerous and potentially abusive and even addicting in their sixties and seventies (47).

Other factors that predispose women to substance abuse are biologic and genetic factors that may account for other psychiatric disorders that co-occur with substance abuse (51). Some data have suggested that many disorders in childhood are linked to the occurrence of alcoholism in adult women (52). Increased risk of substance abuse has been demonstrated in young girls with childhood conduct disorders such as aggression, property destruction, lying, and a severe disregard for authority. Young girls who present these predisposing factors are more than four times more likely to experience substance abuse than their peers who do not demonstrate the predisposing factors (53). It has also been shown that some women may be genetically predisposed to certain destructive behaviors.

Self-esteem and self-confidence can also play an important role in substance abuse. When children enter into middle school, self-esteem declines for both girls and boys, but in girls the decline is more dramatic and thus can affect girls much more than boys (54). In a national survey of girls, it was revealed that high-school-aged girls were more likely to suffer from self-esteem issues than younger girls. Furthermore, teenage girls who report low self-esteem are much more likely to report substance use or abuse. Body image can also affect the self-esteem of younger girls. Girls may use substances such as alcohol and drugs to relieve their negative feelings and also to lose weight that they feel is unattractive (55–57).

Another gender difference that can contribute to a woman's substance abuse is how men and women deal with stress. Women are more likely to internalize the stress of life events, causing them to become more depressed and anxious. Their male counterparts are more likely to externalize stress and anxiety in the form of aggression (58). Girls are more likely to divert stress through substance use; this can ultimately lead to substance abuse (59). This combination of a woman's stress and low self-image can predispose women to depression and the use of substances to self-medicate the symptoms (60).

Child abuse can predispose children to substance abuse, and this effect can be compounded in women. As previously mentioned, women are more likely to internalize stress, sometimes making abuse harder to recognize from a behavioral standpoint. More than one in five high school girls have reported some form of abuse, physical or sexual in nature (55). These young women are twice as likely to use drugs or other substances as are their unabused peers (55).

Substance abuse is often used as a coping strategy to provide escape from the painful emotions of abuse and as a means of self-medicating the internalized anxiety and stress that can continue for a lifetime (61). Teens who have experienced physical or sexual abuse are more likely to experience feelings of isolation, loneliness, and depression, which are all known contributors to substance abuse (62).

In treatment for substance abuse, more than twice as many girls report that they were either physically or sexually abused or that they have endured both physical and sexual abuse compared with boys in treatment (63). The victimizations experienced in childhood do not go away with the passing of adolescence; adult women who were abused as children are significantly more likely to drink to intoxication, experience alcohol-related problems such as alcohol dependency, and to abuse both prescription and illicit drugs compared with their nonabused counterparts (64,65).

Addiction is far more than a disease of the individual but is an epidemic in our society. Although the substance use leading to substance abuse and full addiction begins in the individual, the consequences reach every facet of today's society. Every individual suffering from substance abuse affects the people and family members around them. These effects can range from emotional stress and financial strain on the family, to cases of child and spousal abuse. Addiction transforms from disease into a parasite on our society, further perpetuating its survival through the effects the individual suffering from the addiction has on others. Substance abuse increases the prevalence of child abuse, and, in an effort to cope with the emotional scars of the abuse, abused children are more likely to turn to drugs and alcohol. Once again, the circle of substance abuse in our society is renewed.

Case Study 7.1. The Orchid Model for Treating Women with Drug and Alcohol Addictions

It is well documented that males and females are affected by chemical substances differently through both physiologic and psychological factors. Because addiction affects the sexes differently, it follows logically that they should be treated accordingly. A new therapeutic model of treatment is being used to treat the specific needs of women suffering from drug and alcohol addictions.

The Orchid treatment model is unlike any other because it offers women an approach that is uniquely focused on the recovery needs of the female who suffers from the painful effects of drug addiction, alcoholism, and unresolved trauma. This novel treatment program recognizes that the impact of untreated trauma on women in early recovery can be devastating and often leads to unhealthy choices, a continuing inability to cope without chemical dependence, and chronic relapse. Trauma can be significant or persistent verbal, physical, emotional, or sexual abuse, either past or present, which can affect a woman's self-esteem, her emotional well-being, and her general ability to function.

It is paramount to recognize that substance abuse in women has a distinctive etiology and disease progression that differs from that of men and requires specialized treatment services. As such, the Orchid model combines a variety of holistic healing methods especially designed for women with chemical addiction and trauma. These treatments include acupuncture, healing art, healing sound, meditation and breath work, yoga, and exercise. The therapies utilized are individual, group, and family counseling, relapse prevention, life skills lecture series, daily process groups, family sculpting, and experiential group therapy. It is important that these treatments are provided by an all-female staff in an aesthetically pleasing atmosphere with a low patient to therapist ratio.

Research Basis

The Orchid model combines the latest empirical research on the treatment of addicted women with trauma. Although cognitive-behavioral therapy techniques have traditionally been the standard in the treatment of chemical dependency, this approach alone is not sufficient to treat women with addiction and posttraumatic stress disorder or other trauma issues. Women with posttraumatic stress disorder often have limited skills in developing and maintaining intimate relationships with others and therefore have difficulty experiencing and expressing emotions. With this in mind, the therapy model integrates cognitive-behavioral therapy with dynamic experiential group work, family sculpting, healing arts therapies, and 12 Step recovery tools to offer women maximum therapeutic benefits throughout their treatment experience.

In order for substance-abusing women with trauma injury to be successful and to maintain long-term recovery, both issues must be addressed simultaneously. In order to achieve this, the Orchid model utilizes present-focused therapy but does not seek to elicit the painful traumatic events. The focus of treatment is to provide information and therapy to patients within the context of safe, supportive, and clinically appropriate techniques. By learning how to identify and express feelings, developing healthier boundaries and responsible behaviors, women begin to take control over their lives and their destinies.

Expressive Therapies

A variety of expressive therapies are utilized in the Orchid model to help women heal in mind, body, and spirit. This creates an opportunity for patients to express themselves artistically to improve mind/body energy flow and explore on a deeper level the serenity necessary to improve their prognosis at time of discharge.

Art Therapy

Meaningful art projects assist clients in addressing their chemical dependency and trauma issues through imagery, collage, and mask making, color therapy, and work with clay.

Healing Sound Therapy

Patients learn to reduce stress and create their own sense of safety within and around themselves. Healing sound therapy offers the healing benefits of focused breathing and meditation techniques. The sound vibrations of the "singing bowls" induce a centered state of deep relaxation.

Acupuncture

Auricular therapy is combined with traditional oriental medical techniques to alleviate symptoms of stress, anxiety, and postacute withdrawal.

Yoga

Combined with a healthy diet plan, exercise regimen, and meditation, yoga is another tool that promotes healthy breathing and self-soothing activities for patients. Yoga is used very successfully with women to deal with addiction and trauma.

Meditation and Breath Work

The meditation series assists women as part of their transformation and self-discovery, while breath work is a safe, gentle, yogic breathing process that promotes relaxation, inner peace, and cleansing. Meditation and breath work are holistic aspects of the treatment program.

Experiential Group Therapy and Psychodrama

Patients are able to gain insight and further develop emotional coping skills while participating in various situations through role plays and reenactments. This further promotes the ability to make healthy choices and accept responsibility for decisions while helping themselves and other group members. This can help in decreasing the impact of the trauma, which has often been stored in the body, muscles, and brain.

References

1. Federal Bureau of Investigation. CRIME 2004 in the United States: Uniform Crime Report. Washington, DC: Federal Bureau of Investigation, U.S. Department of Justice; 2004.
2. Office of National Drug Control Policy. The Economic Costs of Drug Abuse in the United States, 1992–1998. Washington, DC: Office of National Drug Control Policy, Executive Office of the President; 2001.
3. Quick facts about the Federal Bureau of Prisons. Federal Bureau of Prisons Web page. Available at: http://www.bop.gov/news/quick.jsp. Accessed June 2006.
4. Clark RE. Family costs associated with severe mental illness and substance use. Hosp Commun Psychiatry 1994;45(8):808–813.
5. The National Center on Addiction and Substance Abuse at Columbia University. Family Matters: Substance Abuse and the American Family. New York: The National Center on Addiction and Substance Abuse at Columbia University; 2005.
6. Kumpfer KL, DeMarsh J. Family environmental and genetic influences on children's future chemical dependency. In Ezekoye S, Kumpfer K, Bukoski W, eds. Childhood and Chemical Abuse, Prevention and Intervention. New York: Haworth Press; 1986:49–92.

7. Hogan DM. The psychological development and welfare of children of opiate and cocaine users: review and research needs. J Child Psychol Psychiatry 1998;39(5):609–620.
8. Smith AE, Jussim L, Eccles J. Do self-fulfilling prophecies accumulate, dissipate, or remain stable over time? J Pers Social Psychol 1999;77(3):548–565.
9. DeBellis MD, Broussard ER, Herring DJ, Wexler S, Moritz G, Benitez JG. Psychiatric co-morbidity in caregivers and children involved in maltreatment: a pilot research study with policy implications. Child Abuse Negl 2001;25:923–944.
10. Dube SR, Anda RF, Felitti VJ, Croft JB, Edwards VJ, Giles WH. Growing up with parental alcohol abuse: exposure to childhood abuse, neglect, and household dysfunction. Child Abuse Negl 2001;25:1627–1640.
11. Chaffin M, Kelleher K, Hollenberg J. Onset of physical abuse and neglect: psychiatric, substance abuse, and social risk factors from prospective community data. Child Abuse Negl 1996;20(3):191–203.
12. Kelleher K, Chaffin M, Hollenberg J, Fischer E. Alcohol and drug disorders among physically abusive and neglectful parents in a community-based sample. Am J Public Health 1994;84(10):1586–1590.
13. National Clearinghouse on Child Abuse and Neglect Information. Substance Abuse and Child Maltreatment. Washington, DC: National Clearinghouse on Child Abuse and Neglect Information, U.S. Department of Health and Human Services; 2003.
14. U.S. Department of Health and Human Services. Blending Perspectives and Building Common Ground: A Report to Congress on Substance Abuse and Child Protection. Washington, DC: U.S. Government Printing Office; 1999.
15. National Center on Child Abuse Prevention Research. Current Trends Abuse Prevention, Reporting, and Fatalities: The 1999 Fifty State Survey. Chicago: Prevent Child Abuse America; 2001.
16. National Center on Addiction and Substance Abuse at Columbia University. Shoveling Up: The Impact of Substance Abuse on State Budgets. New York: National Center on Addiction and Substance Abuse at Columbia University; 2001.
17. Wilt S, Olson S. Prevalence of domestic violence in the United States. J Am Med Womens Assoc 1996;51(3):77–82.
18. Irons R, Schneider JP. When is domestic violence a hidden face of addiction? J Psychoactive Drugs 1997;29(4):337–44.
19. Blume SB. Women and alcohol: A review. JAMA 1986;256(11):1467–1470.
20. Brookoff D, O'Brien KK, Cook CS, Thompson TD, Williams C. Characteristics of participants in domestic violence. Assessment at the scene of domestic assault. JAMA 1997;277(17):1369–1373.
21. Dinwiddie SH. Psychiatric disorders among wife batterers. Comp Psychiatry 1992;33(6):411–416.
22. Bhatt RV. Domestic violence and substance abuse. Int J Gynaecol Obstet 1998;(63 Suppl 1):S25–S31.
23. Gondolf EW, Foster RA. Wife assault among VA alcohol rehabilitation patients. Hosp Commun Psychiatry 1991;42(1):74–79.
24. American Medical Association. Diagnostic and treatment guidelines on domestic violence. Arch Fam Med 1992;1(1):39–47. Erratum in: Arch Fam Med 1992;1(2):287.

25. Smith JW. Addiction medicine and domestic violence. J Subst Abuse Treat 2000;19(4):329–338.
26. Dunnegan SW. Violence, trauma and substance abuse. J Psychoactive Drugs 1997;29(4):345–351.
27. Gilbert L, El-Bassel N, Schilling RF, Friedman E. Childhood abuse as a risk for partner abuse among women in methadone maintenance. Am J Drug Alcohol Abuse 1997;23:581–595.
28. Herman J. Trauma and Recovery. New York: Random House; 1992.
29. Miller BA, Wilsnack SC, Cunradi CB. Family violence and victimization: treatment issues for women with alcohol problems. Alcohol Clin Exp Res 2000; 24(8):1287–1297.
30. Grisso JA, Schwarz DF, Hirschinger N, Sammel M, Brensinger C, Santanna J, et al. Violent injuries among women in an urban area. N Engl J Med. 1999; 341(25):1899–1905.
31. Kyriacou DN, Anglin D, Taliaferro E, Stone S, Tubb T, Linden JA, et al. Risk factors for injury to women from domestic violence against women. N Engl J Med 1999;341(25):1892–1898.
32. Miller BA, Downs WR, Testa M. Interrelationships between victimization experiences and women's alcohol use. J Stud Alcohol Suppl 1993;11:109–117.
33. Wilsnack S, Wilsnack R, Hiller-Sturmhofel S. How women drink: epidemiology of women's drinking and problem drinking. Alcohol Health Res World 1994;18:173–180.
34. Durose MR, Harlow CW, Langan PA, Motivans M, Rantala RR, Smith EL, et al. Family violence statistics including statistics on strangers and acquaintances. Washington, DC: U.S. Department of Justice, Office of Justice Programs, Bureau of Justice Statistics; 2005.
35. Straussner SL, Brown S, eds. The Handbook of Addiction Treatment for Women. San Francisco: Jossey-Bass; 2002.
36. Ellis BJ, McFadyen-Ketchum S, Dodge KA, Pettit GS, Bates JE. Quality of early family relationships and individual differences in the timing of pubertal maturation in girls: a longitudinal test of an evolutionary model. J Pers Social Psychol 1999;77(2):387–401.
37. Tarter R, Vanyukov M, Giancola P, Dawes M, Blackson T, Mezzich A, et al. Etiology of early age onset substance use disorder: a maturational perspective. Dev Psychopathol 1999;11(4):657–683.
38. Tschann JM, Adler NE, Irwin CE Jr, Millstein SG, Turner RA, Kegeles SM. Initiation of substance use in early adolescence: the roles of pubertal timing and emotional distress. Health Psychol 1994;13(4):326–333.
39. Dick DM, Rose RJ, Viken RJ, Kaprio J. Pubertal timing and substance use: associations between and within families across late adolescence. Dev Psychol 2000;36(2):180–189.
40. Harrell JS, Bangdiwala SI, Deng S, Webb JP, Bradley C. Smoking initiation in youth: the roles of gender, race, socio-economics, and developmental status. J Adolesc Health 1998;23(5):271–279.
41. Ellis BJ, McFadyen-Ketchum S, Dodge KA, Pettit GS, Bates JE. Quality of early family relationships and individual differences in the timing of pubertal maturation in girls: a longitudinal test of an evolutionary model. J Pers Social Psychol 1999;77(2):387–401.

42. Kandel DB, Udry JR. Prenatal effects of maternal smoking on daughters' smoking: nicotine or testosterone exposure? Am J Public Health 1999;89(9):1377–1383.
43. Martin CA, Logan TK, Portis C, Leukefeld CG, Lynam D, Staton M, et al. The association of testosterone with nicotine use in young adult females. Addict Behav 2001;26(2):279–283.
44. Stice E, Presness K, Bearman SK. Relation of early menarche to depression, eating disorders, substance abuse, and comorbid psychopathology among adolescent girls. Dev Psychol 2001;37(5):608–619.
45. Crisp A, Sedgwick P, Halek C, Joughin N, Humphrey H. Why may teenage girls persist in smoking? J Adolesc 1999;22(5):657–672.
46. Dawes MA, Antelman SM, Vanyukov MM, Giancola P, Tarter RE, Susman EJ, et al. Developmental sources of variation in liability to adolescent substance use disorders. Drug Alcohol Depend 2001;61(1):3–14.
47. Atkinson RM, Ganzini L, Bernstein MJ. Alcohol and substance-use disorders in the elderly. In Birren JE, Sloane RJ, Cohen GD, eds. Handbook of Mental Health and Aging. New York: Academic Press; 1992:516–556.
48. Montamat SC, Cusack BJ, Vestal RE. Management of drug therapy in the elderly. N Engl J Med 1989;321(5):303–309.
49. Barry PP. Gender as a factor in treating the elderly. In Ray BA, Braude MC, eds. Women and Drugs: A New Era for Research. Rockville, MD: U.S. Department of Health and Human Services, Public Health Service, Alcohol, Drug Abuse, and Mental Health Administration, National Institute on Drug Abuse; 1986:65–69.
50. Braude MC. Drugs and drug interactions in elderly women. In Ray BA and Braude MC (Eds.). Women and Drugs: A New Era for Research. Rockville, MD: U.S. Department of Health and Human Services, Public Health Service, Alcohol, Drug Abuse, and Mental Health Administration, National Institute on Drug Abuse; 1986:58–64.
51. Giancola PR, Mezzich AC. Neuropsychological deficits in female adolescents with a substance use disorder: better accounted for by conduct disorder? J Stud Alcohol 2000;61(6):809–817.
52. Miles DR, Van den Bree MBM, Pickens RW. Sex differences in shared genetic and environmental influences between conduct disorder symptoms and marijuana use in adolescents. Am J Med Genet 2002;114(2):159–168.
53. Disney ER, Elkins IJ, McGue M, Iacono WG. Effects of ADHD, conduct disorder, and gender on substance use and abuse in adolescence. Am J Psychiatry 1999;156(10):1515–1521.
54. Johnson NG, Roberts MC, Worell J. Beyond Appearance: A New Look at Adolescent Girls. Washington, DC: American Psychological Association; 1999.
55. Schoen C, Davis K, Collins KS, Greenberg L, Des Roches C, Abrams M. The Commonwealth Fund Survey of the Health of Adolescent Girls. New York: Commonwealth Fund; 1997.
56. The National Center on Addiction and Substance Abuse at Columbia University. The Formative Years: Pathways to Substance Abuse Among Girls and Young Women Ages 8–22. New York, NY: Center on Addiction and Substance Abuse at Columbia University; 2003.

57. Bellafante, G. When midlife seems just an empty plate. New York Times 2003; 9.1
58. Aneshensel CS, Rutter CM, Lachenbruch PA. Social structure, stress, and mental health: competing conceptual and analytic models. Am Sociol Rev 1991;56(2):166–178.
59. Byrne D, Byrne A, Reinhart M. Personality, stress and the decision to commence cigarette smoking in adolescence. J Psychosom Res 1995;39(1):53–62.
60. Whalen CK, Jamner LD, Henker B, Delfino, RJ. Smoking and moods in adolescents with depressive and aggressive dispositions: evidence from surveys and electronic diaries. Health Psychol 2001;20(2):99–111.
61. Widom CS, Weiler BL, Cottler LB. Childhood victimization and drug abuse: a comparison of prospective and retrospective findings. J Consult Clin Psychol 1999;67(6):867–880.
62. Garnefski N, Arends E. Sexual abuse and adolescent maladjustment: differences between male and female victims. J Adolesc 1998;21(1):99–107.
63. Rounds-Bryant JL, Kristiansen PL, Fairbank JA, Hubbard RL. Substance use, mental disorders, abuse, and crime: gender comparisons among a national sample of adolescent drug treatment clients. J Child Adolesc Subst Abuse 1998; 7(4):19–34.
64. Galaif ER, Stein JA, Newcomb MD, Bernstein DP. Gender differences in the prediction of problem alcohol use in adulthood: exploring the influence of family factors and childhood maltreatment. J Stud Alcohol 2001;62(4):486–493.
65. Jasinski JL, Williams LM, Siegel J. Childhood physical and sexual abuse as risk factors for heavy drinking among African-American women: a prospective study. Child Abuse Negl 2000;24(8):1061–1071.

8
The Pharmacologic Treatment of Alcohol and Drug Addiction

Nikita B. Katz, Olga A. Katz, and Steven Mandel

This chapter is about the pharmacologic treatment of drug and alcohol addiction. The National Institute on Drug Abuse has issued a set of principles of drug addiction treatment as a research-based guide for practitioners. These principles are given in Table 8.1 and make it clear that pharmacologic treatment is only one component in a broad range of treatment modalities (1). This chapter reviews the pharmacologic treatments for (1) alcohol; (2) stimulants: cocaine and amphetamines; and (3) opioids and other narcotics.

Alcohol

There are two steps in the pharmacologic management of alcoholism:

1. Safe detoxification.
2. Pharmacologic interventions to reduce alcohol relapse.

Step One: Alcohol Detoxification

The majority of patients may be safely and effectively detoxified in ambulatory settings using medications such as benzodiazepines and anticonvulsants. Because benzodiazepines differ in their half-lives, there are at least two popular and effective regimens of detoxification. One approach is to use a benzodiazepine with a long half-life, such as chlordiazepoxide (Librium®, half-life up to 25 hours), at a relatively high loading dose and to let the benzodiazepine self-taper. The second approach uses a shorter acting benzodiazepine, such as oxazepam (Serax®, half-life less than 15 hours), in multiple doses that are titrated to the patient's symptoms and overall progress. This may allow the physician to use a smaller total dosage of the drug. Benzodiazepines present a substantial risk to the patient with a history of complex addiction to both alcohol and benzodiazepines; for these patients anticonvulsants are a safer and more effective option (2–5).

Table 8.1. Basic principles of drug treatment.

1. No single treatment is appropriate for all persons. Matching treatment settings, interventions, and services to each person's problems and needs is critical to his or her ultimate success in returning to productive functioning in the family, workplace, and society.
2. Treatment needs to be readily available. Because people who are addicted to drugs may be uncertain about entering treatment, taking advantage of opportunities when they are ready for treatment is crucial.
3. Effective treatment attends to multiple needs of the person, not just his or her drug use.
4. A person's treatment and services plan must be assessed continually and modified as necessary to ensure that the plan meets the person's changing needs.
5. Remaining in treatment for an adequate period of time is critical for treatment effectiveness. The appropriate duration for a person depends on his or her problems and needs.
6. Counseling and other behavioral therapies are critical components of effective treatment for addiction.
7. Medications are an important element of treatment for many patients, especially when combined with counseling and other behavioral therapies.
8. Addicted or drug-abusing individuals with coexisting mental disorders should have both disorders treated in an integrated way.
9. Medical detoxification is only the first stage of addiction treatment and by itself does little to change long-term drug use.
10. Treatment does not need to be voluntary to be effective.
11. Possible drug use during treatment must be monitored continuously.
12. Treatment programs should provide assessment for HIV/AIDS, hepatitides B and C, tuberculosis, and other infectious diseases.
13. Recovery from drug addiction can be a long-term process and frequently requires multiple episodes of treatment. As with other chronic illnesses, relapses to drug use can occur during or after successful treatment episodes.

Source: National Institute on Drug Abuse. Commonly Abused Drugs. NIDA Web site. Available at: http://www.nida.nih.gov/DrugPages/DrugsofAbuse.html. Accessed November 6, 2006.

Anticonvulsants may be used as the alternative to benzodiazepines, especially because they have the practical advantage of no abuse potential and a theoretical advantage of reducing kindling, an aggravation of the withdrawal symptoms often observed in patients who experience multiple episodes of alcohol withdrawal. Drugs that have been successfully used for the purposes of detoxification include valproate (Depakote®, Depakene®), carbamazepine (Tegretol®), and gabapentin (Neurontin®). The combination of valproate with barbiturates has been reported as having the least incidence of spontaneous hostility in the recovering patient. This combination is not indicated for patients with a history of barbiturate abuse (5,6).

Step Two: Reduction of Alcohol Relapse

The aversive agent disulfiram (Antabuse®) has been available for the treatment of alcoholism since 1949. This drug inhibits the liver enzyme that catalyzes the oxidation of acetaldehyde, a toxic by-product of alcohol metabolism, resulting in a strong aversive reaction 5 to 10 minutes after alcohol intake. The patient may experience the effects of a severe hangover such as sweating, difficulty breathing, rapid heartbeat, rash, nausea, vomiting, and headache for a period of 30 minutes to several hours. Disulfiram should not be taken if alcohol has been consumed in the previous 12 hours. There is no tolerance to disulfiram, and because it is absorbed and eliminated slowly, the effects may last for up to 2 weeks after the initial intake (4–6).

Disulfiram is thought to deter drinking by making the negative consequences of drinking more certain, immediate, and aversive than they would be otherwise. At the same time, clinical trials of disulfiram have not shown efficacy in the absence of supervision and positive contingencies. Subcutaneous implants have not yielded better results, as they often fail to produce adequate disulfiram blood concentrations. A rarely used but somewhat less toxic alternative to disulfiram is calcium carbimide (Temposil®). All the potential pitfalls of disulfiram apply to calcium carbimide (7–9).

Two classes of drugs offer the most promise from the standpoint of reduction of the risk of alcohol relapse: opioid antagonists (naltrexone) and gamma-aminobutyric acid (GABA)/glutamate agonist–antagonists (acamprosate). Naltrexone (Revia®, Vivitrol®) is an opioid antagonist that was originally developed for use in the prevention of relapse in detoxified opiate addicts (9,10).

Naltrexone and its active metabolite 6-beta-naltrexol are competitive antagonists at mu and kappa opioid receptors and to a lesser extent at delta opioid receptors. This blockade of opioid receptors is the basis of its action in the management of opioid dependence, as it reversibly blocks or attenuates the effects of opioids. Its mechanism of action in cases of alcohol dependence is not fully understood, but as an opioid-receptor antagonist it is likely to be due to the modulation of the dopaminergic mesolimbic pathway that alcohol is believed to activate (9,10).

Naltrexone has a half-life of approximately 4 hours, and 6-beta-naltrexol has a half-life of 12 hours. The medicine is rapidly absorbed upon ingestion, and blood concentration of naltrexone reaches peak levels between 60 and 90 minutes. In alcohol-dependent patients, adverse events were not common and included nausea (10%), headache (8%), dizziness (4%), nervousness (4%), fatigue (4%), insomnia (3%), vomiting (3%), anxiety (2%), and somnolence (2%), making this drug relatively easy to recommend even to sensitive patients (11).

Because of its mechanism of action, naltrexone is contraindicated for patients who are currently opioid dependent, are in acute opioid withdrawal, or require opioid analgesics for management of pain and those with acute hepatitis or liver failure. Empirical evidence suggests that naltrexone can be easily and safely combined with antidepressants. Naltrexone is approved for use in the treatment of alcoholism in the United States, Canada, and many European and Asian countries (11).

The majority of studies have found naltrexone to be superior to placebo in treatment of alcohol dependence, especially when naltrexone is initiated following a period of abstinence of about 5 to 7 days. In the clinical trials, alcohol-dependent subjects often reported feeling less high and experienced lower levels of craving for alcohol. Most commonly, studies of alcohol-dependent patients taking naltrexone find that this medication reduces the risk of drinking at hazardous levels and reduced the percentage of drinking days. Good treatment compliance and concurrent psychological interventions increase the likelihood of positive outcomes (11,12).

Nalmefene (Revex®) is a newer opioid antagonist that is structurally similar to naltrexone. It has been in clinical trials for a variety of indications, including compulsive shopping and gambling and opioid and alcohol dependence. In several trials, nalmefene has been found to reduce the risk of relapse to heavy drinking (13).

Acamprosate (calcium acetyl-homotaurine, Campral®) is a structural analog of the neurotransmitter GABA that also appears to actively inhibit the N-methyl-D-aspartate receptor of the neurotransmitter glutamate, particularly in the nucleus accumbens, a pleasure and reward area of the brain. The U.S. Food and Drug Administration (FDA) approved acamprosate in July 2004, although in Europe this drug has been legal and widely used since 1989.

The effects of acamprosate appear to be dose dependent, favoring the higher doses of up to 3 g/day. There are no laboratory studies examining the interactions of acamprosate and alcohol, although anecdotally there appears to be no aversive effect. The possibility of combining acamprosate with disulfiram has been evaluated in both small-scale and case studies and at least one large-scale study. It appears that the combined use of acamprosate and disulfiram may lead to the highest number of continuous abstinent days compared with the other treatments, possibly by combining the reduction of desire for alcohol due to acamprosate and the aversive effects of disulfiram that become prominent should a lapse occur (13).

Although antidepressants such as fluoxetine (Prozac®) and sertraline (Zoloft®) are often considered for treatment of alcohol addiction, their efficacy appears to be minimal and may be observed only in patients who have a significant psychiatric comorbidity, such as major depression. Similarly, tricyclic antidepressants such as amitriptyline (Elavil®) or imipramine (Tofranil®) appear to be no different from placebo in the outcomes of reduction of cravings and prevention of relapses (14).

A number of experimental and preclinical studies have been performed in the past decade: various combinations of approved agents, combinations of off-label medications and investigational drugs such as thyrotropin-releasing hormone analogs, the calcium channel blocker isradipine, as well as the serotonergic antagonists ritanserin, buspirone, and ondansetron. At the moment, only two medications stand the test of clinical trials and may be recommended: naltrexone and acamprosate (Table 8.2).

TABLE 8.2. Summary of trials of medications for the treatment of alcohol abuse.

Drug	Dosage	Number of subjects	Reduction of cravings	Time to relapse	Time to first drink	Percentage of drinking days vs. sober days	Type of psychological intervention
Naltrexone (Revia®, Vivitrol®)	50 mg/day	70	Observed	Longer	No effect	Smaller	Intensive multimodal psychotherapy
	50 mg/day	97	Not significant	Longer	No effect	Smaller	Relapse-prevention psychotherapy
	50 mg/day	97	Not significant	Longer	No effect	Smaller	Coping skills psychotherapy
	50 mg/day	44	Excluded from measurement	Marginally longer	No effect	No effect	No psychotherapy offered
	50 mg/day	131	Not significant	Longer	No effect	Smaller	Cognitive-behavioral therapy
Nalmefene (Revex®)	40 mg/day	21	Not significant	Longer	No effect	Smaller	Cognitive-behavioral therapy
	20 or 80 mg/day	105	Not significant	Longer	No effect	No improvement	Cognitive-behavioral therapy
Acamprosate (Campral®)	2 g/day	102	Not significant	Excluded from measurement	Longer	Smaller	No psychotherapy data
		538	Marginal improvement	Excluded from measurement	Longer	Smaller	No psychotherapy data
		127	Not significant	Excluded from measurement	Not significant	Excluded from measurement	No psychotherapy data
		448	Excluded from measurement	Excluded from measurement	Longer	Smaller	No psychotherapy data
		302	Excluded from measurement	Excluded from measurement	Longer	Smaller	No psychotherapy data
		246	Not significant	Excluded from measurement	Longer	Smaller	No psychotherapy data
Fluoxetine (Prozac®)	Varies	111	Not significant	Not significant	Not significant	Smaller in some, larger in others, depending on comorbidity	No psychotherapy data
Buspirone (Buspar®)	Varies	213	Not significant	Not significant	Not significant	Not significant	No psychotherapy data
Citalopram (Celexa®)	Varies	62	Not significant	Not significant	Not significant	Not significant	No psychotherapy data
Sertraline (Zoloft®)	Varies	100	Not significant	Not significant	Not significant	Marginally smaller	No psychotherapy data
Ondansetron (Zofran®)	Varies	321	Not significant	Not significant	Not significant	Marginally smaller	No psychotherapy data

Note: All trials were double blinded and placebo controlled and lasted 12 weeks or more. Most trials of acamprosate were of 1-year duration. Use of the brand and trade names are for identification purposes only.

Source: Data from Howard (9), Garbutt et al. (10), Schurks et al. (11), Myrick and Anton (12), Scott et al. (13), and Goldstein et al. (14).

Stimulants: Cocaine and Amphetamines

Pharmacotherapy may help to initiate abstinence and prevent relapse among cocaine and amphetamine abusers; however, the success rate of pharmacologic therapy is far from spectacular, and there are no medications specifically approved by the FDA for the management of stimulant addiction.

A large number of prescription medications have been investigated for stimulant abuse, traditionally using the cocaine abuser as the target of treatment. A relatively smaller number of studies looked at amphetamine abusers. Although many of these medications have provided certain promise in small-scale, noncontrolled trials, in randomized, placebo-controlled clinical trials no drug has emerged as having sufficient efficacy for stimulant dependence.

Desipramine (Norpramin®), a tricyclic antidepressant that is less sedating than other tricyclics, had shown some efficacy in abusers of relatively low doses of cocaine (1 to 2.5 g/week), particularly from the standpoint of abstinence initiation. It was also significantly more effective than placebo in reducing cocaine use during the first 6 weeks of treatment. Dual-diagnosis patients suffering from major depression have shown much greater response to treatment with desipramine. As many as 40% of cocaine abusers suffer from major depression, and the use of desipramine or a related drug, imipramine, may be strongly recommended as the first-line therapy (15).

Most other antidepressants, including the popular members of the selective serotonin reuptake inhibitor family, such as fluoxetine (Prozac®) and sertraline (Zoloft®), seem to be of only marginal benefit that is also limited to depressed stimulant abusers. Bupropion (Wellbutrin®, Zyban®) is an atypical antidepressant that is usually viewed as an enhancer of both dopaminergic and noradrenergic transmission while having little if any effect on serotonergic transmission. Because of these pharmacologic properties, bupropion is commonly used in the management of nicotine addiction and has been used with moderate-to-marginal effect in both depressed and nondepressed stimulant abusers.

Antipsychotic medications such as haloperidol (Haldol®) and chlorpromazine (Thorazine®) have been extensively evaluated, especially because of the neurobiologic finding of inhibition of euphoria induced by cocaine and amphetamines in limited inpatient clinical trials. Outpatient trials, however, did not produce any measurable positive effect (16).

The rationale for the use of dopamine agonists, such as antiparkinsonian medications, is relatively straightforward: stimulant abuse leads to initial overstimulation of the dopaminergic pathways that is followed by their hypofunction. Dopamine agonists used for the purposes of reduction of drug use in cocaine and amphetamine addicts include bromocriptine, pergolide, amantadine, and selegiline. Of these, bromocriptine is poorly tolerated, although there may be a certain statistically relevant reduction of cocaine use as verified by urine screens. Pergolide appears to have no effect on either cocaine or amphetamine cravings or incidence of use. Amantadine (Symmetrel®) may have paradoxic effects and side effects in some abusers, although statistically, amantadine at 200 to 400 mg/day is linked with significant improvement in the likelihood of being and remaining free of stimulant use for at least 1 month. Selegiline belongs to the class of drugs known as *monoamine oxidase type B inhibitors.* The recently approved rasagiline (Azilect®) specifically inhibits the deactivation of dopamine, thus preserving the normal physiologic levels of this neurotransmitter. Some studies have found reduced cocaine use when selegiline was used at 5 to 10 mg/day. An interesting option is the use of the transdermal patch Emsam®, approved for treatment of depression, that continuously releases selegiline and may improve patient compliance (17).

Other medications that have been investigated and may have provided some positive outcomes include (1) GABA agonists (baclofen), (2) calcium channel blockers (nifedipine), (3) opioids antagonists (naltrexone), (4) antiepileptic/antikindling drugs (carbamazepine, topiramate, and gabapentin), and (5) disulfiram. Of these, baclofen, topiramate, nifedipine, and disulfiram show the most promise, and their potential in the management of cocaine and amphetamine addiction needs to be evaluated in large-scale studies. Currently, some enthusiasm is associated with a combined therapy that uses disulfiram and an antiepileptic drug. It has been shown that blood concentration of cocaine was significantly greater with the use of disulfiram, which may have contributed to the decreased craving and increased negative emotional states in up to 65% of subjects, prompting them to discontinue the use of cocaine. An antiepileptic agent, such as topiramate or gabapentin, may also improve mood stability or serve as anxiety-reducing agents (18).

Cocaine Addiction Treatable with Antibodies and Viruses

One potentially promising strategy is protein-based therapeutics, using proteins designed to bind cocaine, thereby blocking its effects, or to degrade cocaine, rendering it less psychoactive. Over the past decade, several research groups have reported the successful blocking of the psychostimulatory effects of cocaine and nicotine by anticocaine and antinicotine antibodies with both active and passive immunization in animal and human models (19).

Anticocaine antibodies bind to cocaine in the blood circulation, retarding its ability to enter the brain. This strategy reduced cocaine-induced locomotor activity and self-administration in rats. A different antibody-based approach to cocaine addiction treatment uses specially created catalytic antibodies specific for cocaine that facilitate deactivation of cocaine by cleaving its molecule. The efficacy of catalytic antibodies has been demonstrated in rodent models of cocaine overdose and cocaine addiction, but the rate of deactivation is not yet sufficient for such antibodies to be used in human beings.

Several scientific laboratories concentrate their efforts on using butyrylcholinesterase, the major cocaine-metabolizing enzyme present in the blood of humans and other mammals. Researchers have reported that pretreatment with genetically engineered butyrylcholinesterase can mitigate the behavioral and physiological effects of cocaine and accelerate its metabolism (20).

A common drawback to all of these approaches is their inability to act directly within the brain. Success of these interactions depends solely on peripheral contact between the enzyme or antibody and ingested cocaine. Therefore, a bacteriophage-based approach has been proposed. Bacteriophages are viruses that infect bacteria but are safe to mammalian cells, including human cells. They can be produced in large quantities inexpensively and are very stable. These viruses may be genetically engineered to manufacture and display on their surface almost any desirable protein, including a cocaine-binding protein. There has been successful genetic engineering of a bacteriophage that, while remaining harmless to human beings, is capable of penetrating into the brain and binding large amounts of cocaine, thus rendering the brain incapable of responding to intake and abuse of this substance. This genetically engineered virus can access and act directly within the central nervous system as an additional mode of treatment for drug abuse (21).

The Prometa Protocol for Alcohol, Cocaine, and Amphetamine Dependence

The Prometa treatment protocol, developed and copyrighted by Hythiam, Inc., is designed for individuals diagnosed with dependencies to alcohol, cocaine, or methamphetamine, as well as combinations of these drugs. The medical component of the treatment protocol is designed to address neurologic changes caused or worsened by addiction. It comprises nutritional supplementation, as well as FDA-approved medications used off label and separately administered in a unique dosing algorithm (22).

The protocol differs from existing approaches as it does not focus solely on the psychosocial aspects of the dependence. It targets the brain receptors (GABA receptors) that are believed to play a central role in the disease process; attempts to address the physical symptoms of dependence, such as cravings, withdrawal, and anxiety; and can be used as a complement to traditional psychosocial therapies, such as Alcoholics Anonymous. This treatment is not designed for opiate or benzodiazepine dependence or for addictive substances other than alcohol, cocaine, or methamphetamines.

The manufacturer does not provide specific information on the cost of treatment or identify the medications that are used but discloses that these drugs are not specifically approved by the FDA for the purposes of treatment of drug addiction and withdrawal.

A search of the official database of clinical trials (www.clinicaltrials.gov) reveals that trial NCT00262639 at the Medical University of South Carolina is of the Prometa protocol for alcohol addiction. According to the mandatory disclosure, in this trial approximately 60 alcohol-dependent individuals who are drinking heavily up until 72 hours, or less, prior to study participation will be randomly assigned to receive flumazenil (Anexate®) on 2 successive days and gabapentin (Neurontin®) for 39 days or their matching placebos. They also will receive hydroxyzine (an antihistamine and antianxiety medication) and vitamins. Individuals will be evaluated for alcohol withdrawal, their response to acoustic startle, cognitive ability, craving, mood, sleep, and drinking during the first week. They will then be seen weekly for about 6 weeks during which they take gabapentin or placebo and will be provided with counseling once a week or more, as required. Over this period, participants will be evaluated weekly for alcohol consumption, craving, sleep, mood, and biologic markers of alcohol consumption. After the end of treatment, subjects will be followed up at 4 weeks and at 8 weeks after treatment to evaluate alcohol consumption, craving, sleep, and mood. Subjects will also undergo a functional magnetic resonance imaging procedure sometime during the second or third week of study medication to assess cue-induced regional brain activation to investigate the effect of medication on brain response to alcohol-related visual cues, such as photographs of various drinks, alcohol beverages, or parties (23).

It is premature to endorse or oppose this protocol on the basis of unfinished or small-scale clinical trials. At the same time, components of the Prometa protocol have been independently studied, often in large and long-term scientific studies, and has shown some promise. However, it is worth noting that the cost of treatment is several thousand dollars, which is bound to restrict the availability of treatment. As of May 2006, several health insurance companies were evaluating the possibility of at least partial reimbursement for this treatment and at least one drug court (in Gary, IN) has accepted the protocol as an allowable treatment option (24,25).

The Prometa protocol needs a large-scale, multicenter scientific study conducted by physicians with no relationships with the company that developed the protocol. After the results of such scientific study are published and debated, the protocol in question may be considered for wider deployment.

Opioids and Other Narcotics

Opioids, alcohol, barbiturates, and benzodiazepines act on the opioid receptors of the nervous system. There are five recognized classes of these: *mu*, *kappa*, *sigma*, *delta*, and *epsilon*. These receptors are located in the brain as well as in the spinal cord, peripheral nerves, adrenal glands, ganglia, and stomach/intestines. Alcohol is not, strictly speaking, a narcotic; however, addiction to alcohol is exceedingly common because of easy availability and the role it plays in social rituals. The action of alcohol is partially due to its ability to change the micromechanical properties of the cell membranes (especially those of the neurons in the nervous system) and also to its complex agonist–antagonist action in the brain.

Our bodies make natural opioids, such as beta-endorphin (normally binds to the *mu* receptor) and various enkephalins and dynorphins (normally bind to *sigma* and *kappa* receptors). These natural processes may be the reason for the especially high addictive properties of exogenous opioids such as morphine.

Activation of opiate receptors results in changes in neurotransmission (chemical information exchange), particularly in the brain and the spinal cord. The effects of opioids are due to their selective binding to four receptors:

1. *Mu* receptor activation produces pain relief, euphoria, respiratory depression, and miosis (narrowing of the pupil).
2. *Kappa* receptor effects include pain relief, dysphoria (negative mood), miosis, respiratory depression, and sedation.
3. *Sigma* receptors mediate dysphoria, hallucinations, and psychosis.
4. *Delta* receptor activation gradually results in euphoria, analgesia, and seizures.

The opiate antagonists (such as naloxone, nalmefene, and naltrexone) antagonize all of these effects. Most opioids associated with abuse and dependence are *mu* agonists (morphine, hydrocodone, oxycodone, and meperidine). Some partial *mu* agonists, such as buprenorphine, or some that have no obvious *mu* agonism, such as pentazocine, also can possess reinforcing properties through interactions with other opioid receptors and subsequent reduction of dysphoria or increase in reward-related neurotransmission. Rapid development of physical dependence and a long abstinence syndrome (up to 14 days for heroin, 7 days for meperidine) are almost always seen in narcotics abusers.

The death rate of people who use opioids is disproportionately high compared with people who use other intravenously abused drugs, such as cocaine and phencyclidine. The majority of people who abuse opioid narcotics die in their third decade of life (26).

Opioid Detoxification and Maintenance Protocols

Much like with management of alcohol dependence, the management of opioid dependence is twofold. The patient is detoxified, after which the maintenance stage begins. Detoxification may include use of the following:

1. Opioid agonists (methadone, levo-alpha-acetylmethadol [LAAM]).
2. Partial agonists (buprenorphine).
3. Antagonists (naltrexone).
4. Nonopioid alternatives such as clonidine and benzodiazepines.
5. Combinations, such as naloxone with clonidine and a benzodiazepine.

There are several options with regard to the duration of the detoxification process:

1. Long-term: typically 180 days.
2. Short-term: up to 30 days.
3. Rapid: 3 to 10 days.
4. Ultrarapid: 1 to 2 days.

The most commonly performed detoxification protocols are the long-term (typically 180 days) and short-term (up to 30 days) paradigms involving the use of methadone. Unfortunately, these paradigms have a relatively poor record with regard to the incidence of relapses in the detoxified patient. At the same time, despite the propaganda efforts that often come from the practitioners of the rapid detoxification, the rapid and ultrarapid detoxification protocols are not superior in any way and, if not combined with psychological, social, and employment services, may be as ineffective as the long-term detoxification (27).

Most rapid detoxification protocols involve the use of an opioid antagonist, typically naltrexone or naloxone, in combination with clonidine and benzodiazepines to minimize the gravity of the withdrawal syndrome. A major concern regarding rapid, and especially ultrarapid, detoxification is the occurrence of potentially serious adverse effects, such as respiratory distress or other pulmonary and renal complications, during or immediately after the procedure (28).

Opioid agonist therapy includes methadone, LAAM, and buprenorphine maintenance with the goal of replacement of heroin with legally obtained opioid agonists and subsequent mitigation of many risk factors of the drug-abusing lifestyle. Until recently, LAAM was also used in opioid agonist maintenance programs. However, LAAM is associated with cardiologic toxicity, and several cases of cardiac arrhythmia and death have been reported. The drug was subsequently removed from the market in the European Union and was given a black box label by the FDA in the United States (29).

Methadone, a long-acting synthetic opioid agonist, can be given once daily and replaces the necessity for multiple daily heroin doses. As such, it stabilizes the drug-abusing lifestyle, reduces criminal behaviors, and also reduces needle sharing and promiscuous behaviors leading to transmission of the human immunodeficiency virus and other diseases (30).

Methadone maintenance therapy has been the standard of care for more than 30 years. However, methadone is a Schedule II drug that is only available at specialized methadone maintenance clinics. It is estimated that established methadone clinics currently accommodate no more than 180,000 addicts, a scant 15% to 20% of the total population of heroin addicts in the United States.

Buprenorphine is a *mu* opioid partial agonist that, like methadone, suppresses withdrawal and cravings. However, the property of partial agonism confers a ceiling effect, at which higher doses of buprenorphine cause no additional effects. This ceiling effect allows for a wider margin of safety than methadone, which can be lethal in overdose. The increased safety of buprenorphine has allowed it to become available by prescription as a Schedule III medication. Buprenorphine has been combined with naloxone in a 4 : 1 ratio (Suboxone®) in order to alleviate concerns that the sublingual tablet would be dissolved and injected by addicts. Naloxone is an opioid antagonist that is poorly absorbed sublingually and orally but is well absorbed intravenously. As a result, an opioid-dependent patient injecting buprenorphine/naloxone will suffer a withdrawal syndrome secondary to naloxone's occupation of *mu* opioid receptors (31).

Office-based treatment of opioid addiction is possible with buprenorphine maintenance therapy. Physicians can take an 8-hour training course to become certified to prescribe buprenorphine, and, although currently physicians are limited to 30 buprenorphine patients, this restriction may be lifted soon (31).

Published studies indicate that higher dose methadone (60 to 109 mg/day) is more effective in retaining patients in treatment than lower dose methadone (1 to 59 mg/day). Moreover, methadone at flexible doses was more effective in retaining patients in treatment than buprenorphine. Not surprisingly, multiple clinical trials have also shown that low-dose methadone (20 mg/day) was less effective than buprenorphine (2 to 8 mg/d), and high-dose methadone (50 to 65 mg/day and higher) was more effective than buprenorphine (2 to 8 mg/d) (32,33).

A recent, randomized, placebo-controlled trial suggested that an injectable, sustained-release form of naltrexone (Depotrex) increased retention of patients in treatment for opioid abuse. This, combined with the rapid investigational work aimed at the development of the implantable sustained release product of naltrexone, may soon become the gold standard of medical management of opioid addiction (34).

Conclusions

When used in conjunction with other forms of therapy and disease management, pharmacologic methods of drug treatment can introduce a measure of safety to the withdrawal process and reduce the physical discomfort and cravings.

References

1. National Institute on Alcoholism and Alcohol Abuse. Ninth Special Report to the U.S. Congress on Alcohol and Health. Rockville, MD: U.S. Department of Health and Human Services; 1997.
2. Armour DJ, Polish JM, Stambul HB. Alcoholism and Treatment. New York: Wiley Publications; 1978.
3. Stine S, Meandzija B, Kosten R. Pharmacologic therapies for opioid addiction. In Graham AW, Schultz TK, eds. Principles of Addiction Medicine, 2nd ed. New York: Society of Addiction Medicine; 1998:545–555.
4. Castaneda R, Cushman P. Alcohol withdrawal: a review of clinical management. J Clin Psychiatry 1989;50(8):278–284.
5. Hall W, Zador D. The alcohol withdrawal syndrome. Lancet 1997;349:1897–1900.
6. Holbrook AM, Crowther R, Lotter A. Diagnosis and management of acute alcohol withdrawal. CMAJ 1999;160(5):675–680.
7. Mayo-Smith ME. Pharmacological management of alcohol withdrawal: a meta-analysis and evidence-based practice guideline. JAMA 1997;278(2):144–151.
8. Olmedo R, Hoffman RS. Withdrawal syndromes. Emerg Med Clin North Am 2000;18(2):273–288.
9. Howard MO. Pharmacological aversion treatment of alcohol dependence: I. Production and prediction of conditioned alcohol aversion. Am J Drug Alcohol Abuse 2001;27:561–585.
10. Garbutt JC, West SL, Carey TS, Lohr KN, Crews FT. Pharmacological treatment of alcohol dependence: a review of the evidence. JAMA 2000;132:26–40.
11. Schurks M, Overlack, Bonnet U. Naltrexone treatment of combined alcohol and opioid dependence: deterioration of co-morbid major depression. Pharmacopsychiatry 2005;38:100–102.
12. Myrick H, Anton R. Recent advances in the pharmacotherapy of alcoholism. Curr Psychiatry Rep 2004;6:332–338.
13. Scott LJ, Figgitt DP, Keam SJ, Waugh J. Acamprosate: a review of its use in the maintenance of abstinence in patients with alcohol dependence. CNS Drugs 2005;19:445–464.
14. Goldstein BI, Diamantouros A, Schaffer A, Naranjo CA. Pharmacotherapy of alcoholism in patients with co-morbid psychiatric disorders. Drugs 2006;66:1229–1237.
15. Kongsakon R, Papadopoulos KI, Saguansiritham R. Mirtazapine in amphetamine detoxification: a placebo-controlled pilot study. Int Clin Psychopharmacol 2005;20:253–256.
16. Srisurapanont M, Jarusuraisin N, Kittirattanapaiboon P. Treatment for amphetamine dependence and abuse. Cochrane Database Syst Rev 2001;4: CD003022.
17. Grabowski J, Shearer J, Merrill J, Nagus SS. Agonist-like replacement pharmacotherapy for stimulant abuse and dependence. Addict Behav 2004;29:1439–1464.
18. Laqueille X, Dervaux A, El Omari F, Kanit M, Bayle FJ. Methylphenidate effective in treating amphetamine abusers with no other psychiatric disorder. Eur Psychiatry 2005;20:456–457.

19. Carrera MR, Trigo JM, Wirsching P, Roberts AJ, Janda KD. Evaluation of the anticocaine monoclonal antibody GNC92H2 as an immunotherapy for cocaine overdose. Pharmacol Biochem Behav 2005;81:709–714.
20. Pan Y. Gao D, Yang W, Cho H, Yang G, Tai HH, Zhan CG. Computational redesign of human butyrylcholinesterase for anticocaine medication. Proc Natl Acad Sci USA 2005;102(46):16656–16661.
21. Carrera MR, Kaufmann GF, Mee JM, Meijler MM, Koob GF, Janda KD. Treating cocaine addiction with viruses. Proc Natl Acad Sci USA 2004;101(28):10416–10421.
22. ttp://www.prometainfo.com/pi/resources/news-articles/20060620-cpddraa.jsp;jsessionid=4EC6B53F6792AD29A2231B784B4B9E32. Accessed August 21, 2006.
23. http://www.clinicaltrials.gov/ct/show/NCT00260481;jsessionid=77422A8EC6466C5705FF7842F1A9C03C?order=1. Accessed August 21, 2006.
24. Bonnet U, Banger M, Leweke EM, Maschke M, Kowalski T, Gastpar M. Treatment of alcohol withdrawal syndrome with gabapentin. Pharmacopsychiatry (Germany) 1999;32(3):107–109.
25. Chatterjee CR, Ringold AL. A case report of reduction in alcohol craving and protection against alcohol withdrawal by gabapentin. J Clin Psychiatry 1999; 60:617–620.
26. Li L, Smialek JE. Observations on drug abuse deaths in the state of Maryland. J Forensic Sci 1996;41:106–109.
27. Jaffe JH, Jaffe AB. Opioid-related disorders. In Comprehensive Textbook of Psychiatry, 7th ed. Philadelphia: Lippincott Williams & Wilkins; 2000.
28. Teplin D, Raz B, Daiter J, Varenbut M, Zachos CT, Whang P, Herman S, Chaudry S, Yang M. Measurement of symptom withdrawal severity in a 24-hour period after the anaesthesia-assisted rapid opiate detoxification procedure. Am J Drug Alcohol Abuse 2005;31:327–335.
29. Marsch LA, Stephens MA, Mudric T, Strain EC, Bigelow GE, Johnson RE. Predictors of outcome in LAAM, buprenorphine and methadone treatment for opioid dependence. Exp Clin Psychopharmacol 2005;13:293–302.
30. Stimmel B, Kreek MJ. Neurobiology of addictive behaviors and its relationship to methadone maintenance. Mt Sinai J Med 2000;67:375–380.
31. Vigezzi P, Guglielmino L, Marzorati P, Silenzio R, DeChiara M, Corrado F, Cocchi L, Cozzolino E. Multimodal drug addiction treatment: a field comparison of methadone and buprenorphine among heroin- and cocaine-dependent patients. J Subst Abuse Treat 2006;31:3–7.
32. Newman RG. Expansion of opiate agonist treatment: an historical perspective. Harm Reduct J 2006;3(1):20–45.
33. Vocci FJ, Acri J, Elkashef A. Medication development for addictive disorders: the state of the science. Am J Psychiatry 2005;162(8):1432–1440.
34. Johnson BA. A synopsis of the pharmacological rationale, properties and therapeutic effects of depot preparations of naltrexone for treating alcohol dependence. Expert Opin Pharmacother 2006;7(8):1065–1073.

9
Co-Occurring Substance Abuse and Mental Health Disorders

Edward L. Hendrickson and Bert Pepper

Co-occurring substance abuse and mental illness is a condition that is also called *dual diagnosis*. This subject is reviewed from the following standpoints:

1. Historical context.
2. Prevalence of co-occurring disorders.
3. Assessment and classification.
4. Development of a comprehensive treatment plan.
5. Standardized treatment intervention.
6. Common treatment themes.
7. Community corrections issues.
8. An integrated model.
9. Staff training.

Historical Context

Social institutions are created in response to a need. Every society has found it necessary to create institutions that deal with people who disturb the public order, be it by theft, assault, public drunkenness, or bizarre behavior (1). Since the colonial era, the United States has evolved a series of institutional responses to disturbances of the public order. These responses were based on available resources and the generally accepted belief system of the era. Thomas Kuhn argued that we do not change paradigms just because new knowledge becomes available. We only adopt a new paradigm when the old one is no longer functioning (2).

Rough justice was the predominant paradigm during the American colonial period. There were few jails and prisons and no mental hospitals or drug treatment facilities. People were subjected to the stocks, public flogging, banishment, or even burning at the stake as a witch for behaviors resulting from criminal activity, mental illness, or excessive alcohol use.

Around 1790, community responses became more humane and rehabilitation focused. That year, the Quakers of Philadelphia opened the Walnut

Street Jail and coined the term "correctional institution." Inmates were housed in private rooms and were expected to use their removal from society as a time to meditate on and correct their behavior. The next paradigm shift occurred in 1820, when New York State introduced dormitories and prison industries. Inmates were expected to pay society back for the damage they had done and for the cost of their incarceration.

In 1841, Dorothea Dix promoted the establishment of state mental hospitals instead of jails for the placement of the mentally ill. By 1955, the state hospitals reached their peak, and the United States had 559,000 public mental hospital beds for a population of 170,000,000 people. The state hospital paradigm was considered dysfunctional in the 1960s, and deinstitutionalization became the new public policy promoting the establishment of community mental health centers.

By 2001, the number of beds had been reduced to 80,000 and the population increased by 100,000,000 people. Marked reductions in the capacity of the public mental health system to provide inpatient or community treatment to large numbers of mentally ill people brought many of the mentally ill into the criminal justice system. This has been cited as an unintended consequence of good intentions.

The number of incarceration slots in federal, state, and local facilities swelled to about 2,000,000 people. This explains why some researchers refer to the process as transinstitutionalization, from the mental health to the criminal justice system, rather than deinstitutionalization (1).

From the 1970s onward, the combination of deinstitutionalization and the failure to adequately fund community services led to a marked rise in homelessness and other problems for the mentally ill. The mentally ill often turned to alcohol and street drugs in an attempt to self-medicate, survive, and fit in.

The humane treatment of alcohol and other drug disorders was slow in developing. Although a limited patchwork of treatment services did exist for alcohol and other drug disorders by the 1930s, it was not until the 1970s that a national substance treatment system was developed. Before that Alcoholics Anonymous and Narcotics Anonymous were the primary resources for those seeking substance abuse treatment.

Because the criminal justice, mental health, and substance abuse systems evolved separately, their staffs became specialists in only one particular area. Thus the systems were not prepared to address the issues presented by an individual with criminal behavior, mental health symptoms, and substance use. By the late 1970s, the authors of this chapter, along with other clinicians and researchers, began to call attention to the existence of an overlapping population of mentally ill substance abusers who were also involved in the criminal justice system (1).

Few treatment resources existed for this newly identified population until the 1990s, when the term *co-occurring disorders* came into favor. Clinical and research findings indicated that people with co-occurring disorders had improved outcomes when treated by a single treatment team through a process described as integrated treatment. Implementation of the integrated treatment paradigm met financial, jurisdictional, political, training, and stigma obstacles. Slowly and painfully over the past 15 years the substance abuse and the mental health treatment fields have learned to provide integrated treatment and to work effectively with the criminal justice system.

Drug courts were created in response to the awareness that much of the need for the increased capacity of local jails and, to a lesser extent, of state prisons was due to the existence of many people who entered the criminal justice system because of drug abuse. Drug courts have been found to be effective in keeping many such offenders out of jail and prison by enhancing the effectiveness of community correction approaches. Although drug courts are effective in dealing with the offender who has only a drug problem, they are less effective with offenders who also have mental illness.

Prevalence of Co-Occurring Disorders

By the end of the 1980s, it had been well documented that there were significant rates of co-occurring mental health disorders in substance abuse treatment populations. The first study that examined the general population (people who may or may not be in treatment) had the following findings:

1. Twenty-nine percent of people with a mental disorder also had a substance use disorder.
2. Thirty-seven percent of people with an alcohol disorder also had a mental disorder.
3. Fifty-three percent of people with a drug disorder other than alcohol also had a mental disorder (3–6).

The National Co-Morbidity Survey found that 51% of people with a mental disorder also experienced a substance use disorder during their lifetimes, and 41% to 66% of people with a substance use disorder experienced a mental disorder sometime in their lives. Those with alcohol abuse disorder had the lowest level of co-occurrence, and people with drug dependency disorders experienced the greatest (7).

The same study also estimated that about 10 million people are dually disordered. That is, if subjected to diagnostic criteria, they would be found to have at least one mental health and one drug or alcohol diagnosis. Furthermore, in 89% of cases the mental health disorder developed first, at the median age of 11 years. These same people first met the criteria for substance or alcohol abuse somewhere between 17 and 21 years of age. These data support the theory that many of the dually disordered are self-medicating psychiatric distress, making abstinence harder to achieve and to maintain. The further implication is that a focus on emotionally troubled youth might be an effective approach to drug abuse prevention (7).

The National Co-Morbidity Replication Study found that 45% of people with one mental disorder had one or more co-occurring disorders and that the severity of impact of these disorders increased with co-morbidity. Two studies also found that people with co-occurring disorders are much more likely to be in treatment than are people with just one disorder (8–12).

While any of 165 mental health disorders (V codes excluded) identified in the fourth edition, text revision, of the *Diagnostic and Statistical Manual of Mental Disorders* (11) may be present with a substance use disorder, only 22 are found to co-occur frequently with substance use disorders (Table 9.1).

TABLE 9.1. Mental health disorders that occur frequently with substance use disorders.

Mood disorders
Bipolar
Major depression
Dysthymia
Cyclothymia
Personality disorders
Antisocial
Borderline
Histrionic
Eating disorders
Bulimia
Anorexia
Attention deficit and disruptive disorders
Conduct disorder
Oppositional defiant
Attention deficit/hyperactivity
Psychotic disorders
Schizophrenia
Schizoaffective
Anxiety disorders
Panic disorder
Social phobia
Obsessive-compulsive
Posttraumatic stress
Generalized anxiety
Dissociative disorders
Dissociative identity
Depersonalization
Impulse-control disorder
Pathologic gambling

Assessment and Classification

People assigned to a drug court will vary greatly in the following areas:

1. Substance use behaviors.
2. Levels and types of mental health symptoms.
3. Types and reasons for criminal behaviors.
4. Levels of support needed to function independently in the community.

Some people will use only one substance, whereas others will use multiple substances. Some people will have co-occurring mental health disorders, and others will have none. Some people will be significantly impacted by their mental health and substance use symptoms, and others will have minimum impact. Some people will participate in criminal behaviors solely as a result of their substance use or mental health symptoms, whereas others see criminal behavior as a way of life; and some will be able to live independently in the community with minimum supports, whereas others will need significant support services in order to retain their independence. It is essential to use assessment and classification procedures to identify the differences so that appropriate individualized treatment and probation plans can be developed.

It would be expected that a comprehensive substance abuse assessment and classification process is completed on all people assigned to a drug court. However, because significant numbers of drug court clients will also present with mental health symptoms, a comprehensive assessment for those people must also include the following:

1. Identification of their mental health symptoms.
2. Differentiation between true co-occurring disorders and substance-induced psychiatric symptoms.
3. Determination of what effects substance use has on mental health symptoms.
4. Identification of how psychiatric symptoms may promote substance use.
5. Determination of the impact psychiatric and substance use symptoms have on criminal behavior.

Identification of the Mental Health Symptoms

Numerous instruments can be used for identifying psychiatric disorders. However, the purpose of an expanded assessment is to identify the existence of mental health symptoms, not to make a diagnosis. The best way for a substance abuse therapist to identify these symptoms is by observation and report.

Differentiation Between Co-Occurring Disorders and Substance-Induced Psychiatric Symptoms

Substance use can cause psychiatric symptoms. These can range from depression to mania, from anxiety to impulsivity, and from emotional explosiveness to criminal behavior. When psychiatric symptoms are present, it is important to sort out if these symptoms are the result of substance-induced disorders or the result of a co-occurring mental health disorder. Four very useful questions can help with this process:

1. *Did the psychiatric symptoms predate the onset of the substance use?* Although many clients are poor historians, they can still provide valuable information about when the symptoms began, how frequently they occur, and how they affect functioning. Important collateral information can also be obtained from family members and long-time friends.
2. *Is there a history of similar mental disorders in the client's biologic family?* Most mental health disorders have a genetic component and are more common in biologic relatives than in the general population. It is important to find out if other family members have similar symptoms or have been diagnosed with a mental disorder.
3. *Is the onset of the symptoms within the normal age range?* Although there are exceptions, most mental disorders have a normal age range for onset of symptoms. Attempt to find out when the symptoms first began, and then compare that with the normal onset age range.
4. *Is there a significant change in the psychiatric symptoms after 2 or more weeks of abstinence?* Although it normally takes an extended period of time for all the symptoms of a substance-induced disorder to disappear, a significant reduction of symptoms generally occurs within the first few weeks of abstinence. When co-occurring disorders are present, symptoms may actually increase after a period of abstinence because substance use helped to self-medicate some of the symptoms. A good follow-up question is, "Have you ever gone a period of time in the last five years without using and, if so, did your psychiatric symptoms get better or worse?"

Behaviors that result from substance use can also appear to result from a personality disorder. Hence, when these behaviors are present, it is also important to determine if they are substance-induced behaviors or behaviors of an individual with a personality disorder. Three questions can be helpful with this process:

1. *Did the personality behaviors predate the onset of substance use?* Because personality disorders tend to manifest at an early age, one would expect personality disorders normally to appear before the onset of substance use. Most clients with personality disorders will not recognize their behaviors as inappropriate; therefore, this question is best answered by family members or other professionals working with them.

2. *How frequent are these behaviors?* Because people with personality disorders tend to a fixed and rigid view of the world from which their behaviors originate, one would expect behaviors resulting from a personality disorder to be frequent and consistent. Substance-induced behaviors would be expected to be inconsistent and more strongly linked to substance use.

3. *Is there a reported personality change when under the influence of alcohol and other drugs?* A statement such as "he is a nice guy except when he drinks" is common and would indicate a marked personality change resulting from substance use.

None of these questions guarantees diagnostic clarity; only an extended period of abstinence can do that. However, the more questions that can be accurately answered, the greater the likelihood that therapists can make an educated guess about whether they are dealing with substance-induced psychiatric behaviors or a true co-occurring psychiatric disorder. Such an educated guess can help greatly in early treatment planning.

Determination of What Effects Substance Use Has on the Mental Health Symptoms

In almost all cases, any alcohol or drug use increases a person's psychiatric symptoms. However, the exact extent differs greatly among clients. This information may be obtained from the client, but more likely it will be obtained from family members or other professionals who have worked with the client.

It is important that this information be obtained to assess the risk that continued substance use might have for the client and the community. This information will play significantly into treatment planning decisions concerning outpatient, inpatient, or residential treatment settings.

The level of impact can be categorized in three ways:

1. Mild-to-moderate impairment.
2. Major impairment.
3. Severe psychotic decompensation.

Mild-to-Moderate Impairment

Clients experience a mild decrease in cognitive, emotional, or behavior control that may not be readily noticed by either clients or those around them.

Major Impairment

Clients experience a major decrease in cognitive, emotional, or behavioral control that is readily noticeable by clients and those around them. The symptoms of the mental disorder are significantly increased but not to the point where emergency, residential, or hospitalization services are needed.

Serious Psychotic Decompensation

Clients experience a significant decrease in cognitive, emotional, and behavior management to the point that their ability to take care of themselves is greatly diminished. Those around them almost always immediately notice impairment. The intensity of the psychiatric symptoms is such that they require an immediate intervention strategy that may include emergency stabilization in either a residential or a hospital setting.

Identification of How Psychiatric Symptoms May Promote Substance Use

People with mental health disorders often turn to alcohol and other drugs to help them manage their mental disorders. This information can often be obtained directly from the client, although third party report and direct observations can be important sources. It is important to identify the reasons for substance use in order to offer nonsubstance use alternatives to clients.

The most common reasons for substance use among people with mental health disorders are to:

1. Seek symptom relief.
2. Reduce social discomfort.
3. Seek peer acceptance.
4. Prevent self-harm.
5. "Kill" time.
6. Deny the existence of a mental disorder.

Symptom Relief

Often referred to as *self-medication*, the client uses alcohol or other drugs to manage symptoms of a mental disorder. Examples are when people use marijuana to reduce anxiety disorder symptoms or drink alcohol to reduce some of the manic symptoms of bipolar disorder.

Reduction of Social Discomfort

People with mental health disorders such as social phobia often experience discomfort around other people. This may vary from mild anxiety to full-blown paranoia. Using drugs or alcohol may temporarily reduce these symptoms.

Peer Acceptance

Peer acceptance is the use of alcohol or other drugs as a way of establishing contact with or being part of a peer group. Many people with major mental disorders seem odd or strange to others and find themselves isolated, avoided, or ridiculed. However, they may be readily accepted into a drug-using peer group based solely on having drugs to share or the willingness to use them.

Time Management

People with mental disorders such as schizophrenia often find it difficult to join extended social networks, maintain employment, develop and maintain intimate relationships, and retain their interest in even activities of their own choice. As a result, they often have a time void to fill and may turn to using alcohol and other drugs to occupy the time. Finding, obtaining, and managing the altered state and then recovering from the effects of a substance can be very time consuming.

Self-Harm

Many people with mental disorders are unhappy and at times either consciously or unconsciously wish themselves dead. However, for personal or religious reasons, they do not see suicide as an option. The use of alcohol and other drugs can inflict injury or cause danger to self and thus serves as an alternative to suicide.

Seeking to Deny the Existence of a Mental Disorder

For many people, the stigma associated with having a mental disorder is greater than the stigma associated with having a substance use problem. Therefore, alcohol or other drugs may be used to deny the existence of the mental disorder by attributing mental health symptoms to substance use.

Determination of the Impact Psychiatric and Substance Use Symptoms Have on Criminal Behaviors

It is important that clear relationships be identified among substance use, psychiatric symptoms, and criminal behaviors so that appropriate treatment and community protection guidelines can be implemented. Clients being assessed for drug courts can be categorized by their motivation for criminal behavior (1,11). The categories of criminal behavior are the following:

1. Purely criminal acts.
2. Criminal acts caused primarily by substance abuse.
3. Criminal acts caused by mental illness.
4. Criminal acts caused by mental illness and substance abuse.

Purely Criminal Acts

When offenders use alcohol and other drugs to assist them in committing criminal acts to overcome fear or anxiety or when their substance use is part of their involvement in the drug trade, treatment is not indicated.

Criminal Acts Caused Primarily by Substance Abuse

When substance users behave in an emotionally unstable or drug-seeking manner that results in criminal acts, their behaviors may appear to be the result of a mental illness. However, these symptoms dissipate once the substance use is discontinued. Substance abuse treatment would be indicated for these people.

Criminal Acts Caused by Mental Illness

Individuals commit criminal acts as a result of paranoid delusions, hallucination, or other mental health symptoms. Mental health treatment would be indicated for these people.

Criminal Acts Caused by Mental Illness and Substance Use

Criminal behaviors occur because of the interaction of substance use with a mental disorder, and the person's mental health symptoms or substance use alone would not cause criminal behavior. Co-occurring treatment would be indicated for these people.

Developing a Comprehensive Treatment and Probation Plan

Once a comprehensive assessment has been completed, the therapist must decide on the type of treatment that would be most appropriate for the client. This decision is based on three factors:

1. What treatment is needed?
2. What treatment is available?
3. What leverage and influences are available?

What Treatment Is Needed?

The first step is determining the client's functioning level. Some clients are less affected by their mental disorder and have a job, friends, and family and are mostly self-sufficient. Others are much more impacted by their mental disorder and thus have great difficultly maintaining a job or housing, maintaining intimate relationships, or developing a peer network. The clients' levels of functioning help dictate where they should receive their treatment.

Higher functioning clients can be mainstreamed with little difficultly into traditional substance abuse treatment services that are group centered and provide minimal individual and case management services, as long as medication services are available. Lower functioning clients will need more flexible and less demanding treatment services that can also be group centered but will need more individual and case management services. Additionally, emergency services may be called upon.

What Treatment Is Available?

The treatment provider should already have at hand a survey of the treatment options available in the area that are open to drug court clients. A comprehensive list of available resources, payment requirements, entry criteria, and other important pieces of information is critical.

What Leverage and Influences Are Available?

Leverage will be readily available for clients in a drug court system, so the key will be for the treatment component to have available outpatient, residential, medication, and supportive housing treatment options for these clients.

Standardized Treatment Interventions for all Clients with Co-Occurring Disorders

Twelve standardized treatment interventions are discussed that can be used for all people with co-occurring disorders (Table 9.2).

TABLE 9.2. Standardized treatment interventions.

Use leverage to promote treatment
Match treatment demands to what is possible
Set clear treatment goals and expectations early for clients mandated to treatment
Provide information for self-diagnosis
Identify and discuss the positive benefits of substance use and psychiatric symptoms
Connect alcohol and drug use and behaviors resulting from psychiatric symptoms with negative life consequences
Explain the relationship between substance use and psychiatric symptoms
Require clients to be abstinent during treatment sessions
Promote medication compliance
Promote skills needed to achieve treatment goals
Use group treatment as much as possible
Promote self-help involvement

Use Leverage to Promote Treatment

Few people with substance use disorders freely admit to these disorders and still fewer go to treatment willingly. Without experiencing some form of leverage, people with co-occurring disorders would not enter treatment services that address their substance use. Thus it is important that therapists use leverage resources, such as the criminal justice system, family services, and social services, to promote enrollment, attendance, and participation in co-occurring treatment services.

Match Treatment Demands to What Is Possible

Retention in treatment is the strongest variable for long-term treatment success. Thus it is important that clients can be realistically expected to comply with treatment requirements. People with more serious mental disorders will normally not be able to comply with the same treatment requirements as higher functioning people. Making treatment demands realistic allows clients to remain in treatment, thus increasing their chances of learning to effectively manage their co-occurring disorders.

Set Clear Treatment Goals and Expectations Early for Clients Mandated to Treatment

Because treatment is mandated, it is important that what is expected of clients be clearly established at the beginning. These expectations must cover abstinence, length of treatment, attendance, participation, medication compliance, and drug testing requirements, in addition to consequences for noncompliance. When this information is presented to the client at the beginning of treatment, the client has a choice between entering treatment or accepting the alternative. Although consequences for rejecting treatment may be overpowering, clients still have a choice. The ability to choose allows clients to begin to have some sense of power over their lives.

Provide Information for Self-Diagnosis

Most clients entering treatment are still minimizing or denying the existence of their co-occurring disorders. Clients need, therefore, appropriate information and feedback in a variety of formats to help them recognize both the existence and impact of their disorders.

Identify and Discuss the Positive Benefits of Substance Use and Psychiatric Symptoms

It is important to acknowledge what clients already know: that they benefit from their substance use. Alcohol and other drugs often provide some symptom relief to clients with mental health disorders. Psychiatric symptoms can also be helped by the substance abuse. Acknowledging these facts connects with the client's reality and opens a path to more honest discussions about a client's motivations for continued substance use. Of course, this has to be done in conjunction with the next intervention.

Connect Alcohol and Drug Use and Behaviors Resulting From Psychiatric Symptoms with Negative Life Consequences

Although substance use and psychiatric symptoms may have some short-term benefits, they ultimately lead to long-term negative consequences. Pointing out short-term and long-term consequences allows clients to develop a more balanced view of how substances and psychiatric symptoms affect their lives, leading to motivation for behavior change.

Explain the Relationship Between Substance Use and Psychiatric Symptoms

Co-occurring disorders have a reciprocal relationship. It is essential that clients understand how their substance use and psychiatric symptoms interact. Without this knowledge, clients lack understanding of the condition that they must learn to manage.

Require Clients to Be Abstinent During Treatment Sessions

When working with clients who use alcohol and other drugs, it is necessary to refuse scheduled treatment sessions whenever a client is under the influence of these substances. To allow a client to be intoxicated during a session undermines the treatment goal of abstinence, and, because substance use impairs cognitive processes, little of value can be achieved in that therapy session. The purpose of this intervention is not to catch a client using but to set appropriate therapeutic boundaries.

Promote Medication Compliance

Most people with co-occurring disorders will need psychiatric medication at some time during their treatment. Medication compliance promotes psychiatric stability and reduces psychiatric symptoms that increase the desire to use alcohol and other drugs. If clients fail to comply with a medication regimen, the long-term goals of psychiatric stability and abstinence are not likely to be accomplished.

Promote Skills Needed to Achieve Treatment Goals

Few people with co-occurring disorders enter treatment with the skills needed to achieve and maintain abstinence and psychiatric stability. These skills range from refusing drugs to managing such emotions as anger, emptiness, or fear. Often a therapist must initially focus on helping clients develop these building block skills before the longer term goals of abstinence and psychiatric stability can be achieved.

Use Group Treatment as Much as Possible

There are many benefits from the use of group treatment for this population and for the professionals treating them. It is time efficient and cost effective, includes important peer input, allows a client to be in a helping role, promotes social skill development, and helps counter the social isolation experienced by many people with co-occurring disorders. Although some people with co-occurring disorders may initially be too disorganized or paranoid to successfully participate in a group, almost all will eventually be able to participate in groups designed for their specific needs.

Promote Self-Help Involvement

Managing co-occurring disorders is a 24 hours a day, 7 days a week, 365 days a year process. Treatment agencies and families have neither the resources nor the emotional energy to provide all the support that people need for long-term recovery. Self-help programs such as Alcoholics Anonymous and Narcotics Anonymous are designed to provide such support; therefore, it is important that therapists promote client involvement in these programs.

Ten Common Treatment Themes

When treating people with co-occurring disorders, 10 common themes arise during the treatment process. It is important that therapists be aware of these themes and have strategies for addressing them (Table 9.3).

Accepting the Existence of Co-Occurring Disorders

Everyone wants to use alcohol and other drugs without negative consequences, and nobody wants to have a mental disorder. Most clients will enter treatment acknowledging the existence of one disorder and many find acknowledging more than one disorder much more difficult. Therapists must be ready to use psychoeducational and feedback approaches to help clients recognize and accept the presence of all their disorders.

TABLE 9.3. Ten common treatment themes.

Accepting co-occurring disorders
Understanding and accepting the impact of the disorders
Identifying what is normal
Differentiating between medication and substance use
Dealing with negative community and family responses
Dealing with the "victim role"
Dealing with psychiatric symptoms that manifest at self-help meetings
Dealing with relapse and the return of psychiatric symptoms
Dealing with becoming more stable
Dealing with suicidal ideation

Understanding and Accepting the Impact of the Disorders

Acceptance of having a disorder does not necessarily mean understanding and accepting the implications of what having that disorder means. Substance use and mental health disorders place limitations on clients. Part of managing these disorders requires clients to accept these limitations and change some behaviors. Therapists must constantly point out what clients can successfully do but also what behaviors increase the risk of substance use or psychiatric instability.

Identifying What Is Normal

Clients often characterize everything that happens to them as a result of their co-occurring disorders. It is important to help clients differentiate between normal experiences of all human beings and experiences resulting from substance use and mental disorders. Therapists can use feedback from other group members and self-disclosure techniques to promote this differentiation.

Differentiating Between Medication and Substance Use

Clients often misconstrue medication use as just a dependence on another drug. Therapists must help clients differentiate medications that promote stability from alcohol and drug use, which promotes destabilization.

Dealing with Negative Community and Family Responses

Community or family members often view people with co-occurring disorders as willfully bringing on their conditions. They may label them as lazy, unmotivated, or pleasure seekers, which clients often accept as true.

Therapists must help clients understand how their disorders promote such behaviors and refocus clients toward acknowledging the amount of courage and work they must perform to manage their disorders effectively. Such a refocus promotes a positive instead of a negative self-view.

Dealing with the Victim's Role

Clients often see themselves as victims of their disorders and feel that they have lost mastery over their lives. Therapists must help instill hope in the client's worldview. A question that we have found to promote self-efficacy is "How would you have handled such a situation two years ago?" Clients who have been in treatment are almost always more adept at handling life situations. Such a question points out positive change.

Dealing with Psychiatric Symptoms at Self-Help Meetings

Although involvement in self-help groups is critical for long-term abstinence and recovery, people with mental disorders often feel uncomfortable in these groups, making it difficult to fully participate. Therapists must coach clients on how these groups work, how to handle their symptoms when at meetings, what to say and what not to say, and how to handle questions concerning their mental illness and medication usage. Having strategies concerning how to handle certain situations and answers to expected questions ahead of time makes it easier for people with co-occurring disorders to attend these meetings and participate successfully in them.

Dealing with Relapse and the Return of Psychiatric Symptoms

A relapse or the return or intensification of psychiatric symptoms can trigger guilt, thoughts of failure, or a sense that nothing has changed. Therapists must help clients not to focus on returned symptoms but instead to focus on how they can now deal differently with such occurrences.

Dealing with Becoming More Stable

Getting more stable often takes clients into uncharted waters and can create anxiety and fear about their ability to function effectively in that new environment. Therapists must assure clients that they will continue to have their support as they make the transition to stability. Therapists must also point out to clients the strengths they have that will help them make this transition effectively.

Dealing with Suicidal Ideation

The substance-abusing population often struggles with suicidal thoughts, and many will have attempted suicide. Therapists must encourage clients to talk about these thoughts and behaviors, help them manage them effectively, and know when clients are in need of immediate evaluation by local emergency services.

Community Corrections Issues

The task of the drug court team is to protect the community while keeping the client with co-occurring substance abuse and mental health disorders out of jail, out of trouble, and in appropriate integrated or collaborative treatment. Once drug court staff have identified a client and a comprehensive treatment plan has been devised, a member of the drug court team, usually a probation officer or a case manager, will be assigned to arrange for treatment to be provided. Some drug courts will have established a substance abuse treatment clinic within the court's jurisdiction, whereas others will depend on public or private treatment agencies within the community.

The Court Clinic

Drug courts have a substance abuse treatment clinic directly under the court's authority. In this situation, mental health professionals can enhance the staff of the clinic. Ideally, a mental health team, consisting of a part-time psychiatrist or a nurse-practitioner with prescribing privileges, can prescribe and monitor medications. A social worker or other mental health worker trained to maintain cooperation with families can become part of the team. Some clinics may wish to add a psychologist to carry out assessment and evaluation. Any or all members of the mental health component of the clinic team, in partnership with substance abuse counselors, can provide the important group psychoeducation and group therapy components of the treatment program.

Integrated Treatment in the Community

In the ideal situation, community mental health and drug abuse treatment agencies will have already recognized the need for integrated treatment and established a dual diagnosis treatment team. In this situation, the task of the probation officer is relatively simple: make the referral, follow up to ensure compliance, and keep the court informed.

Establishing Collaborative Treatment in the Community

In some communities, referral to community resources is difficult. If separate mental health and substance abuse treatment agencies acknowledge the problematic existence of the dually diagnosed client, but each agency expects the other to provide treatment, the case manager is placed in the role of community organizer and leader.

With the support of and, if necessary, the authority of or participation by the drug court judge, the probation officer may convene meetings with the governmental and nongovernmental agency leaders. On occasion, the use of the court's authority can bring about a new, higher level of cooperation between existing public and private agencies.

Duties of Case Managers or Probation Officers with People Who Have Co-Occurring Disorders

One variable stands out as a predictor of treatment success: *duration of treatment*. Whatever the treatment modality, the longer treatment continues, the better the client outcome is. The effectiveness of a drug court is closely related to the ability of the court to keep the client in treatment, be it in the court's own clinic or in a community agency.

The case manager may be responsible for monitoring the client's attendance and participation in assigned treatment modalities and for checking on abstinence from drug use, usually by periodic or unscheduled urine screens. The case manager carries the authority of the judge and the court as she or he monitors each client. In the case of the dually disordered client, however, the officer can enhance and augment that authority by being perceived as concerned and helpful when, as inevitably happens, the client faces new, unexpected problems. These may involve the usual problems concerning housing, family relationships, money, or employment. The dually disordered client risks relapse to drug or alcohol abuse or psychiatric relapse because of noncompliance with prescribed medications.

An Integrative Model

The Community Client Protection System

The assertive community treatment team (ACT) model has been demonstrated by rigorous research to be an effective approach to maintaining seriously mentally ill substance-abusing clients in the community. First proposed by Leonard Stein and MaryAnn Test in the 1970s as an alternative to the state hospital for mentally ill clients, the ACT model has been modified to treat those with co-occurring disorders, including the homeless. The team usually consists of social workers, substance abuse counselors, case workers, case managers, nurses, and a consulting psychiatrist. A typical team may have between 6 and 10 members and a defined client caseload of high users of addiction, mental health, health, social, and criminal justice services (12).

With the support and encouragement of federal agencies, many communities now have ACT teams providing services on the streets, in the homeless shelters, and in the homes of these high users of services. Some provide alternatives to incarceration, whereas others deal with clients after release from confinement.

In a community served by both a drug court and an ACT team, interaction between them is the norm, and potentials for conflict, cooperation, and integration all exist. The ACT team generally serves clients in a supportive manner, encouraging abstinence from alcohol and drugs and compliance with psychiatric medications, but there is also the potential for coercion; withdrawal of team services may lead to loss of housing and money, because the team may be the representative payee for federal disability financial support.

Relationship Between the Drug Court and the ACT Team

Although the probation officer can never be a full member of the ACT team because the officer is paid by and responsible to the court system, it is possible for him or her to function as a team member. While always a specialist responsible to the drug court judge, the probation officer may be a frequent or regular participant in ACT team meetings and, subject to compliance with confidentiality requirements, may share important information about clients. In this instance, the court's resources augment the resources that the ACT team can offer clients. The sanctions available to the ACT team are markedly augmented by the court's available sanctions. When community treatment resources and the court's resources are fully integrated, the combination is a community client protection system.

A word of caution: Treatment considerations for substance abuse and for mental health conditions may be different and may conflict with each other, even in designing a treatment plan for an individual client. Coercion to stay abstinent and remain in treatment has demonstrated effectiveness in substance abuse treatment when combined with counseling, education, support, and self-help. However, the effects of coercion on the outcome of mental health treatment has not been shown to be as effective and is strongly objected to by many clients, mental health clinicians, and civil liberties groups (13).

Staff Training Needs and Measuring Outcomes

Most substance abuse professionals have developed a philosophy, knowledge base, and skill set that can effectively address substance use disorders. However, many still need to learn more to effectively treat those individuals on their caseload who also have co-occurring mental health disorders. The purpose of this section is to outline those areas of expertise that many substance abuse therapists must add to their treatment toolboxes in order to effectively work with this population and to propose a methodology for measuring treatment outcomes.

Philosophical Approach

Retention in substance abuse treatment is the key variable in predicting long-term, substance use changes. Therefore, a substance abuse therapist must develop a treatment philosophy that promotes treatment retention. The key to treatment retention is matching the treatment plan with what the client can actually do. The therapist must believe that clients bring very different skills and abilities to treatment. Effective treatment requires both flexibility about what is required initially and the understanding that flexibility does not require the therapist to lose sight of the ultimate treatment goal of abstinence. Bringing these viewpoints to the treatment process promotes treatment plans that ensure client success and longer term treatment retention (14–17).

Knowledge Base

There are three areas that most substance abuse therapists must add to their knowledge bases in order to work effectively with people having co-occurring disorders. These are:

1. The ability to identify and treat those mental disorders that cluster frequently with substance use.
2. Knowledge of how these disorders can affect social skills and a client's ability to function independently in the community.
3. Knowledge of the different types of medications used to treat these disorders and what their potential side effects are.

Skill Sets

Five skill sets that most substance abuse therapists need to add to their treatment repertoire include:

1. Providing integrated treatment.
2. Using a competency-based approach.
3. Promoting medication compliance.
4. Helping clients with mental illnesses make use of self-help groups.
5. Modifying clients' approaches to self-disclosure.

The Ability to Provide Integrated Treatment

Integrated treatment is the concurrent treatment of all substance use and mental health disorders; this is the recommended treatment approach for people with co-occurring disorders. This means that the therapist is able to address the specific symptoms of each disorder and the results of their interactions and is able to switch the focus back and forth between the disorders, depending on which symptoms are most problematic at any given time (15).

Competency-Based Approach

Many of the clients have long histories of life failures, so it is important that therapists focus on the clients' competencies and constantly point out their achievements, even when they are minor. Without this infusion of hope, clients cannot see themselves as having the capacity to manage their disorders.

Promotion of Medication Compliance

Most clients will not maintain abstinence if their psychiatric symptoms are not reduced or controlled. Thus, therapists must be able to promote medication compliance that involves helping the clients identify the benefits they receive from the medication, deal effectively with side effects, and learn how to deal with any negative reactions to their use of medication offered by family, friends, or peers at self-help meetings.

Help Clients with Mental Illnesses Make Use of Self-Help Groups

The substance abuse therapist must learn how to help clients who have social phobias, paranoid thoughts, and other mental health symptoms deal with these symptoms while attending self-help meetings. For some clients, attending these meetings will have to be a long-term goal instead of an initial requirement.

Modify Their Approach to Self-Disclosure

Substance abuse therapists, especially if they are themselves recovering, are used to sharing with clients their history of dependency. However, for clients with certain psychotic, anxiety, and personality disorders, too much self-disclosure or even a simple touch on the shoulder can trigger confusion concerning what is intended or really meant. Thus, the substance abuse therapist must learn to be more withholding with such clients.

Measuring Change

It is important that therapists be able to measure the changes their clients are making. There are two models useful for this:

1. The substance abuse treatment scale: This model has eight stages that measure a client's level of participation in treatment and decreases in substance use (18).
2. The five-stage model that we designed for tracking recovery (Table 9.4).

The five-stage model measures changes in behaviors, attitudes, and motivations concerning substance use, mental health, and criminal behavior. Clients are assigned to a stage (see Table 9.4) at the time of intake and again at the time of discharge, thus documenting changes in their substance use, mental health, or criminal behavior status. This model allows therapists to track changes in clients during the normal course of treatment or after

TABLE 9.4. Tracking recovery.

Recovery stage and status		**Substance abuse** status		
Stage	*Status*	*Substance use behavior*	*Attitude about substance use*	*Motivation concerning use*
1	Denial	Using	Does not see use as a problem	Does not desire abstinence
2	Abstinent because of external factor	Abstinent	Does not see use as a problem	Does not desire abstinence
3	Acknowledges substance problem but commitment only to controlling use and limited change	Using	Sees use as a problem	Does not desire abstinence
4	Commitment to total change	Using (may be reduced)	Sees use as a problem	Desires abstinence
5	Commitment to maintaining changes	Abstinent	Sees use as a problem	Desires continued abstinence

Recovery stage and status		**Mental health** status		
Stage	*Status*	*Behaviors to manage mental illness*	*Attitude about mental illness*	*Motivation to manage mental illness*
1	Denial	Takes no actions	Does not accept having a disorder	None
2	Takes management actions because of external factor	Takes only actions that are required	Does not accept having a disorder	None
3	Acknowledges mental illness but limited commitment to managing it	Takes no actions	Accepts having a disorder	None
4	Commitment to manage mental illness	May take some actions	Accepts having a disorder	Is motivated to manage mental illness
5	Commitment to continued management of mental illness	Takes all actions necessary	Accepts having a disorder	Is motivated to manage mental illness

TABLE 9.4. *Continued*

Recovery stage and status		Criminal behavior status		
Stage	*Status*	*Criminal Behavior*	*Attitude about criminal behavior*	*Motivation to discontinue criminal behavior*
1	Denial	Participates in criminal behavior	Does not see criminal behavior as a problem	None
2	Does not participate in criminal behavior because of external factor	Does not participate in criminal behavior	Does not see criminal behavior as a problem	None
3	Acknowledges criminal behavior as a problem but no commitment to change	Participates in criminal behavior	Sees criminal behavior as a problem	None
4	Commitment to discontinuing criminal behavior	Participates in criminal behavior (may be reduced)	Sees criminal behavior as a problem	Is motivated to discontinue criminal behavior
5	Commitment to maintaining a noncriminal lifestyle	Does not participate in criminal behavior	Sees criminal behavior as a problem	Is motivated to discontinue criminal behavior

they have left, on the basis of observable behaviors and verbalizations. Because lifetime treatment for co-occurring disorders usually consists of multiple treatment episodes, we consider any positive changes in any of these stages as a treatment success.

Conclusions

There is consensus among experienced clinicians that clients with co-occurring disorders are more difficult to treat than those with only substance or only mental health disorders. However, the co-occurring disorder client is quite treatable provided that appropriate modifications and additions are made in the treatment process. Therapists providing substance abuse treatment for drug court clients will need to be able to identify co-occurring mental health disorders, modify their treatments according to the clients' levels of functioning, and expand their philosophical approach, knowledge base, and skill sets to provide effective treatment for this population. Doing so will greatly increase success rates.

References

1. Pepper B. Dual Disorders: Substance Abuse and Mental Illness. New York: The Information Exchange, Inc.; 2001.
2. Kuhn T. The structure of scientific revolutions. Chicago: University of Chicago Press; 1962.
3. Powell BJ, Penick EC, Othmer E, Bingham SF, Rice AS. Prevalence of additional psychiatric syndromes among male alcoholics. J Clin Psychiatry 1982; 43:404–407.
4. Ross H, Glaser F, Germanson T. The prevalence of psychiatric disorders in patients with alcohol and other drug problems. Arch Gen Psychiatry 1988; 45:1023–1031.
5. Nace EP. Substance use disorders and personality disorders: comorbidity. Psychiatr Hosp 1989;20:65–69.
6. Regier DA, Farmer ME, Raem DS, Locke BZ, Keith SJ, Judd LL, Goodwin FK. Comorbidity of mental disorders with alcohol and other drug abuse. JAMA 1990;246:2511–2518.
7. Kessler RC, Nelson CB, McGonagle KA, Edlund MJ, Frank RG, Leaf PJ. The epidemiology of co-occurring addictive and mental disorders: implications for prevention and service utilization. Am J Orthopsychiatry 1994;66:17–31.
8. Kessler RC, Chiu WT, Demler O, Merikangas KR, Walters EE. Prevalence, severity and comorbidity of 12-month DSM-IV disorders in the national comorbidity survey replication. Arch Gen Psychiatry 2005;62:617–627.
9. Kelly JF, Finney J, Moos R. Substance abuse disorder patients who are mandated to treatment: characteristics, treatment process, and 1- and 5-year outcomes. J Subst Abuse Treat 2005;28(3):312–323.
10. Onken LS, Blaine J, Genser S, Horton AM, eds. Treatment of Drug-Dependent People With Comorbid Mental Disorders. NIDA Research Monograph 172, NIH Publication No. 97-4172. Rockville, MD: National Institute on Drug Abuse; 1997.
11. American Psychiatric Association. Diagnostic and Statistical Manual of Mental Disorders, 4th ed, text rev. Washington, DC: American Psychiatric Association; 2000.
12. Stein L, Test M. Alternatives to mental hospital treatment. Arch Gen Psychiatry 1980;37:392–397.
13. Substance Abuse and Mental Health Services Administration. Improving Services for People at Risk of, or With, Co-Occurring Substance-Related and Mental Health Disorders. Rockville, MD: Substance Abuse and Mental Health Services Administration; 1998.
14. Simpson DD, Sells SB. Effectiveness of treatment for drug abuse: an overview of the DARO research program. Adv Alcohol Subst Abuse 1982;2: 7–29.
15. Hubbard RL, Marsden ME, Rachal JV, Harwood HJ, Cavanaugh ER, Ginsburg HM. Drug Abuse Treatment: A National Study of Effectiveness. Chapel Hill: University of North Carolina Press; 1989.
16. Hubbard RL, Craddock SG, Flynn PM, Anderson J, Etherridge RM. Overview of 1-year follow-up outcomes in the drug abuse treatment outcome study (DATOS). Psychol Addict Behav 1997;11:261–278.

17. Hendrickson E, Schmal M. Dual Diagnosis Treatment: An 18-Year Perspective. Paper presented at the MISA conference, sponsored by MCP-Hahnemann University. Philadelphia: Hahnemann University; 2000.
18. McHugo GJ, Drake RE, Burton HL, Ackerson TH. A scale for assessing the stage of substance abuse treatment in persons with severe mental illness. J Nerv Ment Dis 1995;183:762–767.

10
Counseling Strategies

Kathy R. Lay and Lucy J. King

The essence of any counseling, regardless of the theoretical approach, is a series of conversations with an empathic counselor who assists a client in developing alternative perceptions of interpersonal interactions in the social environment. These insights provide the client with a new perspective for viewing people and situations and are used to develop alternative behaviors that are more productive and rewarding than previous inadequate or inappropriate coping strategies.

Counseling flows naturally from an initial assessment process that evaluates personal, social, family, medical, and psychiatric history. Assessment is an ongoing process that continues throughout the therapeutic relationship. Information revealed provides insights into issues to be addressed in counseling.

Theories and methodologies, often based on clinical research, have been developed in the fields of psychology, sociology, social psychology, social work, and psychiatry. Principles and practices have been extended from individual therapy to include group therapy, couples therapy, and family therapy. A wide variety of disciplines use these methods, calling their work psychotherapy, psychosocial therapy, case work, or counseling.

Graduate study and opportunities to counsel clients under the supervision of experienced therapists are now required in most fields. Licensure requirements, including examinations, have been established by states and professional organizations. National certifications also offer the alcohol and drug counselor credentials based on education, supervision, and examinations. These professionalize alcohol and drug counseling so that counselors are qualified and service providers have accountability.

To provide the best practice, it is necessary to document and substantiate knowledge and skills. Knowledge must be specific to those practices for which rigorous research has demonstrated efficacy. Skills should include basic counseling competencies, such as the following:

1. Attentive listening.
2. Identifying and connecting perceptions and behaviors in clients' narratives.

3. Recognizing and identifying feelings for the client.
4. Empathically tolerating clients' negative emotions.
5. Providing encouragement.
6. Emphasizing hope for improvement.

This chapter assumes that counselors possess basic skills and focuses on strategies for counseling the substance-dependent client.

Current Trends

Research has shown that treatment for substance abuse and dependence works. More treatment sessions and a longer time in treatment are correlated with more successful treatment outcomes: abstinence, coping with cravings, improved health, and improved functioning in society (1).

Which treatments work best for different clients with substance dependence is not clear (2). Strategically, it is important to understand a variety of approaches and to formulate a treatment plan that addresses a client's needs and motivation for change. Counselors should practice within their areas of expertise and involve appropriate members of the team for other necessary treatments.

Project MATCH (2), a comprehensive and rigorous study funded by the National Institute of Alcohol Abuse and Alcoholism, focused on the efficacy of three treatment modalities:

1. Twelve Step facilitation.
2. Motivational enhancement therapy.
3. Cognitive-behavioral coping skills therapy.

Twelve Step Facilitation

Twelve Step facilitation sessions were designed to educate patients about 12 Step principles and to encourage attendance at meetings. In the sessions, patients recognize that they have alcoholism and cannot control it and that the only effective cure is abstinence. It is understood that the only hope is faith in a higher power as understood by the individual. The importance of the Alcoholics Anonymous (AA) fellowship is emphasized (2).

Motivational Enhancement Therapy

Motivational enhancement therapy incorporates motivational psychology and behavior change and was designed to produce rapid, internally motivated change. The rationale is to motivate a patient to utilize his or her own resources through the stages of change. The patient's personal resources are mobilized in dealing with relationships in his or her own environment (2).

Cognitive-Behavioral Coping Skills Therapy

In cognitive-behavioral therapy in Project MATCH, patients are taught skills such as understanding their own perceptions about alcohol, learning to cope with craving, learning drink refusal skills, handling stressful situations, and avoiding decisions that might lead to relapse of drinking (2).

Summary of MATCH Results

To summarize a multiplicity of results of the study, all three treatments worked with only minor differences. We still do not understand how treatment works, but we have more information about some of the factors. It is clear that more treatment sessions and greater self-efficacy for abstinence predict better outcomes (3–5).

Components of Counseling or Therapy

Twelve step fellowships will not be a focus here because they are discussed in Chapter 12. One strategy for a counselor is referral to AA or other 12 Step programs that use members with stable abstinence as sponsors for newly sober members. The sponsored member studies the 12 steps with a sponsor in a series of informal meetings and attends group meetings with other members. Twelve step sponsorship and psychotherapy are not the same. However, they are complementary and are useful in various combinations for substance-dependent individuals.

Dual Diagnoses

Dual diagnoses (co-occurring disorders) in clients with both substance use disorder and psychiatric illness have been shown to occur frequently in addiction treatment populations. Philosophically, some members of the 12 Step community have been opposed to the use of psychotropic medications. Alcoholics Anonymous encourages use of medications appropriately prescribed by physicians. Fortunately, antidepressants, mood stabilizers, and antipsychotics are not addicting. For those clients dually diagnosed, referral to self-help programs should include education about possible negative perceptions related to psychopharmacologic interventions. "Double trouble" 12 Step groups for dually diagnosed clients are also helpful.

Education of clients should also include clear understanding of their own illnesses and the benefits of appropriately prescribed medications for their quality of life. This will prepare them to respond to negative feedback from an individual who might mean well but does not know or have a full understanding of the dually diagnosed individual.

Working with Involuntary Clients in the Criminal Justice System

Court-ordered clients have been labeled as resistant, hard to reach, hostile, and unmotivated (6). Often the difficulty is not with the client but with approaches that do not take into account where the client is in the change process. We cannot engage a client who is not ready for change in a course of treatment that is designed for an individual who is ready to take action toward a recovery lifestyle. The client who states, "I am only here because the court has ordered it. I'll attend my sessions, and then I am out of here," is clearly not ready to engage in a plan of action (7).

The understanding of change as a process supports strategies that facilitate movement toward recovery in progressive steps. Labeling clients as resistant does not foster empathic engagement and may communicate to the client a confrontational posture that harms not only the therapeutic relationship but also the client's view toward treatment in general. Clients have been coerced into counseling as compensation for what is viewed as poor decision making (8). However, engaging the clients in treatment on their own behalf is the ultimate goal.

In treating nicotine-dependent clients, and later other populations, Prochaska (9) developed an approach that meets a client where he or she is in terms of motivation for changing behavior. "Change is a process that unfolds over time through a series of stages." This perspective, the transtheoretical model of intentional behavioral change, has been applied to substance-dependent offenders (10). An individual might be at any stage when first seen. It is likely that many criminal justice clients are in the early stages.

The Stages of Change

There are six stages of change experienced by people who seek or are ordered into counseling (7).

Precontemplation

The clients do not understand that there is a problem or sees no need to take action to address it. It seems to them better not to think about it. With nonthreatening questions, a counselor helps the clients to see some negative consequences of substance abuse in their lives. Supportive examination of all that is happening leads to understanding consequences such as being in drug court with a potentially very serious outcome such as long-term incarceration.

Contemplation

Clients are now aware not only of the benefits of changing but also of the costs and are ambivalent about change. They intend to take specific actions for change within the next several months. The counselor continues to help them see the benefits of change and the risks of not changing (7).

Preparation

Clients plan to take action within the immediate future and, with the counselor's help, are making specific plans for action. Plans will differ from individual to individual and might involve any combination of any of the treatments discussed in this book (7). This stage is critical to the continuation of change in that without adequate planning it is unlikely that the clients can move toward actions that will ultimately make a difference in long-standing patterns of behavior.

Action

The ultimate goal for substance-dependent clients is abstinence. It might take time and a series of behavioral changes to reach that goal. The counselor remains encouraging and begins to shift from a focus on external motivators (life problems) to support of internal motivators, such as self-efficacy (7).

Maintenance

Clients are clean and sober and much more confident that sobriety can be maintained (self-efficacy). Coping mechanisms to prevent relapse have been developed and are being used. The counselor continues to monitor progress and encourages the clients to assist others in the recovery process (7,8).

Relapse

Relapse is an expected part of recovery in drug courts and might or might not occur at any stage and require return to an earlier stage. Chapter 25 discusses the strong genetic, biologic, and behavioral reasons that make relapse a life-long possibility. These innate factors necessitate progression through stages of change over a period of time in order to learn ways to prevent relapse. Counseling brings about these changes (9,10).

Suggestions for Counselors

The Center for Substance Abuse Treatment (10) provides suggestions for drug court counselors:

1. Show a positive attitude within the limits of honest discussion of the situation.
2. Avoid promises that cannot be kept. If it becomes necessary to break a promise, explain and accept the consequences.

3. Do as you say. Model appropriate attitudes and behaviors that you want participants to implement, including those that participants observe as you interact with colleagues and others.
4. Work to have the clients respect you even if they do not like what you represent.
5. Learn to understand the complex cultural background specific to each individual you counsel. This goes beyond generalities about ethnicity, religion, geographic origin, and the like. Each individual has been influenced by a different, complex combination of many family and social factors.
6. Clearly articulate roles and boundaries. Define your specific role and the limitations. Boundary setting by defining roles is good modeling and establishes credibility. Clients often expect a counselor to be able to solve all problems. Problems are solved only through collaborative counseling processes. Clients who come to counseling via the criminal justice system are likely to have serious problems with the limits set by society. Repeated definitions of the boundaries serve to reinforce roles, expectations, and limitations (10).
7. Be aware that management of clients who demonstrate manipulative behaviors does not require harsh confrontation. Laws provide consequences to reinforce your counseling, and in most situations the court has already specified expectations. The treatment plan should incorporate these expectations.
8. Be firm regarding the consequences associated with a failure to meet requirements such as positive drug tests and missed appointments. A clear and consistent response takes the counselor out of the position of being arbitrary. The client will ultimately benefit from consistency, and the counselor maintains respect of both clients and drug court personnel.

Approaches, Models, and Methods in Addiction Counseling

The Strength-Based Approach

Although treatment in general has tended to focus on problems, in recent years there has been an attempt to emphasize client strengths and how those strengths are utilized in the discovery of solutions. The client may come to the first session clean and sober. The counselor might ask, "What has helped you to remain abstinent?" or "In times past, what has helped you deal with craving without relapsing?" These questions are simply the beginning of building on client strengths.

Rapp (11) has outlined five principles for a strength-based approach to substance dependence:

1. A counselor facilitates identification of abilities and assets so that clients can appreciate and identify their own past efficacy and achieve personal goals.
2. Clients identify their own needs. A counselor assists in clarifying goals, considering alternatives, and identifying resources within the community.
3. The client–counselor relationship becomes important because the counselor is the consistent person who helps the client to navigate all other aspects of treatment and community resources.
4. The community is seen as beneficial rather than as a barrier in terms of needed resources such as housing agencies or training programs. Counselors help clients to learn behaviors to access such resources successfully.
5. When possible, counselors meet with clients in community situations in order to better appreciate clients' challenges. Counselors can model appropriate behaviors for clients in these situations.

A strength-based perspective provides the counselor with a lens through which to view clients, the systems in which they interact, and the community as one with possibility and resources. This in no way negates the challenges clients face, but it does provide a vantage point that facilitates understanding.

Motivational Interviewing

Review of treatment research (12) indicates that:

> Behavioral, cognitive-behavioral, and motivational treatments are among the most well-defined and rigorously studied psychotherapeutic interventions for substance use disorders. These two general approaches and the twelve-step fellowships almost entirely encompass the universe of scientifically validated behavioral therapies for a range of alcohol and drug use disorders and hence should be a component of any substance abuse clinician's repertoire.

Motivational interviewing, designed by Miller and Rollnick (13), uses principles from motivational psychology and patient-centered counseling plus the stages of change model of DiClemente (7) and Prochaska (9). The fundamental approach to motivational interviewing (13) involves the following:

1. Collaboration.
2. Evocation.
3. Autonomy.

Collaboration

A partnership is formed that utilizes the clients' own experience and perspectives as well as their strengths. It is conducive rather than coercive to change (13).

Evocation

Resources for change are presumed to exist within the clients. Their own values and goals are used to develop motivation for change. The counselor believes in the possibility for change and works to bring out that hope in the clients. There is no preaching or lecturing about what needs to be done.

Autonomy

The counselor affirms the clients' right and capacity for self-direction and facilitates informed choice. The participants find the answers while being empathically led to see the discrepancy between present behavior and important personal goals or values (13). Ordinarily, a counselor does not tell the clients what to do (14). Obviously, with drug court participants there are some must-do and must-not-do rules.

Motivational interviewing involves four basic principles (13):

1. Express empathy.
2. Expose discrepancies.
3. Roll with resistance.
4. Support self-efficacy.

Express Empathy

Show concern for the client's situation. For example, recognize and demonstrate that no participant in the criminal justice system enjoys such an experience.

Expose Discrepancies

Gradually develop the clients' realization that their behavior does not match their goals or values. The clients rather than the counselor develop arguments for change.

Roll with Resistance

Do not argue. If an argument begins to develop, try a different approach in what you are saying. Are you really using principles of motivational interviewing, or are you confronting, lecturing, and telling the client how to solve his or her problems?

Support Self-Efficacy

Continue to encourage hope that the clients can change their behavior and that criminal or substance-abuse behaviors can be stopped. It is a difficult, but possible, task that takes time. It is the responsibility of the participants to choose and carry out change. Things do not just happen to them, and everything is not the fault of others. They are in control of their behavior.

Two philosophies have proven important in motivational interviewing:

1. Change talk.
2. Harm reduction.

Change Talk

"Change talk" is an important part of motivational interviewing. A counselor's comments are structured to elicit responses from a client in which the client describes changes to be made. "The process of eliciting and shaping client language in favor of change during therapy sessions has been implicated as a causal mechanism for motivational interviewing" (15).

Moyers and Martin (15) tested this theory by evaluating a random sample of 38 taped MET interviews available from Project MATCH. Trained coders categorized clients' comments as change talk, counter-change talk (reasons not to change), or "other" and whether they followed counselors' motivational interviewing–consistent comments, motivational interviewing–inconsistent comments, or neutral comments.

Motivational interviewing–consistent comments were the most likely to be followed by client change talk. Motivational interviewing–inconsistent comments were the most likely to be followed by client counter-change talk. Thus, using motivational interviewing appropriately led to clients' comments consistent with the idea of their being able to change (15).

Ginsburg and colleagues (16) have addressed special issues in using motivational interviewing in criminal justice populations. Because they are mandated for treatment, "Some clients view a court order as prima facie coercion and an infringement upon their rights and thus steadfastly refuse to consider behavior change." Other offenders might reinforce the idea of refusing treatment recommendations, and offenders themselves might continue to deny that they committed the crime in the first place.

The specific treatments of these clients might also be mandated, giving a client little choice. Counselors might hold to older views that collaborating with offenders is unnecessary. There is always the temptation to tell offenders what they must do in all areas of their lives, above and beyond what the law requires.

With the current use of newer approaches such as drug courts, motivational interviewing is relevant. It is generally brief and inexpensive and can help counselors develop more therapeutic, rather than authoritarian, relationships with clients. Seeking training specific to motivational interviewing is necessary to implement in accordance with protocol.

Harm Reduction

The term *harm reduction* is used in many ways. This chapter considers harm reduction in terms of clients who have difficulty becoming abstinent, the ultimate goal. In this interpretation, drug courts might be considered a method of harm reduction. The harm to be reduced is criminal recidivism. The method is to address problems in all areas of a participant's life in a monitored situation in order to reduce the likelihood that crimes will be committed again. Attendance at drug court lasts only for a prescribed time or until a defined outcome is reached.

Methadone maintenance or use of buprenorphine in the treatment of opiate-dependent clients is harm reduction in that opiates are still being used, but in highly controlled, medically supervised settings. The properties of the medications make use of additional, nonprescribed opiates unlikely. It would be very expensive to get enough heroin to overcome the usual methadone dosage and get high. Using other opiates while taking buprenorphine leads to very unpleasant withdrawal symptoms. Most methadone or buprenorphine clients are able eventually to discontinue the drug with medical supervision.

A client who emphasizes that abstinence will be an impossible goal might be asked to keep a record of use until the next visit. Use examples from the record that emphasize your concern if the client has:

1. Tried to cut down but could not do so (loss of control).
2. Cut down and had unpleasant symptoms (withdrawal).
3. Cut down and felt better (use was causing symptoms).

In other words, any outcome might be used by the counselor to help the client to understand the need for change. Discuss what helped the client to cut down or what made it difficult to do so. Use this information with the client's input to refine the treatment plan, giving encouragement that abstinence is possible.

Another way to view harm reduction is the idea that alcohol-dependent individuals can learn to drink "socially." Vaillant, who has done decades-long studies of alcohol-dependent individuals, addressed this in a thoughtful review of the research literature about "return to asymptomatic drinking." His conclusion: "Stable return to controlled drinking was best predicted by having few severe symptoms of alcohol abuse on admission and not having alcoholic relatives" (17).

In other words, the less severe the illness and the less genetic loading, the more likely an individual with alcohol problems will be able to drink socially. Even then, the majority either relapse or choose abstinence. Those who can drink moderately over time might well have alcohol abuse rather than alcohol dependence.

Vaillant's research confirms the AA principle that only a small percentage of those who are alcohol dependent are ever able to return to social drinking. Abstinence is the safest choice. In addition, those who remain abstinent for 5 years, for whatever reason, are likely to continue in abstinence and thus avoid the consequences of drinking (17).

Cognitive-Behavioral Therapy

Beck and others (18) developed one of the most commonly used effective therapies. It is based on behavioral conditioning models and on Albert Ellis's rational emotive therapy (18), which looks beyond behavior to help clients understand the thoughts and feelings that were associated with particular behaviors. Thoughts, feelings, and behavior are all involved in any response to environmental stimuli. Cognitive-behavioral therapy has been adapted into many approaches to counseling.

As in all other psychotherapies, counseling must be based on thorough assessment of each client and on the development of a positive counselor–client relationship. The Socratic method is used frequently. That is, through a series of questions a client is led to understand his or her distorted patterns of thinking (perceptions) and unproductive behaviors and to develop alternative perceptions and behaviors. Responsibility for behavior belongs to the client (14).

Homework assignments, jointly devised by counselor and client, involve practicing new ways of looking at situations as well as new behavioral responses. Various journals and lists are kept by the clients and discussed in counseling sessions. For example, clients might keep a daily thought record. Problem-solving techniques are devised, and the clients keep records of when these techniques are practiced and the results. Records are then discussed in counseling sessions. Clients learn to schedule their time and to include activities that do not involve addicting substance use and to exclude those associated with craving and use.

One cognitive-behavioral technique involves listing the advantages and disadvantages of particular beliefs and resulting behaviors, such as continuing to use alcohol and drugs. Drug-related beliefs are identified, that is, perceptions such as "I really need to drink" and "It isn't causing any harm."

Ellis used the concept of "catastrophizing," which Beck and colleagues address by a series of questions in the "downward arrow technique." In one example, after each client statement the counselor asked a question such as, What would the implications of that be? What would be the consequences of that? The client's series of catastrophizing statements: If I don't drink, I won't have fun at parties → People won't hang around me → That means they wouldn't like me → My career would suffer → I would lose my home and family → My life would be ruined. At this point the counselor asked, "All this would happen because you weren't drinking alcohol at social events?" and the client answered, "Well, when you put it that way, I guess it's pretty unlikely" (14).

Clients might be taught relaxation techniques and, when relaxed, use imagery to visualize situations in which they exercise self-control or other positive behaviors. In role playing during sessions, the counselor takes the part of someone the client has to deal with and the client practices new ways to respond. In reverse role playing, the counselor takes the role of the client, and the client plays someone in his life.

In a study of male inpatients in a veterans' hospital alcohol and addiction programs (19) those in programs identified as more "purely" cognitive-behaviorally oriented were compared with those in programs identified as more "purely" 12 Step oriented. Programs that used both approaches to treatment were excluded.

Rating scales administered to patients at the end of treatment measured understanding of 12 Step theories (disease concept of alcoholism) and cognitive-behavioral theories (self-efficacy). These were compared with substance use outcomes 1 year later. The goal was to see what perceptions and behaviors present immediately after treatment predicted longer term outcome (19).

Patients from both programs whose later substance use outcomes were good had developed similar perceptions about drinking and similar behaviors to cope with craving and drinking-related behaviors. That is, regardless of program orientation, patients positively rated concepts of both 12 Step and cognitive-behavioral approaches and used coping techniques promoted by each (19).

Continuing care was a predictor of good outcome in both groups. After inpatient treatment, patients had outpatient visits at Veterans Administration mental health clinics or were involved in 12 Step work. These findings are consistent with Project MATCH results described earlier (19).

Beck and colleagues (14) discuss problems with cognitive-behavioral therapy in clients who have antisocial traits. They are, of course, common in criminal justice populations. They rarely come into treatment unless forced to do so. In their own view, these clients have no problems; rather, their problems are all the fault of others. Any counselor is seen as part of an oppressive system.

Such clients try to seize control of the counseling situation. The authors give an example of a client who complained about having to see a "shrink." The counselor replied that he understood because he was not there by choice either. He had been assigned to see this client, adding, "So, since we seem to be stuck with each other, how are we going to make this a tolerable experience for both of us?" A counselor in this situation is "energetic, innovative, and just a little bit confrontational" (14).

The client who is antisocial will win a few arguments. That is all right. The counselor should not focus on always being one up but rather on keeping the client interested in therapy. An example is a patient who was complaining that his buddies denigrated his manhood if he did not drink heavily. After the counselor's comments on what to say, the client replied, "That s–t might work in your neighborhood, but not in mine." The counselor replied, "Yeah, you're right. I'd probably get my ass kicked if I said that" (14). Then the counselor asked the client to suggest responses to his buddies that might work.

Because clients with multiple antisocial behaviors are more likely than other substance-dependent clients to keep using addicting substances during treatment, counselors must make an effort to catch their lying about use. Beck and colleagues (14) suggest that this can best be done if a counselor keeps extensive notes.

A client's comments at different sessions can be compared and the client confronted with discrepancies in his explanations. For example, "You missed that appointment last month because your wife was sick and you had to take her to the emergency room? My notes suggest that at our last session you said it was because you had to attend your grandmother's funeral. How does that work?" A detailed record can be used as well as urine screens and other specific demonstrations of a client's prevarication.

"Antisocial patients are not altruists" (14). Motivation for this client comes not from satisfaction in doing the right thing but from seeing that it is in his best interest to do a certain thing. For example, a client might eventually come to understand that heavy addicting substance use was connected to getting arrested. Abstinence would help to avoid the oppressive (in his eyes) legal system. The listing of advantages and disadvantages is a helpful technique in developing this perspective.

Homework is valuable, but teaching clients with an antisocial perspective ("others are at fault, not me") can be a long, slow process. For example, one client read in a newspaper that the drug court had received a monetary grant from the state. He accused the counselor of keeping him in treatment just to make money. The counselor noted calmly that her salary remained the same with or without the state grant.

Participants in Counseling

All of the methods and theories discussed in this chapter can be applied to:

1. Individual therapy.
2. Couples therapy.
3. Group therapy.
4. Family therapy.

Although counseling individuals, couples, clients in groups, and families are all important in treating substance dependence and can be employed by counselors at any level of training, extensive psychotherapy in any of these modalities, especially with dually diagnosed patients, requires professional training in the particular treatment.

Individual Counseling

Guidelines for working with individuals include the following (20):

1. Recovering clients usually require structure. Counseling is best when used in a structured program that provides other methods and services.
2. Clear goals are formulated and discussed early in treatment. The client knows that all members of the team are aware of his or performance in all aspects of the program and that the team works together as a unit.
3. Substance dependence is often chronic and relapsing. Compliment the client on improvements. Do not expect a magic cure.
4. Consider appropriate referral for pharmacotherapy. Be aware of any pharmacotherapy and work with the client to encourage contact with the prescribing physician if side effects occur or expected therapeutic effects do not occur.
5. Be familiar with the medications used and testing results so that you can explain them to clients. If you are unsure about something in these areas, check with appropriate drug court team members, "Let me ask Dr. ______ about that and get back to you at our next meeting."
6. Be familiar with the pharmacology of abused drugs, the subculture of addiction, and self-help programs.
7. Acknowledge the importance of urine drug testing and alcohol breath testing with prompt feedback to the patient.

Using urine screens and breathalyzer testing does not mean that a counselor is undermining the therapeutic relationship with a client. Evidence of use and resultant consequences can be presented in a matter-of-fact manner. This also means that if a client catches a counselor in a mistaken statement, the counselor acknowledges it without defensiveness or excuses. If tests are negative, a client can be complimented and the strengths used in achieving abstinence discussed. A counselor should understand urine tests and when there might be false-positive results.

Group Counseling

Some groups include all new clients as they enter the program. Closed groups include only the same patients, and a new group is started when enough new patients enter the program. In any group, group contracts or specific rules for participation are set up to ensure respect for other group members and prompt attendance.

Groups may have any number of clients but seem best when small numbers participate, such as 6 to 12. A group might include clients of any demographic background or be homogenous, restricting membership to men, women, alcoholics, drug abusers, adolescents, adults, or any other category to achieve specific purposes. A group might continue for a specified number of sessions or be open ended, with clients entering or leaving depending on their individual needs.

All group approaches share an appreciation of the healing power of connection with others. Clients with substance dependence benefit from participation in a group because of their frequent difficulty maintaining good relationships (21). Pregroup preparation might well involve motivational techniques to encourage a client to attend a particular group. Cognitive-behavioral methods might be used in the group. Understanding of addiction expressed by other members often influences a client.

The task of a counselor who leads, or facilitates, a group is to guide group members in verbalizing their own perceptions and in discussing among themselves appropriate behaviors to maintain abstinence or deal with relationships. Group counselors need to avoid being put into the role of referee to determine which group member is "correct." The group facilitates group members discussion of the pros and cons of a particular viewpoint. Often, comments by other group members have greater effect on a client than comments or guidance from the counselor.

Family Counseling

Substance dependence is a family disease. The behaviors of intoxicated individuals inevitably affect everyone in their environments, most especially those closest to them. Family therapy, if at all possible, is imperative for adolescents or young adults living at home. Family counseling not infrequently uncovers substance dependence in members other than the client. Techniques similar to those described here are used to help that family member through the stages of change.

Recovery, itself, might affect family interactions when the family system has been altered to deal with an intoxicated family member. For example, a wife who has learned particular ways to cope with a husband who drinks heavily might feel abandoned when he begins to attend a lot of counseling and 12 Step meetings. Family counseling and groups such as Al-Anon can be helpful.

Inclusion of family members during assessment of a client clarifies the clinical picture. Early involvement of the family increases engagement and participation of a client in the program, and family participation not only improves the client's substance use outcome but leads to increased marital satisfaction and family stability (22).

Cognitive-behavioral family counseling involves clear, easily learned steps. Families learn how some family behaviors maintain addiction and how specific reinforcement techniques can diminish substance use and improve coping skills. The family becomes involved in planning ways to help a client maintain abstinence (23). The entire family learns alternative perceptions of addiction and alternative behaviors to reinforce abstinence.

Therapies and so-called psychoeducation theories that label family members or pathologize behaviors have not proven to be effective and can serve to alienate family members from professionals and the treatment community. Most behavior of family members has been an effort to survive difficult circumstances and should be acknowledged as such. Family can be a source of support for the client who exhibits motivation toward recovery, and the counselor is in the position to facilitate this process. Discussion of the process of family interactions, rather than the content (who-said-what) is the key to positive reinforcement of the substance-dependent client and family. The client may be ready to take on roles in the family that have not been fulfilled in times past because of the disease process; however, family members may be quite reluctant to accept new roles. This is to be expected. Listening to the family's narrative, providing support, and encouraging patience are key to restoration of hope.

Couples Therapy

The same theories and techniques used in group or family therapies can be used with spouses or partners. In complicated situations, clients and spouses or partners might be seen separately in individual therapy until their interactions become less tense. Then they can be seen as a couple or in a small group of three or four couples.

Conclusions

In summary, the same counseling strategies that research has proven valuable in other counseling situations can and should be used in drug court settings. Although there are limitations imposed by the law, counselors can be empathetic, work with clients to help each find what treatment modalities are best, encourage motivation for change, and reinforce the reality that there is hope for behavioral changes that will be to a client's advantage.

References

1. McLellan AT, McKay JR. Components of successful treatment. In Graham AW, Schultz TK, Mayo-Smith MF, et al., eds. Principles of Addiction Medicine, 3rd ed. Chevy Chase, MD: American Society of Addiction Medicine; 2003:327–343.
2. Project MATCH Research Group. Project MATCH: rationale and methods for a multisite clinical trial matching patients to alcoholism treatment. Alcohol Clin Exp Res 1993;17:1130–1145.
3. Ilgen M, Moos R. Deterioration following alcohol-use disorder treatment in Project MATCH. J Stud Alcohol 2005;66:517–525.
4. Project MATCH Research Group. Matching alcoholism treatments to client heterogeneity: Project MATCH posttreatment drinking outcomes. J Stud Alcohol 1997;58:7–29.
5. Bogenschutz MP, Tonigan JS, Miller WR. Examining the effects of alcohol typology and AA attendance of self-efficacy as a mechanism of change. J Stud Alcohol 2006;67:562–567.

6. O'Hare T. Court-ordered versus voluntary clients: problem differences and readiness for change. Social Work 1996;41(4):417–422.
7. DiClemente CC. Addiction and Change: How Addictions Develop and Addicted People Recover. New York, NY: Guilford Press; 2003.
8. Institute of Medicine, Committee on Crossing the Quality Chasm. Adaptation to Mental Health and Addictive Disorders. Improving the Quality of Health Care for Mental and Substance-Use Conditions. Washington, DC: Institute of Medicine; 2006.
9. Prochaska JO. Enhancing motivation to change. In Graham AW, Schultz TK, Mayo-Smith MF, et al., eds. Principles of Addiction Medicine, 3rd ed. Chevy Chase, MD: American Society of Addiction Medicine; 2003:825–837.
10. Center for Substance Abuse Treatment. Substance Abuse Treatment for Adults in the Criminal Justice System. Treatment Improvement Protocol (TIP) Series 44. DHHS Publication No. (SMA) 05-40Rockville, MD: Substance Abuse and Mental Health Services Administration; 2005.
11. Rapp RC. Strengths-based case management: enhancing treatment for persons with substance abuse problems. In Saleebey D, ed. The Strengths Perspective in Social Work Practice, 3rd ed. Boston, MA: Allyn and Bacon; 2002:128–147.
12. Carroll KM, Ball SA, Martino S. Cognitive, behavioral, and motivational therapies. In Galanter M, Kleber HD. Textbook of Substance Abuse Treatment, 3rd ed. Washington, DC: American Psychiatric Publishing; 2004:365–376.
13. Miller WR, Rollnick S. Motivational Interviewing: Preparing People for Change, 2nd ed. New York: Guilford Press; 2002.
14. Beck AT, Wright AD, Newman CF, Liese BS. Cognitive Therapy of Substance Abuse. New York, NY: Guilford Press; 1993.
15. Moyers TB, Martin T. Therapist influence on client language during motivational interviewing sessions. J Subst Abuse Treat 2006;30:245–251.
16. Ginsburg JID, Mann RE, Rogers F, Weekes JR. Motivational interviewing with criminal justice populations. In Miller WR, Rollnick S, eds. Motivational Interviewing: Preparing People for Change, 2nd ed. New York: Guilford Press; 2002:343–352.
17. Vaillant GE. The Natural History of Alcoholism Revisited. Cambridge, MA: Harvard University Press; 1995.
18. Ellis A. Reason and Emotion in Psychotherapy. New York: Lyle Stuart; 1962.
19. Johnson JE, Finney JW, Moos RH. End-of-treatment outcomes in cognitive-behavioral treatment and 12-step substance use treatment programs: do they differ and do they predict 1-year outcomes? J Subst Abuse Treat 2006;31:41–50.
20. Mercer D, Woody GE, Luborsky L. Individual psychotherapy. In Galanter M, Kleber HD. Textbook of Substance Abuse Treatment, 3rd ed. Washington, DC: American Psychiatric Publishing; 2004:343–352.
21. Khantzian EJ, Golden-Schulman SJ, McAuliffe WE. Group therapy. In Galanter M, Kleber HD, eds. Textbook of Substance Abuse Treatment, 3rd ed. Washington, DC: American Psychiatric Publishing; 2004:367–378.
22. Steinglass P, Kutch S. Family therapy: alcohol. In Galanter M, Kleber HD, eds. Textbook of Substance Abuse Treatment, 3rd ed. Washington, DC: American Psychiatric Publishing; 2004:379–388.
23. Kaufman E, Brook DW. Family therapy: other drugs. In Galanter M, Kleber HD, eds. Textbook of Substance Abuse Treatment, 3rd ed. Washington, DC: American Psychiatric Publishing; 2004:389–402.

11 Client Life Skills Training

Jerri E. Thompson, Rick A. Thompson, and James E. Lessenger

Client life skills training is an integral part of the drug court process and is typically part of the probation agreement that clients must sign. Client life training is generally provided by groups and classes designed to extinguish drug-using behaviors and reinforce behaviors consistent with a non–drug-using culture. The skills taught to the clients are designed to prepare them for a sober, noncriminal life. Client life training teaches life, family, and occupational skills and helps the client stay off drugs.

Client life training strategies include educational programs, employment assistance, dress and behavior training, and family life training. Some clients may already have degrees and jobs, but many clients have never been taught how to act, dress, and behave on a job, in school, or within a family.

Looking at the drug court client population, five types can be identified. By identifying these client types, counselors can tailor a program to better meet clients' needs (1):

1. Clear sailors: Clients are compliant throughout their tenure in the program.
2. Late bloomers: Clients initially have some episodes of noncompliant behavior but later demonstrate compliance, except for perhaps a brief period during the last several months of participation.
3. Occasional stumblers: Clients are mostly compliant but exhibit a period of noncompliance in the middle or end of their tenure in the program.
4. Chronic stumblers: Clients are noncompliant at times throughout their period of participation but are nevertheless sufficiently compliant to graduate.
5. Noncompliant: Clients repeatedly fail to meet the requirements of the probation agreement, miss counseling sessions, and fail drug tests. These people most often are terminated from the program and sent to jail or prison.

Case Management

In a drug court, the key to a successful outcome, measured as decreased criminal and drug recidivism, is the case management concept. Often the case manager will also be the counselor responsible for the client. The initial task of the case manager is to eliminate initial barriers to sobriety and rehabilitation, such as:

1. Lack of transportation.
2. Lack of child care.
3. Lack of a clean and sober support environment.
4. Mental and general health needs.
5. Denial of drug or alcohol addictions.

Case managers work best within the treatment structure. They typically have experience in drug addiction and may be former addicts themselves. They may also have degrees in counseling, social work, or psychology. The case manager is responsible for:

1. Performing psychosocial evaluations to assess needs.
2. Obtaining releases of information from inpatient or other treatment programs to provide seamless care.
3. Creating customized treatment plans.
4. Coordinating individual and group therapy.
5. Recommending and, in some cases, arranging for psychiatric or medical evaluations and treatment.
6. Providing client life skills training.
7. Listening to the clients' complaints and problems and guiding them through solutions.
8. Organizing counseling.
9. Reporting to the courts on the client's behavior, attendance, cooperation, and accomplishment in the programs.

Role Models

Counselors, case managers, educators, and office staff must remember that they are role models for clients. Appropriate dress, hygiene, speech, and behavior are as important for the counseling and educational staff as for the clients. Furthermore, each counselor needs to understand the behavior necessary in the courtroom and the respect due to court officers.

Overloading the Client (Piling on)

Many drug court clients have legal cases with family courts that require counseling and child care classes, drunk driving or driving under the influence cases that require counseling, or other court cases requiring classes or counseling. It is easy to overload the client with too much work, especially if the counseling or education is redundant and the clients struggling with sobriety are also trying to work. Coordination of court-ordered programs is essential.

Client Life Skills Training Components

Components of the client life skills training include housing and transportation, education, employment, dress and behavior, family life, and perinatal programs (Table 11.1).

Housing and Transportation

The basic level of any program is to make sure the client has a place to stay and a means of getting to court, counseling, and employment. In choosing a place to stay, the client, with the assistance of the counselor, needs to remain separated from friends and family who may reinforce the client's drug use and culture.

Education

Educational level was found to be a significant predictor of successful graduation from Florida's Broward County Dedicated Drug Treatment

TABLE 11.1. Client life training strategies.

Type of program	Subprograms
Housing and transportation	Referrals to appropriate programs
	Bus passes and other transportation aids
Education	High school diploma
	GED equivalent
	Trade and technical training
	Education about the disease
Employment	Job placement
	Curriculum vitae preparation
	Appropriate dress and behavior
	Interview training
Dress and behavior ("charm school")	Dress, speech, behavior
Family life	Child rearing
	Family relationships and changing roles
	Blended families
Perinatal programs	Nutrition
	Self-image enhancement
	Exercise programs
	Self-help programs

Court. (2) Most drug courts have some type of education requirement, typically the completion of high school or the equivalent. If a client is in a full-time educational or vocational program, the best practice is to waive the employment requirement until the educational requirements are completed. Education is the key to employment, and employment is the key to preventing recidivism. Education can take the form of:

1. High school.
2. High school completion courses.
3. General education development (GED) equivalent courses.
4. Vocational education.
5. Degree programs (3).

The process begins with an assessment, followed by advice to the client on where and how to register. Most counselors will argue that it is better to let clients go through the registration process on their own. Accomplishing this task requires that the counselor knows the educational facilities available in the area, the costs, the courses offered, and the entrance requirements (Table 11.2).

Accountability is important. The counselor can either obtain a release to obtain the records directly from the educational institution, or the client can provide monthly reports or attendance cards.

It is also important to educate clients about their disease. Classes provided by the counseling organization include the following:

1. The disease concept of addiction.
2. Relapse prevention.
3. Self-esteem, guilt, and shame.
4. Information on the physical and mental consequences of drug abuse.

Skills important to relapse prevention include refusal skills, identification of relapse signs prior to use, the process of identifying and expressing feelings, and facing up to fears.

Employment

Many drug court probation agreements require that the client obtain a job. Exceptions may occur when the client has a documented disability. The drug court schedule of regular court appearances, weekly group counseling, Alcoholics Anonymous or Narcotics Anonymous meetings, and random drug screening conflicts with 9 am to 5 pm work schedules. Therefore, it may be necessary for the client to obtain a job with an evening or flexible work schedule or an employer who understands the drug court process and is willing to allow the participant to work on a schedule that will mesh with court activities. Requirements that the client obtain stable employment should allow seasonal or part-time jobs but encourage permanent, full-time employment.

TABLE 11.2. Educational advice for clients.

Preparation
1. Get the education and experience needed to succeed in your chosen field.
2. Research prospective employers.
3. Tailor your resume to each job opening.
4. Memorize details for your resume.
5. Rehearse your interview; anticipate what you will be asked.

Focus
1. Analyze your interests and skills. Match them to your job search.
2. Set realistic goals.
3. Develop a specific course of action and a job search timeline.
4. Do not let distractions sidetrack your search.

Exploration
1. Utilize community resources such as libraries, employment agencies, career centers, and job fairs.
2. Take advantage of the Internet to post resumes and search for job openings.
3. Conduct informational interviews to learn more about particular occupations.
4. Remember, most jobs are never advertised. Be proactive in finding out about unadvertised openings.

Networking
1. Tell everyone you know about your job search.
2. Seek advice and ask for leads from people in your field of interest.
3. Attend trade shows, seminars, and workshops relating to your line of work.
4. Use online newsgroups, chat rooms, and forums to make contacts and develop leads.

Attitude
1. Convey enthusiasm through body language, speech, and your cover letter.
2. Show professionalism in your appearance and in the presentation of your resume.
3. Do not let self-doubt defeat you. Believe that you *can* and *will* get the job.
4. Stress positive aspects of your qualifications and of previous jobs. Avoid negatives.

Persistence
1. Treat your search as a full-time job.
2. Follow up cover letters with phone calls and interviews with thank-you notes.
3. Constantly strive to improve your job search materials and to hone interviewing skills.
4. Do not let rejection dampen your resolve. Keep trying.

Employment of drug court clients and the pretreatment employment of clients have been associated with a positive outcome in drug courts (4,5). For clients, regular employment provides the following benefits (6):

1. Enhances self esteem.
2. Provides a stable source of income (especially if the client is paying for the drug court services).
3. Offers an environment removed from a substance-using subculture.
4. Decreases substance use and criminal activity (especially high-quality jobs).
5. Keeps the client occupied and on a regular schedule.

6. Prevents needless physical and mental disability by keeping the client employed and taking advantage of the healthy worker effect (i.e., people who are at work are healthier).

Barriers that must be overcome when obtaining a job for drug court clients include the following (7):

1. The client's criminal record, including felony convictions.
2. Inadequate education.
3. Lack of work experience.
4. Lack of public transportation (many clients either cannot afford their own car or have had their driver's licenses revoked).
5. Limited or no child care.
6. Tattoos, body piercing, branding, or scarification that may evoke repugnance in the potential employer.
7. Inappropriate dress, behavior, or speech (especially profanities).

Preparing the Client for the Job Market

Drug court clients relate that there are many jobs out there if only they had the skills and training to do them (Table 11.3). The process of preparing the client for the job market includes the following:

1. Identifying the type of work the client is physically, mentally, and emotionally capable of performing.
2. Identifying the skills and experience the client already possesses (this can be accomplished through the completion of a skills assessment inventory; several are available commercially).
3. Providing vocational training.
4. Teaching and reinforcing specific skills of punctuality, dress, speech, and behavior.

For women, classes teach proper makeup, hair care, posture, and deportment. Many retail establishments will donate makeup, accessories, and clothing, especially after Christmas; these can be provided to clients. It is important to help the client select an appropriate outfit for interviews and for the job. Women are briefed that in many, if not all, job locations, heavy fragrances are inappropriate and discouraged.

Men also need help in creating a job-appropriate appearance, including appropriate shoes, clothing, and deodorants. The male use of fragrances at the workplace is discussed as are little things like proper care for shoes and boots when coming in from fields or shops.

Job-Seeking Skills

Most clients already have a lot of experience in looking for jobs. Fewer have experience in obtaining and keeping them. Training and assistance in job-seeking skills include the following:

TABLE 11.3. Job search and life skills workshops.

Number	Subject	Content
1	Orientation	Grooming, hygiene, speech Dress for job interviews
2	Setting vocational and educational goals	Short and long term
3	Assessment of personal skills	Create a personal employment record Create job descriptions of past employment Review applications
4	Job search techniques	Review and assess employment short-term goals Apply goals to job search Review employment classified advertisements Perform Internet job search Access community resources Incorporate short-term goals with long-term goals
5	Resume writing	Create and review resumes
6	Interviewing techniques	Mock interviews Job search assignments
7	Review and discuss results of job search	Mock interviews Job search assignments
8	Review and discuss results of job search	Mock interviews Job search assignments
9	Personal budgeting	Goals Savings accounts Checking accounts Household planning Credit cards
10	Apartment and other rental applications	
11	Resolving past budget disasters and legal responsibilities	Planning debt payment Clearing bad debt

1. Finding jobs through newspapers, public and private employment services, and resource centers (finding jobs through family contacts and word of mouth may be a problem if the client is trying to escape friends or family who reinforce substance abuse).
2. Locating employers who do not mind that the client is in drug court or may have a criminal record (some employers *prefer* drug court clients because their behavior is managed by the courts and they are tested frequently).
3. Assistance in filling out employment applications.
4. Assistance in writing cover letters.
5. Preparation of resumes.
6. Job interview training, especially in how to deal with tough questions about the client's past or employment gaps that may be difficult to explain because the client was in jail or prison.
7. Completing skills assessment instruments.

Retaining a Job

The client needs to have the job meet certain requirements in order to remain employed. These factors include the following:

1. A stable income.
2. Health insurance benefits for children.
3. An employer who understands the drug court schedule and makes allowances for demands.
4. Enjoyment and challenge in the job.
5. Enjoyment in being kept busy and receiving recognition.

Keeping a job is different for drug court clients than for the regular workforce for the following reasons:

1. Employment is monitored through employer contacts and payment receipts.
2. When clients leave a job, a new job must be prearranged and approved by the counselor.
3. If a client leaves a job, he or she can temporarily meet the employment requirement through community service, thus keeping busy and accountable to the program.

Appropriate Dress and Behavior (Charm School)

If the goal of drug court is to reintegrate clients into the non–drug-using community and to decrease recidivism, many of the clients will have to be taught how to act, talk, and dress in a manner that does not identify them with the drug-using community. Service groups can be especially helpful in programs that:

1. Teach proper dress for the workplace.
2. Help to purchase clothing that does not identify the client with gangs or the drug culture.
3. Help to purchase protective clothing or uniforms.
4. Teach table manners.
5. Teach etiquette, particularly for men in dealing with women.

The basic role of the counselor is to set limits on the client's behavior within and outside the treatment venue, condemn inappropriate behavior, and serve as a role model for appropriate dress and behavior.

Proper etiquette is extremely important. It is important to teach men how to act appropriately with a woman on a date, in the home, and in the workplace. They learn how to speak appropriately, how to avoid profanity, and how to act, such as when to hold the door open for a woman and allow her to enter a room first. Instruction for men in how to appropriately act with a female supervisor is especially important.

For women, proper etiquette training requires instruction in how to walk and sit appropriately, speak appropriately, and maintain appropriate body language. Appropriate interactions with male supervisors and coworkers is important, but equally important is the proper interactions with female coworkers on the job.

Education also includes teaching appropriate courtroom behavior. Early in the drug court process, counselors instruct clients on the proper dress and behavior in court. Instruction includes the following:

1. The proper way to address the judge and court officers.
2. Proper interaction with law enforcement.
3. Appropriate professional interaction with attorneys.
4. Appropriate, clean, and modest dress.

Family Life

About 75% of drug court participants have children (1). Along with employment, family ties strengthen the clients' identification with and participation in the community (4). The types of programs offered to clients, depending on their needs, include the following:

1. Child care.
2. Parenting classes for fathers and mothers.
3. Batterer's school for men who have been physically or emotionally abusive to their wives or girlfriends.

In designing and implementing these programs, it is important to involve the spouse or significant other of the client and sometimes the children as well. If only one member of the family is involved in rehabilitation classes, there is growth in that person that can upset the status quo of the relationship.

Families in drug addiction often drift into a pattern where one member may be using drugs while the other maintains the family cohesiveness. As the one member gets into the program, obtains counseling, and learns vocational and social skills, the roles within the family become unraveled with the other family members feeling surpassed. For that reason, it is important that the whole family be drawn into the program and receive education and treatment as a unit. Blended families in particular need assistance in maintaining family relationships, especially as former husbands and wives regain sobriety and try to reenter the unit.

Women in Drug Court

Many women in drug court have led lives similar to prisoners-of-war. Many have been beaten, tortured, raped, sold into prostitution, and abused mentally. Some have seen their children abused. Others have had children taken away from them by the courts. A large number of these women are the victims of incest and have sold their bodies to support their habits.

Many, if not all, of the women in drug court suffer from a posttraumatic stress disorder not unlike a soldier who has survived combat and for which they have medicated themselves with drugs. These women benefit from parallel counseling sessions, one with a woman and another with a man. The female counselor can discuss intimate sexual issues, while the male counselor can serve as a role model to reestablish trust and allow women to express their feelings about the abuse they have endured.

Perinatal Programs

The health problems of the pregnant and addicted offender are complicated; many of these women need intensive and specialized assistance to ensure a healthy childbirth. Programs include nutrition counseling, referrals to meals programs, self-image enhancement programs, prenatal and postnatal exercise programs to strengthen the core body functions, and enrollment in self-help programs whereby the mothers can work with other women who are facing or have faced similar problems and challenges. It may be necessary to teach the new mothers the simplest of things, such as how to clean and care for a baby, how to feed a baby, and how to hold and sing a lullaby to a baby.

Program Examples

Drug courts provide client life training in various forms depending on the demands of the probation agreement and the courts and their resources of time, money, and personnel. Three examples are given below.

Tulare County, California

The probation officer assigns on a rotating basis a private drug treatment program that is close to where the client lives. That program provides case management, counseling, educational, and other services to the client and reports back to the court on the client's progress (Table 11.4). A separate company is responsible for all urine drug screens and reports the results to counselors, who then report them to the court. The drug collection and testing company has on its staff a certified physician medical review officer to assist in evaluation, if necessary.

Riverside County, California

The day treatment program called the Recovery Opportunity Center (ROC) is a unique feature of the program. The ROC counselors, mental health professionals, educators, and social workers see participants 5 days a week for the first 6 months of their drug court experience. Screening for the program is done by ROC program staff in concert with court personnel (5).

TABLE 11.4. Sample drug court life skills training protocol.

I. Screening
II. Intake
  A. Release of information, HIPPA, etc.
  B. Basic registration information
III. Assessment (face-to-face with case manager)
  A. Chemical dependency assessment
  B. Psychosocial assessment completed to determine suitability for outpatient treatment
  C. Treatment compliance issues: ability to stay clean, test results, 12 Step involvement, and ability to function in society
  D. Physical needs: prenatal, medical, dental
IV. Treatment planning
  A. First plan: completed within 30 days of admission
    1. Information that has been obtained in the assessment is included in the first treatment plan
    2. Short and term goals will be consistent with legal issues that need to be resolved
    3. The primary focus is on treatment and building a new support system
    4. The client should be consulted in the development of the treatment plan so he or she takes ownership of the treatment goals
    5. The counselor identifies deficiencies in the client's behavior and attitudes
    6. Client life training programs are initiated, with an emphasis on hygiene
    7. Refer the client to Narcotics Anonymous or Alcoholics Anonymous
    8. Make sure the client understands the discipline of the program:
      a. Keeping appointments
      b. Being punctual
      c. Maintaining appropriate behavior and dress
      d. Paying for services
  B. Second treatment plan: completed 90 days from initial plan and every 90 days thereafter
    1. Goals that were not reached in the first plan are carried over to the next, and new issues that have surfaced are included.
    2. When going over the new treatment plan, it is also important to look at the goals that have been completed and completion dates. This should be reviewed with the client so that he or she can see progress and feel positive about his or her accomplishments.
    3. The treatment plan can be used as a barometer for the client's progress when making recommendations to the court.
V. Reports are made to the courts in a timely fashion when the client
  A. Fails appointments
  B. Engages in illegal or grossly inappropriate behavior
  C. Fails to meet goals
  D. Completes goals and programs
  E. Pays all bills

State of Idaho

Idaho funds treatment and counseling for drug court clients through a preferred provider network. The program includes a detailed application and a performance contract that lays out the curriculum for the program through the phases of the drug court. The contract can be accessed at www.isc.idaho.gov/dc5thapp.pdf.

References

1. Wolf E, Colyer C. Everyday hassles: barriers to recovery in drug courts. J Drug Issues 2001;31(1):233–258.
2. Schiff M, Terry W. Predicting graduation from Broward County's dedicated drug treatment court. Justice Syst J 1997;19(3):291–310.
3. Belenko S. Research on Drug Courts: A Critical Review 2001 Update. New York: The National Center on Addiction and Substance Abuse at Columbia University; 2001.
4. Makkai T, Veraar K. Final Report on the South East Queensland Drug Court. Technical and Background Paper Series, No. 6. Canberra: Australian Institute of Criminology; 2003.
5. Sechrest DK, Shicor D. Determinants of graduation from a day treatment court in California: a preliminary study. J Drug Issues 2001;31(1):129–148.
6. American College of Occupational and Environmental Medicine. Preventing Needless Work Disability by Helping People Stay Employed. Evanston, IL: American College of Occupational and Environmental Medicine; 2005.
7. Staton M, Mateyoke A, Leukefeld C, Cole J, Hopper H, Logan TK, Minton L. Employment Issues Among Drug Court Participants. Lexington: University of Kentucky, Center on Drug and Alcohol Research; 2005.

12
Self-Help and Mutual Aid Organizations

Anne M. Herron and Dee S. Owens

In the early 1900s, there was little understanding of addiction as a disease. People who suffered addictive disorders were often considered mentally ill, criminals, or morally corrupt. Often they were institutionalized. There was no generally accepted treatment, the medical community did not recognize addiction as a disease, and persons with addictive disorders were treated in what we would now consider an inhumane manner (1). By the late 1930s, there were limited options for individuals with addictive disorders or for their families. A small group of alcoholics came together to offer each other support, encouragement, and hope for a life without addiction. This small group of visionaries formed a fellowship that became known as Alcoholics Anonymous (AA), the best-known and most widely attended self-help or mutual aid program ever developed (2).

Alcoholic Anonymous describes itself as "a fellowship or society of men and women for whom alcohol had become a major problem. We are recovering alcoholics who meet regularly to help each other stay clean" (2). This self-help program features:

1. Support.
2. Encouragement.
3. Hope for the daily lives of the members.

It accomplishes these goals with:

1. No professional intervention.
2. No leader.
3. No planned series of interventions.
4. No dues.
5. Only one requirement for membership: the desire to quit drinking.

Many members or prospective members of AA experience a host of other problems in addition to alcoholism. Alcoholics Anonymous recognizes this and publishes a pamphlet entitled "Problems Other Than Alcohol." Although persons with multiple problems, including drug addiction, are welcome to attend and become members of AA, there is the expectation that alcoholism is the primary problem being addressed.

Because of the success of AA, many additional programs have been modeled on its practices, traditions, and guiding principles. Groups have developed to address a wide variety of specific issues and to include all manner of addictive disorders, eating disorders, and other syndromes or diseases with a behavioral component. The professional treatment system has had a longstanding and closely cooperative relationship with these self-help programs. Because there are no financial obligations and no time limit for involvement, self-help programs have been encouraged as a long-term and ongoing support for individuals receiving and completing treatment. In addition, many of the principles of these self-help programs have been incorporated into the professional treatment system (3).

There sometimes is confusion about the differences and similarities between the professional treatment system and self-help programs. They are complementary but provide very different resources and services to the individual who is struggling with addiction. There are three characteristics generally present in self-help groups (3):

1. The common experience shared by group members.
2. The free nature of the participation.
3. The willingness of the members to accept each other as equals.

Most self-help groups are voluntary, nonprofit associations open to anyone with a similar need or interest. However, groups also exist to meet the needs of particular special interests, for example, the elderly, women, or persons of specific ethnic or cultural backgrounds. Usually, groups are led by peers, have an informal structure, and are free except for voluntary small donations to cover meeting expenses. However, a variety of professionals lead some self-help groups (4).

In the past 30 years, the number of self-help organizations and groups operating in communities throughout the United States has dramatically risen. Some organizations operate in several countries, primarily in the developed world. One of the reasons for the rapid proliferation of groups focusing on health problems may be the widespread increase in interest and attention to self-care. In addition, for individuals with insurance plans offering limited substance abuse and mental health coverage, self-help groups are an economical way to find ongoing emotional and social support (4).

Self-Help Groups and Professional Treatment

Results of the most recent membership survey of AA confirm growing trust and transparency in the relationships between alcoholics and their health care givers (doctors, nurses, counselors, and others) who, in turn, appear to be more informed about AA. Seventy-seven percent of members' doctors know they are in AA, and 39% of members said they had been referred to AA by a health care professional. Sixty-four percent said they had received some type of treatment or counseling before coming to AA, and, of these, 74% said it had played an important part in directing them to AA (5).

Because of the peer-led, informal and democratic, as opposed to hierarchical and medical, structure, professionals consider self-help groups to be an adjunct to therapy. The primary value of self-help groups is in the mutual aid offered by members to one another. The therapeutic aspects associated with participation include intimacy as a result of self-disclosure, personal growth in response to others' role modeling, and erosion of denial as a result of social confrontation. Although the nature of self-help groups is outside of the medical realm, doctors and therapists see participation as a way to improve the outcome of ongoing or future formal treatment.

The variety of groups is extensive. Groups may include advocacy groups with a focus on legal or social remedies, groups organized around housing or employment needs, and groups focusing on racial or gender issues. Additionally, the self-help movement shares some characteristics with volunteerism. In general, members who remain involved have experience with other voluntary organizations and believe in the value of donating time and service. In addition, members may be viewed as consumers who participate in their own care and who have experience and knowledge of relevant goods and services (6).

Types of Self-Help Groups

Twelve Step Groups

The most popular type of self-help group is based on the 12 Steps and 12 Traditions of AA, which was founded in 1935 by a stock advisor and a physician. The 12 Steps are a simply described and easy-to-follow guide to recovery from alcoholism, whereas the 12 Traditions are a code of values or ethics. The 12 Steps are listed in Table 12.1 (2).

Twelve Step programs are based on the spiritual premise that turning one's life and will over to a personally meaningful higher power, such as God or spirit, is the key to recovery. Another essential idea is that sobriety or recovery (but not cure) depends on the admission of powerlessness with respect to alcohol or the substances abused. This idea is offensive to critics of 12 Step groups, but others believe that this admission accurately reflects the contemporary view of addiction as a disease. Furthermore, members are asked to closely examine their behaviors and characteristics, looking specifically for evidence of self-deception or rationalization.

Although the dropout rate for AA groups during the first 3 months is high, alcoholics who persevere have a good chance of attaining and maintaining sobriety or abstinence. This is especially true if a person regularly

TABLE 12.1. Twelve steps of Alcoholics Anonymous.

1. We admitted we were powerless over alcohol—that our lives had become unmanageable.
2. Came to believe that a Power greater than ourselves could restore us to sanity.
3. Made a decision to turn our will and our lives over to the care of God as we understood Him.
4. Made a searching and fearless moral inventory of ourselves.
5. Admitted to God, to ourselves and to another human being the exact nature of our wrongs.
6. Were entirely ready to have God remove all these defects of character.
7. Humbly asked Him to remove our shortcomings.
8. Made a list of all persons we had harmed, and became willing to make amends to them all.
9. Made direct amends to such people wherever possible, except when to do so would injure them or others.
10. Continued to take personal inventory and when we were wrong promptly admitted it.
11. Sought through prayer and meditation to improve our conscious contact with God as we understood Him, praying only for knowledge of His will for us and the power to carry that out.
12. Having had a spiritual awakening as the result of these steps, we tried to carry this message to alcoholics and to practice these principles in all our affairs.

Source: The 12 Steps are reprinted with permission of Alcoholics Anonymous World Services, Inc. (AAWS). Permission to reprint the 12 Steps does not imply that AAWS has reviewed or approved the contents of this publication or that AAWS necessarily agrees with the views expressed herein. Alcoholics Anonymous is a program of recovery from alcoholism *only*. Use of the 12 Steps in connection with programs and activities that are patterned after AA but that address other problems, or in any other non-AA context, does not imply otherwise.

attends a home group for 90 meetings in the first 90 days, then slowly decreases to two or three times per week for years thereafter, and finds an experienced and sympathetic sponsor who also is in recovery (7).

Recent research demonstrated that those alcoholics who attended either AA or another of the related self-help groups after treatment had higher rates of abstinence from use and, if relapse occurred, fewer drinks were consumed. There is a marked dose–response effect: go to fewer meetings, and outcomes are the worst; go to many meetings, and the outcomes are best (8).

In addition to AA and organizations modeled after it, such as Narcotics Anonymous (NA) and Cocaine Anonymous (CA), a number of 12 Step organizations exist for a variety of disorders, such as Gamblers Anonymous (GA), Schizophrenics Anonymous (SA), Emotions Anonymous (EA), and Overeaters Anonymous (OA). The 12 steps for NA are given in Table 12.2.

Other Groups for Health Problems and Interests

Self-help organizations also provide support for individuals who are ill or have health problems. For example, support exists for people coping with weight management, HIV/AIDS, multiple sclerosis, muscular dystrophy, cancer, and incontinence and for the families of individuals who suffer from these conditions. Also, support exists for people who share interests or circumstances, such as groups for women who breast-feed (La Leche League), singles, older adults, and new parents.

Self-Help Groups for Families

Self-help groups for family members are available because illness, addiction, and distress affect the entire family. Family members are impacted by living with and loving a person who is addicted to alcohol and other substances and may find themselves unwittingly reinforcing illness or addictive behaviors. Moreover, family members often find that once the person with an addiction starts recovery, the person behaves and functions very differently.

Al-Anon, an organization for friends and families of alcoholics, is a companion organization to AA, as is Alateen, a program for teenagers who have been hurt by the alcoholism of significant people in their lives.

Support groups for caregivers of individuals with life-threatening or terminal illnesses such as cancer often meet at treatment centers and hospitals. One popular club for people with cancer, as well as for their friends and families, is Gilda's Club, founded by the actor Gene Wilder, Gilda Radner's widower. Radner, the well-known comedienne from *Saturday Night Live*,

TABLE 12.2. The twelve steps of Narcotics Anonymous.

1. We admitted that we were powerless over our addiction, that our lives had become unmanageable.
2. We came to believe that a Power greater than ourselves could restore us to sanity.
3. We made a decision to turn our will and our lives over to the care of God as we understood Him.
4. We made a searching and fearless moral inventory of ourselves.
5. We admitted to God, to ourselves, and to another human being the exact nature of our wrongs.
6. We were entirely ready to have God remove all these defects of character.
7. We humbly asked Him to remove our shortcomings.
8. We made a list of all persons we had harmed and became willing to make amends to them all.
9. We made direct amends to such people wherever possible, except when to do so would injure them or others.
10. We continued to take personal inventory and when we were wrong promptly admitted it.
11. We sought through prayer and meditation to improve our conscious contact with God as we understood Him, praying only for knowledge of His will for us and the power to carry that out.
12. Having had a spiritual awakening as a result of these steps, we tried to carry this message to addicts and to practice these principles in all our affairs.

Source: Reprinted by permission of NA World Services, Inc.

died at age 40 from ovarian cancer. Gilda's Clubs can be found in almost all cities in the United States.

Online Groups and Clearinghouses

A growing trend in the self-help movement includes online support communities as well as online resource centers and clearinghouses. Chat rooms, bulletin boards, and electronic mailing lists all provide convenient, around-the-clock access to peer support. Many large-scale, consumer health care Web sites provide forums for discussions on numerous diseases and disorders, and major online commercial services such as America Online (AOL) provide sites for health care and patient support. In some cases, professionals moderate online groups, although many are exclusively organized and populated by peers. There are self-help groups, such as AA, that hold some meetings online, often at their own Web sites (9).

Features of Self-Help Groups

There are 11 features of self-help groups that make them so successful in recovery from drug and alcohol addiction:

1. Accessibility.
2. Anonymity.
3. Equality.
4. Social support and mutual aid.
5. Self-esteem and self-efficacy.
6. Introspection and insight.
7. Spiritual recovery.
8. Advocacy.
9. Lack of professional involvement.
10. Awareness of vulnerability in early recovery.
11. Members are at varying stages of recovery.

Accessibility

Accessibility and economy are appealing features of self-help groups. Because the groups are free, organizations such as AA and NA are very cost-effective. In addition, meetings are easy to locate through local newspaper announcements, hospitals, health care centers, churches, school counselors, and community agencies. For AA and other organizations that encourage frequent attendance, hundreds of meetings may be held each week in large metropolitan areas. Furthermore, with the proliferation of online support communities and growth of connectivity to the Internet, self-help groups are becoming as accessible for individuals in rural areas as they are for those in large cities.

Anonymity

An important characteristic of 12 Step groups is the preservation of anonymity by revealing first names only and by maintaining strict confidentiality of stories shared during meetings. Online self-help groups offer even more anonymity because the exchanges are not face to face. The virtual anonymity of online experience helps to reduce social discomfort, discrimination, or stereotyping otherwise associated with real-life perceptions of age, disabilities, race, gender, or culture.

Equality

Equality consists of accepting one another and behaving as equals by setting aside differences that are generally considered superficial and irrelevant. Often the feeling of equality results from the common experience of enduring pain and suffering. To guard against the development of relationships based on superiority or inferiority, most of the self-help groups have developed traditions or principles of interaction between new members and the existing group.

Social Support and Mutual Aid

Self-help groups provide an intact community and a sense of belonging. The social support and mutual aid available in a group may be critical to recovery, rehabilitation, or healthy coping. This is especially true for socially isolated people or people from dysfunctional families who may have little or no emotional support. Participating in a social network of peers reduces social and emotional isolation and supports healthy behavior. Group members can offer unconditional support and, collectively, are a repository of helpful, experiential knowledge.

Self-Esteem and Self-Efficacy

Self-help groups promote self-esteem or self-respect by encouraging acceptance of members as equals, giving each the attention and time to share experiences, and by engaging in nonjudgmental interactions. The concept of self-efficacy, or the belief that one is capable, is promoted by reinforcing appropriate behavior and beliefs and by sharing relevant information regarding the disease or condition. For example, there may be an exchange of information regarding how to cope with failed or disrupted relationships, about what is reasonable to expect from health care professionals, about how to manage pain or public embarrassment, and about where to go and to whom for a variety of needs. In groups such as AA, self-efficacy also is promoted by sponsors who act as mentors and role models and by encouraging rotating leadership roles.

Introspection and Insight

Introspection, or contemplation, is another fundamental feature of many self-help groups, particularly for groups that follow a 12 Step program of recovery. For example, the fourth step of AA states that members make a searching and fearless moral inventory of themselves, and the tenth step states that members continue to take personal inventory and admit wrongdoing. Introspection is particularly beneficial to individuals who are not entirely aware of the moral repercussions of and motivation for their behavior. Working through some of the 12 steps allows the person to begin to understand how he thinks and why behaviors do not always follow thoughts, even intentions. Continued step work supports personal growth and development as maladaptive ideas and behaviors are transformed.

Spiritual Recovery

The final step in a 12 Step program recognizes that recovery entails a spiritual awakening and an emphasis on giving back to others who are suffering from addiction. Recovery depends on giving up both injurious self-will and denial of maladaptive behavior and turning to a higher power. Members are urged to seek guidance or inspiration from this higher power. For many addicts, the key to recovery is a spiritually guided movement away from self-centeredness or self-absorption and a turning toward the power greater than oneself through contemplation and meditation.

Advocacy

Some self-help groups meet to advocate or promote social and legislative remedies with respect to the issue of concern. For example, HIV/AIDS groups have lobbied for improved access to prescription drugs. Groups lobby for reforms by identifying key legislators and policymakers. They submit papers or suggestions for more equitable laws and policies to these key people. They also conduct public education programs, including programs meant to redress the harm of stigmatization. There are groups that advocate for more funds for research and for improved services for people who suffer from one of many diseases or mental disorders. The most important grassroots organization of families and consumers of psychiatric services is the National Alliance for the Mentally Ill. This organization was founded in 1979 and blends self-help with advocacy efforts for the improvement of research, services, and public awareness of major mental illnesses. Its advocacy efforts target both the federal and state levels.

Lack of Professional Involvement

Because the groups are made up of equals operating in a democratic process, there can be a concern about ensuring the health and safety of members. The absence of professional guidance may mean that a member in need of formal medical or psychological intervention or treatment may not be encouraged to seek professional help as soon as might be possible if a professional were present.

Awareness of Vulnerability in Early Recovery

There is a well-known risk associated with attending any social and supportive group, because some members may be more interested in power relationships or control and will prey on the more vulnerable members. Women new to the groups, especially young women, are most vulnerable in the early stages of recovery. Predators who attend meetings could take advantage of the atmosphere of intimacy and mutual trust. To cope with the possibility of exploitation, new members are encouraged to attend meetings with a family member or a trusted friend. There are also meetings set aside by members for "women only" or professionals; vulnerable new members can choose these groups for an additional measure of safety. Finally, new members are encouraged not to become involved in new relationships for 1 year so that they can become centered and focused on recovery. Involvement in romantic relationships can be a significant distraction from recovery and frequently leads to relapse to drug use, particularly when the relationships terminate unhappily. People struggling with early stages of recovery are changing rapidly and are frequently unable to deal with the emotional aspects of romance. It is unlikely that two individuals in such an accelerated state of flux will form an enduring attachment. One common saying among AA and NA members is that relationship is an acronym, standing for "real exciting love affair, turns into nightmare, sobriety hangs in peril."

Members at Varying Stages of Recovery

New members should be aware that self-help groups have members at different levels of recovery, that there is likely to be a mix of persons with more and less time in recovery, and, problematic to some, persons who may be actively involved in the abuse of alcohol or drugs. The only requirement for membership is a desire to quit using. Newcomers need to realize that not all members are interested in supporting their recovery and that people in later stages of recovery may be more reliable. Furthermore, some members are required to attend by disciplinary entities, such as employers or correctional authorities.

One criticism of self-help groups, especially 12 Step groups, is that in the eyes of families and friends, members who persevere and faithfully attend the seemingly endless number of meetings can become addicted to the program. However, professionals and researchers who support self-help groups point out that because addiction is a disease, addicts are particularly vulnerable to relapse and that ongoing involvement with a self-help community assists in maintaining recovery (8).

Effectiveness of Self-Help

Over the past several decades, there has been significant research on the effects of self-help groups on participants. The research has examined a wide variety of variables, including self-help as an adjunct to professional treatment, self-help involvement alone, face-to-face self-help, and electronic self-help. Although there are some differences in outcomes for specific groups, there is no question about the benefits that accrue to the individual and to the family from participation in self-help. The majority of the studies have found important benefits of participation for the members, including both personal growth and development as well as support in the maintenance of treatment outcomes (10). Generally, members found that participation resulted in significant improvements over a period of time in areas such as employment, alcohol and other drug use, legal involvement, self-esteem, family relationships, and reduced physical symptoms (11).

Self-Help Literature and Resources

Literature for the major addictive disorder self-help groups, including AA and NA, is available at any meeting, via mail, or through online sources. Publications are very inexpensive, covering only the basic costs to publish and distribute, and they deal with many issues faced by those in recovery, including recovery and relapse, family issues, and work problems. Additionally, literature for professionals who work with persons in recovery is available.

References

1. American Psychiatric Association. Practice Guidelines for the Treatment of Patients With Substance Abuse Disorders: Alcohol, Cocaine, Opioids. Washington, DC: American Psychiatric Association; 1995.
2. Alcoholics Anonymous, Inc. The Big Book. New York: Alcoholics Anonymous, Inc.; 2006.
3. Katz AH, Bender EI. The Strength in Us: Self-Help Groups in the Modern World. New York: New Viewpoints; 1976.
4. Powell TJ. Self-Help Organizations and Professional Practice. Silver Spring, MD: National Association of Social Workers; 1987.
5. Alcoholics Anonymous, Inc. The 2004 Membership Survey. New York: Alcoholics Anonymous, Inc.; 2005.
6. Gartner A, Riessman F, eds. The Self-Help Revolution. New York: Human Sciences Press; 1984.

7. Emrick ED, Tonigan JS. Alcoholics Anonymous: what is currently known? In McCrady BS, Miller WR, eds. Research on Alcoholics Anonymous: Opportunities and Alternatives. New Brunswick, NJ: Rutgers Center of Alcohol Studies; 1993:209–232.
8. Kelly JF, Stout R, Zywiak W, Schneider R. A 3-year study of addiction mutual-help group participation following intensive outpatient treatment. Alcohol Clin Exp Res 2006;30(8):1381–1392.
9. Alemi RL, Mosavel M, Stephens R. Electronic self-help and support groups. Medical Care 1996;34(Suppl):OS32–OS44.
10. Kyrouz E, Humphreys K, Loomis C. A review of research on the effectiveness of self-help mutual aid groups. In White BJ, Madera EJ, eds. American Self-Help Clearinghouse Self-Help Group Sourcebook, 7th ed. New York: American Self-Help Clearinghouse; 2002: 1–16.
11. Moos RH, Moos BS. Paths of entry into alcoholics anonymous: consequences for participation and remission. Alcohol Clin Exp Res 2005;29(10):1858–1868.

13
Building Supportive Services in Drug Courts

Dennis A. Reilly

Many drug courts focus on the provision of treatment services and only over time become involved in accessing and coordinating supportive services for clients. Because many clients lack a basic foundation for community reintegration, identifying supportive service needs in the early stages of participation helps to treat the person, not just the disease. Supportive services include housing assistance, educational and vocational training and skills development, physical health and testing services, prenatal services, entitlement counseling, debt counseling, financial health, family and domestic violence counseling, child care and parenting, recreational and expressive therapies, mentoring, and other necessary social services.

Supportive services are often referred to as *ancillary services* or *supplemental services*, which suggests that they are secondary to substance abuse treatment. These services enhance relapse prevention, improve self-esteem, and address family needs that help to stabilize the client. Drug court practitioners understand that supportive services eventually become primary services, especially for clients who are young or who have less intensive histories of addiction. If clients become quickly stabilized in their recovery, then supportive services need to receive earlier attention in the program. Courts and treatment providers must be careful to provide supportive services to all clients, not just the clients who have earned it, for these services may engage resistant clients and bring stability to newly won recovery.

Drug courts often leave the job of providing or accessing supportive services to the community organizations that provide primary substance abuse treatment services. Most substance abuse agencies provide access to supportive services to enable clients to stabilize themselves in recovery and meet their treatment goals. Courts have a role in identifying needed supportive services and coordinating and accessing those services to ensure a continuum of care. A key component of drug courts is forging partnerships with public agencies and community-based organizations to generate local support and enhance program effectiveness (1). This chapter identifies the basic challenges in engaging the community and describes effective strategies to link with supportive services to enhance program participation and to fulfill the drug court mission.

The Debate on Engaging the Community

Despite the historical record of judges acting as leaders in the community, there has been a debate as to whether the court can maintain integrity and independence when acting in this role. The Constitution mandates that the courts are formed for the purpose of resolving legal issues, which suggests that they should limit themselves to the role of the neutral trier of the facts. Some argue that court personnel lack the necessary training and resources to effectively assess service needs, to identify services to address those needs, and to evaluate the delivery and effectiveness of the services provided. These arguments have been countered by the recognition that the courts maintain an executive function to ensure that cases are given individual attention and that courts have an oversight role to ensure that the terms of service and supervision orders are met. Casey and Hewitt (2) suggest that "A well performing court must interact with other public institutions, including the network of service providers on which the court relies, to achieve quality in its performance." The fear of the courts and their officers becoming too closely involved with clients and the community providers who serve them should be no more of a concern than the involvement resulting from regular interaction with attorneys and agency representatives.

Canon number 1 of the American Bar Association Model Code of Judicial Ethics describing the court's professional responsibility to remain independent has been addressed in the drug courts' key components formulated by the National Association of Drug Court Professionals. Key components 6 and 10 discuss the drug courts' coordinated service strategy and the need to forge partnerships to improve the effectiveness of their treatment mandate (3). The National Association of Drug Court Professionals suggests that coordinated strategies do not impinge on the courts' ethical responsibilities if, after interaction with treatment partners regarding the proposed response to client compliance, the final decision for action rests with the court (4). The drug court judge may engage the community at arm's length by serving as the primary educator and the ultimate decision maker in the program. When partnerships are formed to improve access to services, such as in the development of a clinical advisory board, the specifics of particular cases are not discussed. The court's role in interacting with community providers is to improve the understanding of the court's needs and expectations with regard to the services and supervision required and to provide the client with the tools necessary to complete the drug court program.

Community treatment providers are asked to address the issues included in a comprehensive treatment plan. However, the drug court may be in a position to assist and coordinate significant pieces of that plan or provide access to other services that the individual treatment provider does not provide. Many clients are unaware of supportive services and treatment, and supportive service providers may be unaware of each other. As the primary referral source, the drug court may be better able to coordinate services among providers who do not normally work together. Additionally, drug courts may be aware of services not provided by the treatment agencies or may be able to identify and help resolve special needs such as civil legal services.

Drug courts may also be in a better position to bridge agency requirements and to create statewide interagency partnerships. They may be able to access services or funding streams to which treatment providers do not have access. Likewise, linkages with criminal justice systems can improve supportive service providers' potential to access additional funding for clients with unique needs. In this way, the drug court can help supportive service providers achieve their mission, fulfill grant requirements, or expand capacity for existing programs.

Connecting with Nonprofit Organizations

Community partnerships provide resources and create the network of community and political support to access supportive services. As drug courts accept larger numbers of clients, they become major referral sources. This may result in treatment programs becoming more economically viable and better able to provide services and effective treatment. The unmet needs of clients can be the basis for grant applications to build program enhancements. Drug education programs and prevention programs can assist the court by providing education services. Prisoner reentry programs can assist program clients in finding employment. Local colleges and universities can provide enhanced student services to drug court participants and offer internships to support staffing in the court.

Drug courts have received financial support from local corporations, faith-based organizations, foundations, and service organizations. These organizations may have mission statements and community outreach goals that can be fulfilled by supporting a drug court. Community service organizations have been instrumental in building meaningful incentive systems and community service opportunities. Corporations may provide matching funds for fundraisers or donate incentives to recognize client and community achievements. Citizens' councils, community antidrug coalitions, and prevention groups facilitate access to services. The existence of foundations and other support systems boosts a court's ability to demonstrate sustainability to funding agencies. Partner organizations can also assist drug court practitioners to focus resources and to create broad support.

Strategic Planning

In 1998, the State Justice Institute investigated the relationship between drug courts and the community. This study found that "engaging communities is a new task for most drug courts, requiring a new set of skills and resources" (5). On a state level, officials from the various state agencies may meet with representatives from community agencies, service providers, and professional associations to craft a comprehensive plan for building support systems for clients. This planning approach takes a high level of coordination and may be more easily done at the local agency level to address local issues. Drug courts can utilize their advisory boards and team members to build a strategic plan to develop treatment and supportive service linkages. Broadening the discussion to include multiple perspectives can result in identifying unforeseen opportunities and new partners.

Strategic planning for drug court support systems involves communicating the identified needs of clients. Providing cumulative client information and creating a demographic profile of clients can help define a service provider's target population, create opportunities to fulfill grant requirements, and realize organizational requirements for corporate outreach.

Planning to build sustainable supportive services may initially mean reducing resistance among potential partners. A common approach to conducting service development is to implement a pilot program to demonstrate the potential effectiveness of a new linkage. Pilot programs allow time to amass resources, refine policies and procedures, and build experience and training before working with a larger population. However, drug courts that rely solely on grant funding may fail to build the support necessary to sustain the service. Therefore, program planning must include sustainability.

When preparing for drug court outreach activities, the program should:

1. Start with an assessment of the strengths and weaknesses of the court.
2. Analyze the community environment in which they are operating to see if there are sufficient resources and supervision to address the needs of the clients.
3. Evaluate the political climate and community support for alternatives to incarceration before venturing out into the community to develop resources.
4. Evaluate other agencies to determine which government offices can contribute to the development of the court's support system.
5. Review the obstacles that the drug court team will face in maintaining the operations of the court and the provision of supervision and services.
6. Review the ongoing need for program development.
7. Plan for staff turnover and transition that may impact the development process.

Community Mapping

Community mapping is the process of identifying treatment and supportive services. It may also be conducted as needs for services arise that are not covered by the court or partner treatment providers. It is beneficial to formally gather interested parties together to identify additional resources that may be needed.

Drug court staff and community providers can jointly identify the need for supportive services, identify the time frame for their implementation, and determine which party can access these services most effectively. Social service and treatment resources can then be collected into referral guides in which services are identified, and sometimes rated, to allow the courts and treatment providers to quickly access the appropriate resource. The results of an initial community mapping exercise and the resource guide should be made available to all the parties involved.

The Role of the Drug Court Team

The court's ability to coordinate service activities is enhanced through the program's staffing structure (1). Judicial leadership is universally acknowledged as a pivotal element of effective court operations. Operational effectiveness hinges on judicial involvement in direct client supervision, ongoing planning, resource development, and outcome tracking and information dissemination. Effective judicial leadership can overcome bureaucracy and skepticism through positional authority and personal relationships.

Team members can also act as leaders for their agencies and speak to the community about how drug courts achieve many agency missions and goals. A successful team effort can provide the community with the factual basis for sustained services. Presentations on reductions in recidivism and systemwide cost savings can set the stage for long-term community commitment and sustainable services.

The drug court team must be engaged in action planning to acquire resources and agree in writing on the goals for service development. Attached to these goals should be a timeline for their achievement and a plan that assigns tasks to different team members and supports organizations based on their abilities. Finally, there needs to be some form of accountability to the assigned tasks and timelines.

Many drug courts include a coordinator who acts as an intermediary between the court and the community providers to address particular service issues. This coordinator has the following responsibilities:

1. Oversees community supervision and serves as an interagency coordinator of services.
2. Works on behalf of the court to serve as the hub of a network of providers offering a full range of services.

3. Manages the interagency and community linkages necessary to ensure the integration of treatment within a continuum of supportive services.
4. Implements development strategies to organize the court's provider network.
5. Ensures a continuum of care and comprehensive treatment planning that may span multiple providers and time frames during the lifetime of each client's mandate to a drug court.
6. Conducts quality assurance of the services provided.
7. Ensures accountability of the client to make sure that linkages are not strained because of a client's failure to follow through with a referral.
8. Assists in the provision of information to determine eligibility for supportive services by accessing client criminal information and by providing court documentation for financial aid, certifications, licenses, and driving privileges.
9. Works to improve the speed of the delivery of services and thus improve their effectiveness by working to overcome barriers to entry.

Creating the Link

A drug court staff member should be designated to collect information on identified resources and present that information to the remainder of the team. A simple way to collect information about a service provider is to call the provider and develop a fact sheet including services provided, a contact person's name, and a phone number. Another useful tool is to invite providers to conduct educational sessions with staff and the judge. Drug courts should conduct site visits to gain a more intimate understanding of community service providers. Development staff should check certifications, oversight by state agencies, and any ratings systems that may be included in resource guides or findings of monitoring organizations.

The next step is to identify who should make the first contact. The drug court team can discuss with their advisory board or community leaders the best approach to engage identified resources. It is imperative that the team be notified of the intent to form the linkages so they can identify any concerns they may have or provide background or suggestions as to how the linkage should be developed.

Maintaining Community Relationships

Once the drug court program is initiated, ongoing monitoring and adjustments are required to ensure continued effectiveness. Drug court target populations evolve over time as arrest patterns or funding sources change. State intervention approaches and laws may change eligibility requirements or availability of services. The program may experience changes in community support that will affect its ability to access services. Community organizations also experience significant change over time because of the inconsistencies in funding systems and staffing.

Drug court teams must be in tune with the changes in the laws, community, referral strategies, and delivery plans to meet the needs of new clients in the new provider environment. Methods that can be used to keep current include the following:

1. Review criminal statistics and offender profiles.
2. Review information from court staff, supervision officers, and judges to identify common challenges in serving different populations.
3. Compare the assessments done by the treatment providers to identify the level and type of services and supervision required.
4. Monitor accumulated data and conduct regular analyses to identify trends and the specific need for services.
5. Regularly review client needs.
6. Continue to determine which organization may best address specific needs.
7. Join or build community coalitions having common goals and purposes with the program.
8. Review the federal and state grant awards, follow newspaper and newsletter announcements, and ask community partners and the advisory board about new funding sources established in the community.
9. Establish a consistent, formal process of program evaluation.

Much of the work in maintaining strong community linkages must be done by an assigned staff person. Drug courts may be able to obtain some immediate services in the preplacement stages by having established good relationships with providers. This often means that clients receive services even though they have not yet received the appropriate entitlements to pay for them. In these instances, it is helpful if the court staff can provide information on subsequent approval of entitlements so the service providers can conduct retroactive billing of services delivered prior to entitlement acquisition.

Staff should meet regularly with the providers to obtain feedback on the effects of the linkage on the provider and any ongoing issues that the provider is experiencing. It is necessary for the drug court to maintain a good working relationship with social service providers to ensure sustainability of the service and the relationship. Drug courts can build a history of reliability through proper assessment of a client's eligibility, the client's appropriateness for the identified services, and the client's ability to follow through with a referral for services. The court's response to a client's failure to follow through with referrals for services can impact the sustainability of the resource.

When a disruptive incident occurs at a service provider, the court staff must be willing to listen to how that incident not only affects the client's compliance with the court but also to how it affects the remainder of the clients in the program and the credibility of the program itself. Carefully reasoned responses to client behavior require intensive communication skills, effective case management, and consistent judicial monitoring.

Court staff must monitor the resource usage, quality, and effectiveness. Staff must determine if the resources are being used as planned and if different resources are needed than were originally planned. Court staff must be organized and track multiple funding sources and reporting requirements, local matching funds, and the rate of expenditures. The coordinator must understand how the court's financial system operates and how grants are managed and must build a system of accountability. Tracking of data is essential to compile the necessary financial and narrative statements in anticipation of reporting requirements. The responsible staff person should regularly involve the drug court team to make sure that they understand the budgetary rules, grant requirements, regulations, and timelines for the use of the secured resources.

The drug court can participate in a structurally accountable community coalition. In a presentation titled "Community Anti-Drug Plans: Building Structural Accountability for Program Effectiveness," the founder of the National Association of Drug Court Professionals, Judge Jeffery Tauber, spoke to the United Nations Conference on Communities in the Global Drug Problem about building structurally accountable coalitions in which participating agencies share program responsibilities and are accountable to each other for program effectiveness (6). At this conference, Judge Tauber described the theory of "Co-Funding of Anti-Drug Systems" as a structurally accountable partnership in which resources are allocated to the whole coalition, relying on the system clients to coordinate the distribution within the system using a steering committee made up of the partners. The value of building an interdependent system of services is evident. "Because continued funding depends on the success of the system as a whole, the success of the entire system becomes a priority for all," Tauber notes. The Co-Funding of Anti-Drug Systems creates institutional commitment to a broader mission than departments and agencies have traditionally embraced. This model of service has significant ancillary benefits, because broad-based, multiagency partnerships enhance credibility.

Ultimately, coalition partners may recognize the value of becoming interdependent with each partner providing the service or supervision that they can offer best. Clearly this vision does not account for competition between equally qualified organizations that provide identical services. The drug court should produce sufficient volume to fill available program capacity, but each court must make reasoned evaluations of which providers and services best meet the needs of each client as part of the program's decision-making process.

Public Relations

The drug court can build an educational and awareness campaign to develop support from community leaders and to engage community providers in the effort to secure services. Any drug court outreach effort must utilize the strengths and contacts of the team and advisory board members. These individuals have communication skills that are an asset to the court in this process. Team members must also act as leaders for their own agencies to provide education and build support for the program. Some team members have a unique ability to reach certain audiences; for example, prosecutors are effective when addressing law enforcement. Judges have a unique ability to communicate with the legislators and the media.

Local political support can be garnered through presentations by the drug court judge to educate decision makers on the process and to persuade individuals that the drug court's approach is not soft on crime but a thoughtful process using proven methodologies to reduce crime and improve the chances of recovery and assimilation back into the workforce.

Drug court team members can build community understanding by inviting law enforcement, community leaders, and the media to planning sessions, courtroom hearings, graduations, and alumni events. It is important to communicate not only research and evaluation results but also individual stories that powerfully personalize the message. This can be achieved by having program graduates describe their experience. Graduation ceremonies are positive events that allow members of the community to see results. Influential community members, including law enforcement officials, prosecutors, legislators, and city and county officials, should routinely be invited to attend and have personal contact with the graduates to understand their achievement.

References

1. National Association of Drug Court Professionals. Defining Drug Courts: The Key Components. Alexandria, VA: Drug Courts Program Office, Office of Justice Programs, U.S. Department of Justice; 1997.
2. Casey P, Hewitt WE. Courts Responses to Individuals in Need of Services: Promising Components of a Service Coordination Strategy for Courts. Williamsburg, VA: National Center for State Courts; 2001.
3. American Bar Association's Model Code of Judicial Conduct, 1998 Edition, Standing Committee on Ethics and Professional Responsibility and Judicial Code Subcommittee. Washington, DC: American Bar Association; 1998.
4. National Association of Drug Court Professionals. Ethical Considerations for Judges and Attorneys in Drug Court. Alexandria, VA: National Association of Drug Court Professionals; 1998.
5. Harrell AV, Bryer S. The Process Evaluation of Project Connection Lessons on Linking Drug Courts and Communities. Washington, DC: Urban Institute; 1998.
6. Tauber J. Community Anti-Drug Plans: Building Structural Accountability for Program Effectiveness. New York: Speech to the United Nations Conference on Communities in the Global Drug Problem, May 18, 1994.

14 Drug Testing Methods

Karl Auerbach

The challenge in drug testing is to have a reliable, reproducible, and economical test that can be used to make critical decisions about peoples' lives. The choice of which material to test is often a matter of which specimen is accessible and how people feel about how the sample is obtained. Testing methods depend on whether laboratory equipment is available and how well the methodology holds up to legal challenge. A concern expressed by some is that "any test with less than 100% accuracy is likely to produce a high percentage of false positives" (1). To date, there is no evidence that this is a valid concern with the testing procedures currently in place.

Basic Terms

The following basic terms are used when planning, conducting, and evaluating drug tests (2,3):

Adulterant: something added or done to the sample so that the drug of abuse present in the sample is not detected.

Adulterated specimen: a specimen that contains a substance that is not naturally present in human urine or contains a substance expected to be present but is at an unnaturally high concentration.

Alcohol concentration: the alcohol in a volume of breath expressed in terms of grams of alcohol per 210 liters of breath as indicated by a breath test.

Blind specimen or blind performance test specimen: a specimen submitted to a laboratory for quality control testing purposes with a fictitious identifier so that the laboratory cannot distinguish it from a collected specimen.

Breath alcohol technician: a person who instructs and assists donors in the alcohol testing process and operates an evidential breath testing device.

Cancelled test: a drug or alcohol test that has a problem identified that cannot be or has not been corrected. A cancelled test is neither a positive nor a negative test.

Chain of custody: the procedure used to document the handling of the specimen from the time the donor gives the specimen to the collector until the specimen is destroyed after laboratory analysis.

Confirmation (or confirmatory) drug test: a second analytical procedure performed on a specimen to identify and quantify the presence of a specific drug or drug metabolite.

Confirmation (or confirmatory) validity test: a second test performed on a specimen to further support a valid test result.

Cutoff: an agreed on level representing a positive test. It must be above the level of detection. Typically it reflects a level at which there is no doubt that the test is showing the drug and not background substances. It is arbitrarily set depending on the testing program.

Dilute specimen: a specimen with creatinine and specific gravity values that are lower than expected for human urine.

Dilution: the addition of some material to the sample so that the drug level goes below a cut-off level or the level of detection.

Direct observation: the sample is obtained with a collector witnessing that the individual is actually the source of the sample.

Initial drug test: the test used to differentiate a negative specimen from one that requires further testing for drugs or drug metabolites.

Initial validity test: the first test used to determine if a specimen is adulterated, diluted, or substituted.

Interfering agent: something added to the sample that interferes with the testing method so that a reliable test cannot be done. Agents that interfere with one method do not necessarily interfere with other methods.

Invalid drug test: the result of a drug test for a urine specimen that contains an unidentified adulterant or an unidentified interfering substance, has abnormal physical characteristics, or has an endogenous substance at an abnormal concentration that prevents the laboratory from completing or obtaining a valid drug test result.

Level of detection: the lowest level that can be reliably detected by the testing method.

Matrix: the biologic substance being tested, such as urine or hair.

Medical review officer: A licensed physician who is responsible for receiving and reviewing laboratory results generated by the drug testing program and evaluating medical explanations for positive drug test results.

Screen or screening test: a series of initial tests designed to distinguish negative from presumptive positive samples.

Sensitivity: the proportion of those cases having a positive test result to all samples with the drug present tested.

Shy bladder: a term used in urine sample collection to indicate the inability of the person to provide a urine sample.

Specificity: the proportion of true negatives to all the negative samples tested.

Split specimen: a part of the specimen that is sent to a first laboratory and retained unopened and that is transported to a second laboratory in the event that the donor requests that it be tested following a verified positive test of the primary specimen or a verified adulterated or substituted test result.

Substituted specimen: a specimen with creatinine and specific gravity values so abnormal that they are not consistent with human urine.

Substitution: the replacement of the sample with some other material that does not contain the drug.

Reasons for Drug Testing

Drug users frequently seek to conceal their drug use. When they are involved in legal proceedings or are subject to adverse consequences such as incarceration, the likelihood of concealment increases. Thus, drug courts may not rely on self-admission to determine if drugs are present. Many studies have shown that self-reporting of drugs, even when the stakes are not high, is a poor predictor of finding drugs in a biologic sample. Even when it would be advantageous for the person to report drug use so that treatment can be provided, reporting rates are still low. Counselor evaluation of drug use by a client is also unreliable. Even when questionnaire screening tests are done, drug use reports are poorly correlated with the drugs actually found (4).

Drug testing is also essential when legal drugs such as methadone are prescribed and usage of illegal drugs is a concern. Studies demonstrate that chronic pain patients frequently provide incorrect information on illicit drug use and that combining behavioral monitoring with drug testing is more effective than either alone (5). Fishbain and associates (6) performed drug tests on chronic pain patients admitted to a pain treatment program. Concordance between drug use reported in a psychiatric examination and urine toxicology results was poor. For cocaine, the concordance was only 20%. For marijuana it was 57% (6). In a study of cocaine abusers in outpatient treatment, researchers found there was substantial underreporting of cocaine use during treatment and retrospectively but that self-reports could be of more value if urine collection is frequent (7).

However, other researchers found that in a setting of dual diagnosis patients, self-reports were highly valid. It should be noted that this study was done in a treatment setting where substance abuse was a given, the subjects knew they were being urine tested, and there were no negative consequences for reporting drug use (8).

Similarly, a study of veterans seeking treatment reported that only 8% of the cases had a positive urine screen but denied drug use. They did have a high rate of participation in voluntary drug testing, and over half of those refusing drug tests admitted to illicit drug use. There were no negative consequences of having a positive drug test or admitting to drug use (9). In contrast, based on prison intake data relative to drug abuse, researchers concluded that prisoners who need help but think that asking for help is unlikely to result in treatment are not likely to be truthful about their substance abuse (10).

In a study of known substance abusers after admission to a 3-month cocaine treatment program, 33% reported use and 67% reported no use. Of the "no use" responders, 32% had cocaine-positive urine drug screens. Of the treatment completers who reported "no use," only 16% had positive tests compared with 40% of the "no use" responders who dropped out early (11).

Timing of drug use is another factor. In a study of U.S. Post Office hires, researchers demonstrated that a positive drug test at hire was significantly associated with absenteeism and involuntary separation. The study did not evaluate accident rates. Rates of positive drug tests were lower than would be expected, and the authors postulated that drug users did not apply for the job knowing they would be tested (12).

Testing Settings

Most drug tests done in the United States are associated with employment. The federal government mandates testing in a number of industries, most notably the transportation and nuclear industries. The military has done drug testing for over three decades. A number of federal agencies require testing of their employees (2). These testing programs have strict rules for when and how testing can be done. It has been said that "only the feds can take 22 steps to pee in a cup" (3). This level of detail is needed to ensure that the rights of the donors are protected and that the tests will stand up to administrative or legal challenges.

Less regulated but often following the same model as the federal programs, many companies have adopted drug testing programs for their employees. Testing can be done in a variety of settings. The ones on firmest legal grounds are those done for safety-sensitive situations, such as law enforcement and fire personnel. On less firm ground are general drug testing programs for all employees. Unless there are state or local laws against such testing, they usually can be implemented without restrictions (12–15).

Schools at various levels have started testing students, typically the members of athletic teams. In addition to testing for recreational drugs, such programs often include testing for performance-enhancing substances, including stimulants and steroids. Drug testing has been used in various British boarding schools for several years (16).

The Olympic athletic system has tested for drugs for over three decades. The Olympics ban a number of medications that in most employment systems would be legal but because of performance-enhancing aspects are tightly controlled. Doping agents such as recombinant human erythropoietin (a substance that increases red blood cell numbers in the blood) present challenges to testing protocols because they are naturally occurring substances in the body that require a combination of methods to detect (17).

Because of the adverse impact of drugs on developing fetuses and on the newborn, the Medical University of South Carolina developed a policy of testing pregnant women and involving the police to enforce mandatory treatment. This policy was ultimately found to be unconstitutional by the U.S. Supreme Court and was discontinued in 1994 (18).

Drug testing has been used by the Correctional Service of Canada to monitor offenders who are on work release or parole. Participation is mandatory and uses urine drug testing. Most offenders provide acceptable samples, but 7% of samples in one study were either dilute or cancelled because of problems with the test process. Twenty-seven percent of the tests were positive for cannabinoids (43%), opiates (22%), or cocaine (10.6%) (19).

Frequency and Patterns of Testing

Testing can be preparticipation, periodic, random, or for cause. In addition, once drug use is discovered, a condition of employment or reinstatement can involve periodic or random testing at increased frequency.

One benefit of any pattern of testing is deterrence. Random testing is particularly useful for deterrence. To identify most of the drug users in a population, testing must be relatively frequent, considering the time a drug is present in the system. Random testing should be unannounced (20). Within drug courts, random tests, with less than 1 day advance notice, are the most effective pattern.

Periodic, announced testing has less value in deterrence. Except in highly addicted individuals, users can abstain for a short period of time to pass the test. Detection can still take place for drugs that remain present for a long time, and drug users frequently misjudge how long it takes for their body to clear the drug. Some testing systems have long windows of detection, so decreased frequency of periodic testing can be feasible and still have high rates of detection and deterrence.

A weakness of frequent testing is determining whether a positive result represents old or new drug use. If tests are done frequently and the drug remains in the system for a relatively long period of time compared with the frequency of testing, old drug use may be detected. Ehrman and associates (7) found that with testing every few days for cocaine (with a detection period of several days), old use likely accounted for some of the positive tests. Cocaine from use a few days earlier, already detected by testing, was still present in the samples. Thus, there is a need both for rational sampling strategies based on how long the drug remains detectable and for a process for dealing fairly with such situations. Marijuana, with its relatively long detection time, is particularly problematic (7).

Test Modalities

Commercial tests are available for most drugs of abuse. However, as designer drugs evolve, there may be a lag in availability of an appropriate test for the substance.

Drug tests can be done as a standard panel or tailored to the specific situation. Modern kits use relatively small amounts of the matrix so multiple tests can be done on the same sample. However, there are obviously a finite number of tests that can be done on a given sample. Furthermore, it is sometimes necessary to reserve an adequate sample to repeat a test if there is a challenge to the results.

The federal government defined a panel that includes marijuana, opiates, amphetamines, phencyclidine, and cocaine. This came to be known as the *NIDA 5* after the National Institute on Drug Abuse. The tests represent the most common drugs of abuse at the time the laws were written, but the panel does not necessarily represent all of the current common drugs of abuse. For example, in the opiate panel only morphine and heroin are tested. Prescription drugs such as oxycodone, which is frequently abused, do not show up on this panel. Other drugs with legitimate therapeutic roles that are often abused are also excluded from the NIDA 5 panel.

Depending on the setting, nongovernmental test panels add a variety of drugs. For example, a hospital might add oxycodone, barbiturates, and benzodiazepines, drugs typically abused in hospital settings. Care should be given to include any drug preferred by a subject in a drug court setting to the testing protocol.

Testing can impact drug use patterns. People may switch to drugs that clear the body faster and are therefore less likely to be detected, such as alcohol (1).

What Sample to Test: The Matrices

The matrix is the body substance being tested. Considerations of which matrix to use include the following (21):

1. The biologic material should be easily obtainable and collection as noninvasive as possible.
2. The drug or its metabolite must be present in the material.
3. A test is available that can accurately identify the suspect drugs in the chosen material.
4. The drug must appear at a level that can be detected after a single dose (i.e., have a low false-negative rate).

TABLE 14.1. Drug testing matrices.

Biologic matrix	Drug detection time	Major advantage	Major disadvantage	Primary use
Urine	2–4 Days except marijuana and long-acting barbiturates, which may be up to 30 days	Mature technology, onsite use methods available. Tested in courts	Only detects recent use. Potential for adulteration or dilution	Detection of recent drug use
Saliva	12–24 Hours	Easily obtainable. Samples "free" drug fraction and parent drug presence	Short detection time. Oral contamination. Collection methods influence pH. Newer technology	Linking positive drug tests to behavior and impairment/ performance
Sweat	1–4 Weeks	Cumulative measure of drug use	High potential for environmental contamination. Newer technology	Detection of recent drug use over a period of time
Hair	Months	Long-term measure of drug use. Similar sample can be re-collected	Concern about environmental contamination. Newer technology	Detection of drug use in the recent past (1–6 months)

Source: Data from Cone (21).

5. The relationship between the concentration of the drug and the dosage should be carefully plotted through experimentation.
6. The drug must have time to appear in the material and remain long enough to be detected.
7. The risk of false-positive results from environmental contamination should be extremely small.
8. The methodology should be completely unbiased toward all populations and ethnic groups.

Table 14.1 summarizes the various matrices used and their major advantages and disadvantages.

Urine

Urine is the preferred matrix in most settings. Many drugs are eliminated from the body in the urine, so it is a good place to look for presence of a drug. Urine provides the potential for a sample size that is adequate for laboratory testing. The technology used in urine testing is well developed and has withstood legal challenges. Urine collection does not require an invasive method, and urine can be collected by nonmedical personnel. Relatively little equipment is needed to make the collection. It is a matrix

TABLE 14.2. Cut-off values and detection times for the more common drugs of abuse in urine.

Drug	Screening cutoff (ng/mL urine)	Confirmation cutoff	Urine detection time
Amphetamines	1,000	500	2–4 Days
Barbiturates	200	200	2–4 Days for short acting; up to 30 days for long acting
Benzodiazepines	200	200	Up to 30 days
Cocaine	300	150	1–3 Days
Codeine, morphine	300	300	1–3 Days
Heroin	300	300 morphine 10 for 6-monoacetylmorphine	1–3 Days
Marijuana	100, 50, 20	15	1–3 Days for casual use; up to 30 days for chronic use
Methadone	300	300	2–4 Days
Methamphetamine	1,000	500 (200 for amphetamine)	2–4 Days
Phencyclidine	25	25	2–7 Days for casual use; up to 30 days for chronic use

Source: Data from Cone (21).

that remains relatively stable over time and can be frozen to maintain the integrity of the sample. Detection times with urine vary by drug and the screening cut-off level (Table 14.2) (21).

Disadvantages of urine testing include the perception of donors that the sampling process is intrusive in a personal body function and an aversion to handling a body waste product with attendant potential for transmitting diseases. The major disadvantage of urine is the lack of sample integrity resulting in false-negative results. Urine is subject to adulteration by adding material. It is subject to dilution by either increased fluid intake or addition of fluid to the sample. Unless the sample is obtained under direct observation, substitution of another person's urine is possible. Even with direct observation, donors have been known to substitute samples through such devices as "the wizinator," an artificial penis, or even by injecting urine into their bladder by catheter (22). Web sites sell a kit that includes a tube to be worn to dispense urine during a drug test, vials of pretested, sex-specific, clean urine, and heating pads to warm the sample. At least one state, Arkansas, bans the sale of clean urine designed to beat drug tests (23).

To determine if a substituted sample meets the temperature requirements in the U.S. Department of Transportation regulations, researchers had volunteers strap condoms containing water to their body for 2 hours, which is within the time allowed to get to the collection site, and measured the temperature of the water. There was considerable overlap into the range considered acceptable for urine samples. The study concludes that someone trying to thwart the temperature test with a substituted sample could easily meet the temperature requirement (24).

By analyzing several parameters of submitted urine samples, Kapur and associates (25) showed that patients in a methadone treatment program would resubmit their known negative urine samples on different days and that multiple patients might submit the same sample on the same day. They proposed testing urine sodium, chloride, creatinine, and pH to develop chemical fingerprints of the samples to prevent substitution (25).

In the prison system testing program in Canada, correction for dilution using urine creatinine or specific gravity adjustments has resulted in higher rates of detection of several drugs. Similar results were obtained with experimental programs in the general population (26).

The U.S. Department of Transportation programs do not allow for adjustment of cut-off levels based on low creatinine or specific gravity. However, when the sample creatinine and specific gravity meet certain criteria, the sample is flagged as dilute and may result in a retest. If the degree of dilution appears to be extreme, the test is repeated under direct observation and is considered substituted unless the donor can demonstrate the ability to produce such a dilute specimen under direct observation (27,28). In drug courts, evidence of adulteration or substitution is grounds for sanctions.

Blood

Blood is an excellent fluid for determining the presence of drugs. The major disadvantage is that obtaining a sample is invasive and carries with it a small but not negligible risk of injury to the donor. It may be difficult to obtain blood from veins scarred by repeated heroin injections. The time window for detection in blood is shorter than in urine. This difference can be significant. For example, at a given dosage of cocaine, blood testing can detect use for 12 hours while urine testing can detect use for 48 to 72 hours (29,30). The advantage of blood is that, absent collusion with the collector, substitution and dilution are not possible.

Hair

Hair has been used for over 100 years to detect drugs and arsenic in the body. In the past 15 to 20 years, various drugs of abuse have been reported as reliably detected in hair. One distinct advantage of hair is that, depending on which portion of the hair is analyzed, drug use can be evaluated at different points in time. In studies comparing hair and urine, hair testing detected drug use 35% more effectively than urine testing (31,32).

The time window for which drug use can be assessed is much longer with hair than any other matrix. Hair has been used to show freedom from drug use for up to 1 year in cases in which individuals had to show long-term abstinence for driver license revocation hearings. Hair has been used to show presence of date rape drugs after the time for urine detection has past. Hair is particularly useful in heroin detection because 6-monoacetylmorphine, a unique heroin metabolite, is measurable, which allows legal use of morphine or codeine to be distinguished from heroin use. The methodologies used to analyze hair are generally the same as for urine (31–34).

There are concerns about racial differences in drug deposition in the hair. Rates of hair growth can impact the results, especially regarding timing of drug use. Hair also tends to concentrate drugs (35–37). Hoffman (36) analyzed the data from police candidates who were tested using both urine and hair. Hair samples had higher rates of positive results, and there was no statistically significant difference between black and white candidates. Although blacks had a higher positive rate, drugs were found in both urine and hair. However, other studies are reported as showing higher binding in hair from blacks than hair from blond, white men (35–37).

A major concern about hair testing is external contamination. There are reports of hair absorbing cocaine when cocaine base is vaporized or when contamination from another person's sweat occurs. By using washing techniques and looking for metabolites that are not deposited on the outside of the hair but rather incorporated in the hair shaft, these concerns can be addressed. Another concern is the potential inability to detect very recent use because the drug or its metabolites have not yet been deposited in the hair outside the hair follicle (37–39).

Saliva

Saliva is increasingly used for drug testing because the concentrations of many drugs in saliva correlate well with blood concentrations. This makes it an excellent material for determining the current degree of exposure to the drug at the time of sampling. Saliva is also easy to collect, can be done with close supervision to prevent adulteration or substitution, and is noninvasive. Amphetamines, cocaine, opioids, nicotine, and cannabis can be detected in saliva (35,40).

The main disadvantage of testing saliva is the short window of detectability. Cocaine, for example, is detectable in saliva for 5 to 12 hours compared to 48 hours or more in urine. The very characteristic that makes it excellent for determining very recent use makes it poor in detecting use over time (30).

Nails

Drugs are deposited in the nails by absorption into the root of the growing nail bed. Initially used in postmortem studies for drug detection, nails have become a source of material for testing antemortem. The same issues that exist for hair (long time frame, problems with external contamination) also impact the use of nails for drug testing (41).

Sweat

Even low levels of drug use can be detected by using patches to collect sweat. Patches have been used as adjuncts to urine testing in some drug rehabilitation programs. Methods can be used to minimize external contamination (35). Sweat samples are difficult to collect, although newer patches are being developed that can collect the sample more efficiently. The high acceptability by subjects and long time frame during which monitoring can be conducted are advantages. Care must be taken in handling the patches during application and removal (32).

The Testing Process

Consent

Typically drug tests are obtained only with the consent of the person being tested. In employment situations, the potential employees can decide if they want to pursue the job and if they are willing to be tested. In drug court situations, the agreement to be tested is part of the probation agreement. In treatment situations, agreement to be tested is likewise part of the process (42,43).

Confidentiality

In drug court, it is important to maintain confidentiality and to obtain consent in writing. Dissemination of the information should be limited to those who need to know it (44).

Collection Security

To ensure the integrity of the process, predefined procedures should be followed precisely. A model for drug courts is the federal testing program. When the sample is not urine, some variation may be necessary (45). Basically, obtaining a sample for testing includes the following:

1. Ensuring privacy of the collection area (including when same-sex observers are used).
2. Identifying the person giving the sample.
3. Removing outer garments and being sure that there are no obvious materials that could be used to tamper with the sample.
4. Removing material that can be used to adulterate, substitute for, or dilute the sample.
5. Checking the integrity of the sample when presented by temperature, pH, and appearance.
6. Processing the sample under a strict chain of custody.

Some programs request those being tested to indicate what medications they are taking, whereas others specifically prohibit asking this question. The reason for asking is to be able to determine if the drug found is a result of a valid medication. In most programs, prescription drug use has to be confirmed by documentation from the provider scripting the medication. Some programs do not inquire into medication on the premise that the process is less invasive into personal history and the issue of medication need only be raised in the face of a positive test (27,45).

Collectors must be trained and should undergo proficiency testing to demonstrate the proper procedures. If an error is made, retraining may be necessary. There should be zero tolerance for errors in this process because of the outcome implications (46).

Problems in Testing

Problems in testing arise in two major forms: adulteration and substitution (Table 14.3).

Adulterants

As long as there have been drug tests, there have been substances added to the sample to try to cause false-negative results. Micklesen and Ash (47) studied the enzyme immunoassay test using known positives and adding various adulterants. They found that there were various mechanisms by which the adulterants impacted testing but that if specific gravity, pH, and appearance were checked, many were detectable. They found that Visine™ was the only thing they could not detect at that time (47).

Since then, the holy grail of drug test manufacturers has been to demonstrate that their particular test is not impacted by adulterants (48–50). Drug test manufactures are also developing systems for the rapid detection of adulterants. The goal of some drug users has been to find new materials

TABLE 14.3. Problems in testing.

Forms	Types	Manner
Adulteration	Dilution	Excess drinking Diuretics
	Breaking down the drug	Oxidizing agents
	Interference with the ability of the test to detect the drug	Changes the pH
Substitution	Precollection	Replace the urine in the bladder with a substitute
	Collection	Bladder systems Secreted container
	Postcollection	Tampering

that will adulterate the test without being detected. A number of Internet-based companies sell materials that they claim will thwart the test. Currently, in most testing programs, pH, specific gravity, creatinine, and oxidizing agents are checked (51–54).

Adulterants are of three basic types:

1. Those that decrease the concentration of the drug without altering the drug (dilution).
2. Those that break down the drug itself, typically using oxidizing agents.
3. Those that interfere with the ability of the assay to detect the drug (pH).

Dilution

Dilution remains the most common method. Water or other liquids added to a urine sample will dilute a drug to a low concentration that is undetectable with the screening test or, if detected, is below the cut-off level. Dilution can be achieved by drinking fluids or taking diuretics to increase urine flow and produce urine that is more dilute than it would otherwise be. It can also lead to water intoxication if carried to extreme. The best way to deal with dilution is to minimize the amount of time the person has to drink fluids prior to the test. In drug court, for example, minimal advance notice should be given.

Dilution by adding exogenous fluid to the specimen is minimized by not having a source of flowing water in the test room. Any standing water, such as in toilet bowls, should have a color additive in it (27).

Oxidizing Agents

Oxidizing agents are often added to a sample by drug users seeking to avoid a positive test. Some oxidizing agents will break down marijuana and morphine metabolites that are the basis for the screening tests.

Bleach, nitrite, hydrogen peroxide-peroxidase, chromate, iodate, periodate, and persulfate are examples of oxidizing agents. Iodine proved to be particularly problematic because it was not detected by older drug testing systems. The problem of oxidizing agents is typically addressed by testing for them in the sample if there is the presence of some unknown interfering agent with the screening test (55,56).

Urine is not the only matrix subject to adulteration. Several mouthwash products are being advertised as having the ability to confound saliva tests. These products clear the residual drug through rinsing but do not directly impact the drug. Ordinary mouthwash would likely do the same (57).

Interference with the Assay Process

The primary way that clients may interfere with the assay process is through alteration of the acidity (pH) of the urine. This is commonly done by taking vitamin C or drinking acidic fruit juices, both of which will acidify the urine, in the hours before the test is done. The method to counter this is to check the urine pH directly after the sample is collected.

Substitution

Substitution is the replacement of the donor's urine with another substance. The most common substitution substance is urine from another person who is presumably drug free. Other substitution substances such as Visine™, saline, and water have been tried.

Substitution may occur:

1. Before the urine is collected by introduction of the substance into the client's bladder by catheter or syringe.
2. During collection by use of a bladder system or secreted container.
3. After collection by tampering.

Substitution can be minimized by the careful training of collectors and the introduction of systems to prevent it.

Chemical Factors

Tests for drugs are chemical reactions. They work in certain ranges of temperature, pH, and concentrations of other materials. Drug test manufacturers make assumptions about these ranges and design the tests accordingly. If the donor adds something to the matrix, these factors may be changed, resulting in an inability to run the test (an invalid test) or in a false-negative result. By checking these parameters and defining acceptable ranges, interference with the test can be reduced, although not totally eliminated.

Testing Systems

There are two levels of testing:

1. Screening.
2. Confirmatory.

Screening Tests

Screening tests are highly sensitive. They may react with a number of substances and detect a variety of substances other than the desired drug. For example, a nonsteroidal antiinflammatory drug, oxaprozin, has been shown to result in a positive drug screen with certain systems (58). Quinolones (antibiotics) can cause false-positive urine screening results in a number of assay systems (59). As these interfering agents are recognized, tests are often further refined to minimize the problem.

Drug testing methods of any type should have high validity. Validity is a function of chemical factors that influence the test outcome (specificity, sensitivity, and accuracy) and pharmacologic considerations including dose, time of administration relative to the test, and route of drug administration. Validity can be considered to include confirmation of initial test results by a different chemical method. When litigation is a possibility, the methods must be highly accurate, reliable, and specific for the drug (21).

Colorimetric

A colorimetric test is a simple screening test where the drug causes a color change in an indicator. This tends to be the most rapid and inexpensive of the screening tests. It is qualitative; the presence of the drug is indicated by the formation of a colored chemical compound (29). One system that has been used in pediatric practice screens high-risk children for drug abuse in the clinic (point of service) using a colorimetric system called "TRIAGE" and following up positive tests with a confirmatory test. However, colorimetric tests have low specificity and are subject to interpretation, especially if the color change is subtle or faint. The potential for both false-negative and false-positive results exists (60). This system used alone would be problematic for settings in which a positive test has negative consequences.

Spectrophotometry

Ultraviolet or visible spectrophotometry is another colorimetric test that can be used for screening. Each substance has its own absorption spectrum that is determined by its structure. By measuring the absorption against the spectrum, a determination of what is present can be made. When used as a screening test, this has problems of yielding false-positive results similar to other colorimetric tests. This screening level should not be confused with the gas chromatography–mass spectrometer systems used for confirmation (29).

Immunoassays

Immunoassays use antibodies that attach to drug molecules. Various immunoassays are used (29):

1. The EMIT test (enzyme multiplied immunoassay technique).
2. The ELISA test (enzyme linked immunosorbent assay).
3. The RIA test (radioimmunoassay).
4. Fluorescent polarization immunoassays (not in common use because they can show false-positive results for barbiturates and benzodiazepines after ibuprofen is taken).

Chromatography

Chromatography is a separation process in which different materials dissolved in a common solvent are separated from each other by differential distribution of the solute between two phases. Once separated, the drug is measured by various means.

Thin-layer chromatography is one such method used for screening drug tests. It is generally inexpensive and simple to perform. A relative migration factor (movement of the material in question) is calculated by comparing it with a known material. The relative migration determines the substance. Although rapid and low cost, thin-layer chromatography lacks the sensitivity and specificity of immunoassays and is also highly operator dependent (29).

Gas chromatography is used to separate materials by vaporizing them and carrying the vaporized mixture with an inert gas and measuring the mixture by one of several methods. Various detectors are used, including flame ionization, electron capture, and nitrogen phosphorus (29).

Confirmatory Tests

Although screening tests are gaining better specificity, they are inherently designed to detect a wider range of substances to be further tested. Drug programs should never rely on the results of a screening test alone. A positive screen should always be followed by a more specific test system that is at least as specific as a gas chromatography–mass spectrometer (GC-MS). Gas chromatography–mass spectrometry meets the requirements for accuracy and precision and quickly became the method of choice for confirming screening results. When a screening test and GC-MS confirmation are used, false-positive rates are very low (60,61).

When errors in the combined screening and GC-MS systems occur, they are usually false negatives. Ibuprofen can also cause a false-negative result in some GC-MS systems. Other adulterants, including benzalkonium chloride or other antimicrobial preservative in Visine™, vinegar, lemon juice, goldenseal tea, lye crystals, and liquid soap, can all cause false-negative results in immunoassays (22). Falsely screened negative tests in most practical situations are not confirmed with the GC-MS portion (61–63).

References

1. Grinspoon L, Bakalar JB. The war on drugs: a peace proposal. N Engl J Med 1994;330(5):357–360.
2. National Institute on Drug Abuse. Urine Testing for Drugs of Abuse. NIDA Research Monograph Series 73. Washington, DC: National Institute on Drug Abuse; 1986.
3. Smith D. Medical Review Officer Course. Evanston, IL: American College of Occupational and Environmental Medicine; 2000.
4. Barnaby B, Drummond C, McCloud A, Burns T, Omu N. Substance misuse in psychiatric inpatients: comparison of a screening questionnaire survey with case notes. BMJ 2004;184:439–445.

5. Katz NP, Sherburne S, Beach M, Rose RJ, Vielguth J, Bradley J, Fanciullo GJ. Behavioral monitoring and urine toxicology testing in patients receiving long-term opioid therapy. Anesth Analg 2003;97:1097–1102.
6. Fishbain DA, Cutler RB, Rosomoff HL, Rosomoff RS. Validity of self-reported drug use in chronic pain patients. Clin J Pain 1999;15(3):184–191.
7. Ehrman RN, Robbins SJ, Cornish JW. Comparing self-reported cocaine use with repeated urine tests in outpatient cocaine abusers. Exp Clin Psychopharmacol 1997;5(2):150–156.
8. Weiss RD, Najavits LM, Greenfield SF, Soto JA, Shaw SR, Wyner D. Validity of substance use self-reports in dually diagnosed outpatients. Am J Psychiatry 1998;155(1):127–128.
9. Calhoun PS, Bosworth HB, Hertzberg MA, Sampson WS, Feldman ME, Kirby AC, Wampler TP, Tate-Williams F, Moore SD, Beckman JC. Drug use and validity of substance use self-reports in veterans seeking help for posttraumatic stress disorder. J Consult Clin Psychol 2000;68(5):923–927.
10. Mason D, Birmingham L, Grubin D. Substance use in remand prisoners: a consecutive case study. BMJ 1997;315(7099):18–23.
11. Lundy A, Gottheil E, McLellan AT, Weinstein SP, Sterling RC, Serota RD. Underreporting of cocaine use at post-treatment follow-up and the measurement of treatment effectiveness. J Nerv Ment Dis 1997;185(7):459–462.
12. Normand J, Salyards SD, Mahoney JJ. An evaluation of preemployment drug testing. J Appl Psychol 1990;75(6):629–639.
13. Kaye DL. Office recognition and management of adolescent substance abuse. Curr Opin Pediatr 2004;16(5):532–541.
14. Weinberg NZ, Rahdert E, Colliver JD, Glantz MD. Adolescent substance abuse: a review of the past 10 years. J Am Acad Child Adolesc Psychiatry 1998;37(3):252–261.
15. Fretthold D. Drug-testing methods and reliability. J Psychoactive Drugs 1990; 22(4):419–428.
16. Kilvert P, Bryant R. Drug testing has been used in schools for several years. BMJ 1996;312(7047):1671.
17. Kazlauskas R, Howe C, Trout G. Strategies for rhEPO detection in sport. Clin J Sport Med 2002;12(4):229–235.
18. Annas GJ. Testing poor pregnant women for cocaine: physicians as police investigators. N Engl J Med 2001;344(22):1729–1732.
19. Fraser A, Zamecnik J. Substance abuse monitoring by the Correctional Service of Canada. Ther Drug Monit 2003;25:723–727.
20. Osterlo JD, Becker CE. Chemical dependency and drug testing in the workplace. West J Med 1990;152:506–513.
21. Cone EJ. New Developments in Biological Measures of Drug Prevalence. NIDA Research Monograph Series 167. Washington, DC: National Institute on Drug Abuse; 1997:108–129.
22. Lessenger JE. Drug programs and testing. In Lessenger JE, ed. Agricultural Medicine: A Practical Guide. New York: Springer; 2006:98–112.
23. Josefson D. Arkansas bans selling of clean urine to beat drug testing. BMJ 2003; 326(7384):300.
24. Drury DL, Masci V, Jacobson JW, McNutt RA. Urine drug screening: can counterfeit urine samples pass inspection. J Occup Environ Med 1999;41(8): 622–624.

25. Kapur B, Hershkop S, Koren G, Gaughan V. Urine fingerprinting: detection of sample tampering in an opiate dependency program. Ther Drug Monit 1999; 21(2):243–250.
26. Fraser AD, Zamecnik J. Impact of lowering the screening and confirmation cutoff values for urine drug testing based on dilution indicators. Ther Drug Monit 2003;25(6):723–727.
27. U.S. Department of Transportation. Procedure for Transportation Workplace Drug and Alcohol Testing Programs. Fed Reg 2004;69(216):64865–64868.
28. Barbanel C, Winkelman J, Fischer G, King A. Confirmation of the Department of Transportation criteria for a substituted urine specimen. J Occup Environ Med 2002;44(5):407–409.
29. Ostrea E. Understanding drug testing in the neonate and the role of meconium analysis. J Perinat Neonat Nurs 2001;14(4):61–82.
30. Verstraete AG. Detection times of drugs of abuse in blood, urine, and oral fluid. Ther Drug Monit 2004;26(2):200–205.
31. Moeller MR. Hair analysis as evidence in forensic cases. Ther Drug Monit 1996;18(4):444–449.
32. Kintz P. Drug testing in addicts: a comparison between urine, sweat, and hair. Ther Drug Monit 1996;18(4):450–455.
33. Kintz P, Villain M, Ludes B. Testing for the undetectable in drug-facilitated sexual assault using hair analyzed by tandem mass spectrometry as evidence. Ther Drug Monit 2004;26(2):211–214.
34. Miller M, Donnelly B, Martz R. The Forensic Application of Testing Hair for Drugs of Abuse. NIDA Research Monograph Series 167. Washington, DC: National Institute on Drug Abuse; 1997:146–159.
35. Kintz P, Samyn N. Use of alternative specimens: drugs of abuse in saliva and doping agents in hair. Ther Drug Monit 2002;24(2):239–246.
36. Hoffman BH. Analysis of race effects on drug-test results. J Occup Environ Med 1999;41(7):612–614.
37. Cone EJ. Mechanisms of drug incorporation into hair. Ther Drug Monit 1996; 18(4):438–443.
38. Vinner E, Vignau J, Thibault D, Codaccioni X, Brassart C, Humbert L, Lhermitte M. Neonatal hair analysis contribution to establishing a gestational drug exposure profile and predicting a withdrawal syndrome. Ther Drug Monit 2003;25(4):421–432.
39. Ostrea EM Jr, Knapp DK, Tannenbaum L, Ostrea AR, Romero Al, Salari V, Ager J. Estimates of illicit drug use during pregnancy by maternal interview, hair analysis, meconium analysis. J Pediatr 2001;138(3):344–348.
40. Toennes S, Steinmeyer S, Maurer H, Moeller MR, Kauert GF. Screening for drugs of abuse in oral fluid—correlation of analysis results with serum in forensic cases. J Anal Toxicol 2005;29:22–27.
41. Palmeri A, Pichini S, Pacifici R, Zuccaro P, Lopez A. Drugs in nails. Clin Pharmacokinet 2000;38(2):95–110.
42. Forrest A. Guidelines are needed if drug testing those arrested by the police becomes compulsory. BMJ 2000;320(7226):56.
43. Gore SM, Bird AG. Mandatory drug tests in prison. BMJ. 1995;310(6979):595.
44. Gentilello LM, Samuels PN, Henningfield JE, Santora PB. Alcohol screening and intervention in trauma centers: confidentiality concerns and legal considerations. J Trauma Inj Infect Crit Care 2005;59:1250–1255.

45. U.S. Nuclear Regulatory Commission. Fitness for duty programs. Fed Reg 1989; 54:24494.
46. Swotinsky RB, Smith DR. The Medical Review Officer's Manual: MROCC's Guide to Drug Testing, 3rd ed. Beverly Farms, MA: OEM Press; 2006.
47. Milkelsen S, Ash KO. Adulterants causing false negatives in illicit drug testing. Clin Chem 1988;34(11):2333–2336.
48. Cooper G, Wilson L, Reid C, Baldwin D, Hand C, Spiehler V. Validation of the Cozart® microplate EIA for analysis of opiates in oral fluid. Forensic Sci Int 2005;154(2–3):240–246.
49. Cirimele V, Kintz P, Lohner S, Ludes B. Enzyme immunoassay validation for the detection of buprenorphine in urine. J Anal Toxicol 2003;27:103–105.
50. Cirimele V, Etienne S, Villain M, Ludes B, Kintz P. Evaluation of the One-step™ ELISA kit for the detection of buprenorphine in urine, blood and hair specimens. Forensic Sci Int 2004;143(2–3):153–156.
51. Dasgupta A, Chught O, Hannah C, Davis B, Wells A. Comparison of spot tests with AdultaCheck 6 and Intect 7 urine test strips for detecting the presence of adulterants in urine specimens. Clin Chim Acta 2004;348(1–2):19–25.
52. Peace M, Tarnai L. Performance evaluation of three on-site adulterant detection devices for urine specimens. J Anal Toxicol 2002;26(7):464–470.
53. Dasgupta A, Wahed A, Wells A. Rapid spot tests for detecting the presence of adulterants in urine specimens submitted for drug testing. Am J Clin Pathol 2002;17:325–329.
54. Wu A, Bristol B, Sexton K, Cassella-McLan G, Holtman V, Hill D. Adulteration of urine by "Urine Luck." Clin Chem 1999;45(7):1051–1057.
55. Paul BD, Jacobs A. Spectrophotometric detection of iodide and chromic (III) in urine after oxidation to iodine and chromate (VI). J Anal Toxicol 2005;29:658–663.
56. Paul BD, Jacobs A. Effects of oxidizing adulterants of detection 11-nor-delta9-THC-9-carboxylic acid in urine. J Anal Toxicol 2002;26(7):460–463.
57. Wong R, Tran M, Tung J. Oral fluid drug tests: effects of adulterants and foodstuffs. Forensic Sci Int 2005;150(2–3):175–180.
58. Pulini M. False-positive benzodiazepine urine test due to oxaprozin. JAMA 1995;273(24):1905.
59. Lindsey RB, Horowitz G, Jacoby H, Eliopoulos G. Quinolones and false-positive urine screening for opiates by immunoassay technology. JAMA 2001;26:3115–3119.
60. Valentine JL, Komoroski EM. Use of a visual panel detection method for drugs of abuse: Clinical and laboratory experience with children and adolescents. J Pediatr 1995;126(1):135–140.
61. Peat MA. Analytical and technical aspects of testing for drug abuse; confirmatory procedures. Clin Chem 1988;34(3):471–473.
62. Nordgren HK, Beck O. Multicomponent screening for drugs of abuse. Ther Drug Monit 2004;26(1):90–97.
63. Taylor PJ, Forrest KK, Landsberg PG, Mitchell C, Pillans PI. The measurement of nicotine in human plasma by high performance liquid chromatography-electrospray-tandem mass spectrometry. Ther Drug Monit 2004;26(5):563–568.

15
The Drug and Alcohol Testing Process

Richard L. McIntire, James E. Lessenger, and Glade F. Roper

This chapter describes the organization and operation of drug and alcohol testing for drug court clients. The focus is on a program in which the clients pay for their own testing. However, grant- or government-financed programs can be operated in much the same manner.

Goals

Drug testing is done primarily to hold drug court clients accountable for the truth related to their recent sobriety and use or abstinence from the use of drugs. It also gives clients a powerful reason to abstain from drug use and can furnish them with a ready excuse for abstinence when approached by drug-using associates. Because honesty with the court, counselors, friends, and family is a critical element of sustained recovery, the goal in operating an effective drug testing program is not just randomly testing and reporting results. It must also include an integrated and complicated process that complements the recovery program efforts put forth by the participants.

The drug testing process must:

1. Provide unannounced testing on a random schedule.
2. Ensure a reasonable frequency of testing according to client need.
3. Prevent adulteration, tampering, and substitution.
4. Provide same-day reporting of results to key program participants, such as counselors and the court.
5. Ensure accuracy.
6. Ensure reliability.
7. Be affordable for the clients.

Random Drug Testing

An ideal testing program would involve testing daily or several times a day. Such a program would have the advantages of rapidly detecting all drug use and serve as a constant deterrent. In practice, such a system would be prohibitively expensive and unduly intrusive on the lives of the participants. The reasonable alternative is periodic random testing. For testing to be optimally effective, it must be random, with appropriate frequency, on any of the 365 days of the year. The clients must have minimal prior notification of when they will be tested. This chapter describes a testing program that has proved successful in a drug court for over 10 years. With modifications and improvements, the system has become an essential component of the functioning drug court.

Group Card

Upon entry into the drug court program, each client is provided with an orientation about the drug testing process by the drug testing agency. The clients are issued a "group card" that contains a summary of the information they learned from the orientation. On the front of the card is the identification of the testing group to which they have been assigned. Clients in Phase 1 are issued a group testing number, such as "51" or "41." The digit identifies their gender (male or female), and the second digit identifies their drug court phase.

The phase identification also determines the frequency with which they will be tested each month. In the early phase, testing is more frequent, and in subsequent phases (2, 3, and aftercare), testing is less frequent. The frequencies are established by the drug court steering committee and administered by the drug testing agency.

Numbers are preferred over colors or symbols because of the flexibility, recorded announcement clarity, and expandability a numbering system serves. Using "group orange, red, and blue" can work well in smaller programs. However, as the number of clients grows, adding groups "magenta, cyan, puce, and fuchsia" can become confusing when announced on a recording, and the number of colors available is limited. A large segment of the male client population may have some degree of color deficiency. A numbering system allows sufficient flexibility to insert special group numbers with different testing frequencies needed to serve the unique circumstances of a group of clients who, for example, will be tested only for alcohol or tested for additional (expanded) drugs of abuse.

In addition to the group identification number on the front of the card, the message telephone number is provided as well as a summary of the testing hours of operation. Testing hours can be modified to suit the needs of each drug court. However, after experimenting over a 9-year period, expanding hours of testing to include early morning and early evening hours produced little if any appreciable benefit to the program or the clients. Often, clients who complained that they were unable to complete their testing because of their job or other daily activities and used this excuse for missing tests, continued to miss their testing requirements when testing hours were expanded.

Operating during regular weekdays from 9:00 am to 5:00 pm and from 9:00 am to 12:00 noon on weekends and holidays has proven over time to be the most effective and efficient testing schedule, and very few people have been inconvenienced by it.

The key to operating during these regular business hours is being able to process each client in less than 2 minutes, which enables them to complete their testing requirements on a rest or a lunch break from their job. The clients are best served if they can complete the testing requirements without causing a major disruption in their normal daily routine of work or school.

The back of the group card contains a summary of the instructions for the client. These instructions are as follows:

1. Every day (7 days a week), you are required to call (phone number) AFTER 7:00 am and listen to the entire recorded message.
2. If your assigned group number is announced, you are required to go to your testing site and submit to the testing process.
3. You must arrive at the test site between the hours of 9:00 am and 5:00 pm Monday through Friday or 9:00 am to 12:00 noon on weekends and holidays.
4. You may be tested any day, even 2 or 3 days in a row.
5. When you arrive at the test site, you are required to pay $(fee amount) cash BEFORE your sample will be taken.
6. Failure to follow any of the above instructions will be reported immediately to the drug court judge and to your counseling provider.

The requirement to call the testing announcement number after 7:00 am every day is an important element in the testing program that should be strictly enforced. The more notification time clients are given, the more time they will have to attempt to frustrate the testing process by consuming large quantities of water (flushing or diluting their urine) or devising a method of substituting "clean" urine for their own. Recording a fresh announcement every day at 7:00 am to announce the testing group(s) that is required to test that day has proven to give ample time for the clients to arrange their day to include their testing requirement.

A standard testing announcement might sound something like this: "Wednesday, August third, Groups 41, 42, 44, 51, and 59 must test today." On occasion, informational announcements are added to the message that might include something like: "Clients are reminded to arrive at the collection site ready to provide a sample" or "Clients are reminded not to smoke in or around the testing facility." These occasional announcements are designed to encourage improved social behaviors and to help the clients learn to follow the drug court rules. On holidays, the announcement includes a reminder that holiday hours will be observed and that they must test before noon.

Necessity of a Completely Random System

The instruction that the clients may be tested on any day, even 2 or 3 days in a row, is important to keep the clients from thinking that they can safely use drugs shortly after their testing because the drugs will likely clear from their system in 2 to 3 days and they will be clean for the next test day. Often, clients will create a calendar and track the past testing days looking for patterns or standard frequencies from which they can plan their drug use. This is why it is critical to develop a completely random testing system that has no identifiable patterns or standard frequencies. At least once a month, it is important to test the clients "back-to-back" on a Friday and then Saturday because weekend drug use is a common pattern. Often, after having been involved in the program for more than a month, clients will leave the testing facility and say "see you tomorrow" to the testing facility collector, who will respond "see you tomorrow," both acknowledging that the client fully understands that they have no idea when their next testing day will be and that it may be the next day. This is a significant milestone of achievement in the mind set of the clients who clearly understand that they cannot beat the random testing system by studying past practices. If planned properly, there will never be any recognizable pattern to detect.

Confidentiality of the random calendar is critical to maintaining this system of random testing. The fewer people who know when and what groups will be tested, the greater the likelihood of maintaining an effective random testing program.

Holiday testing is an important element in the random testing program. However, actually testing on the day of the holiday is not necessarily the best practice. As an example, July 4th may be a potential "party day" on which relapse has a greater likelihood of occurring. In this case, testing on July 5th or 6th would be more appropriate to identify a relapse than testing on the 4th.

Testing frequency is used to maintain an effective random program and should be based on a monthly frequency range rather than a weekly one. In other words, establishing a rule that the clients must test at least twice a week is detrimental to an effective random program, whereas establishing a rule that the clients must test six to eight times per month allows for a much more random program. This gives the option of testing back to back and then again just 2 days later. This also allows for a period of 8 or 9 days to elapse before the next random test occurs. Experience has shown that allowing as many as 8 or 9 days to elapse without testing is effective on occasion. After about 4 or 5 days of not testing, clients believe that the next day will be a testing day, then the next day, and the next, which tends to keep them from relapsing if presented with the opportunity.

Allowing these occasional spans of days in which no random testing takes place provides opportunities to complete back-to-back testing and occasional testing 3 days in a row. It is recommended that more than 10 days without testing be avoided and that spans of 2 to 6 days be the norm, with each day of the week being used for testing. Having clients test on fixed days of the week is both ineffective and inefficient in promoting abstinence from drug use. Equally ineffective is only testing clients a fixed number of times per month (two or three), because after the second or third test the clients will know that they will not be testing the remainder of the month.

An effective random testing program with adequate frequency that includes weekends and holidays can be a powerful service to the drug court program and especially to the clients, who learn to appreciate that while they achieve levels of trust as they work through the drug court program, there will always be verification required by the court to ensure that they are being honest.

The Collection Process

The collection of urine samples from drug court clients is clearly as important, if not more important, than the laboratory testing process. If the urine sample is adulterated in any way, it will frustrate the testing process and invalidate the results. If clients are successful in beating the system through some creative means of adulterating or substituting their submitted urine sample, they will delay their recovery. The importance of administering a tightly controlled collection process cannot be overstated, because it is clear that once the clients realize they cannot beat the system, they begin to embrace the important steps toward sobriety and recovery.

The collection process is most effective when collection personnel of the same gender directly observe the deposit of urine into a collection cup. An absolute rule should be adopted that if the urine is not seen flowing directly from the urethra it is not the client's urine and should not be accepted. When the collector observes the collection, the clients will find it extremely difficult to add substances to their urine sample after it has left their body. There are many clever methods of adding foreign substances into a urine sample. However, most, if not all, of these methods cannot be accomplished under effective direct observation.

Collection Steps

Each client is required to present a government-issued photo identification card at each drug test. Further security may be afforded by requiring a thumbprint on the collection form. However, the most important security point is that the collection personnel get to know the clients by sight.

After clients are processed and present themselves to have a urine specimen taken, they are required to wash their hands under direct supervision (Table 15.1). This procedure is intended to remove any substances on their hands or under their fingernails. This activity prevents them from urinating

TABLE 15.1. Steps in the collection process.

1. Register the client: photo identification, fingerprints, personal identification.
2. Have the client wash his or her hands to remove adulterants.
3. Observe the donation:
   a. Observation must be by same-sex personnel.
   b. Clothing that might hide devices must be observed.
   c. The genitalia and urine stream must be observed.
4. Check the urine temperature. If outside the range of 90° to 100°F, then collect a second sample.
5. Send the specimen to the laboratory.
6. Save a frozen sample if the specimen returns positive.
7. Transmit results to the court, probation officers, and counselors.

across their hands or fingertips and introducing a foreign substance (adulterants) into the sample cup.

The next step is to enter a urinal collection area for males and a toilet collection area for females along with a same-gender collector who controls the collection cup. The collection areas should have installed mirrors that provide visual access to all areas of the client's body from all angles. This not only provides clear viewing of the voiding process by the collector but also serves as an effective deterrent for those clients inclined to attempt an adulteration or substitution activity. An effective urine sample collection is best accomplished when a clear view of the genital area of the client is created while the void is taking place. Anything less allows the clients to creatively conceal various devices that, if undetected, will frustrate the testing process and delay the client's recovery process.

A same-gender collector should be immediately present during the collection process, anywhere from 12 to 36 inches from the client, and adjust themselves as necessary in order to directly view the sample collection. If necessary, the clients should be required to remove certain items of clothing that block the genital area from view while the void is taking place.

Once the client is clearly in view of the collector, the client is instructed to provide a midstream sample. The client is instructed to start the urine stream and then stop. At that point, the collector hands the client the collection cup (labeled with the client's information) and the client is instructed to continue the void into the cup with a minimum of 30 mL of urine. After filling the collection cup, the client hands the cup back to the collector and finishes voiding into the urinal or toilet. While the collector checks the temperature of the sample to ensure that it is within 90° to 100°F (valid temperature), the client is allowed to wash his or her hands and leave the facility.

A midstream urine collection (start, stop, start) is important in order to demonstrate a normal level of urine stream control; it also optimizes the prevention of a client substituting a sample. In addition, the midstream sample allows the draw of urine from the middle or bottom of the bladder where drug metabolites can settle. In the event a substituted sample is detected by the collector (no device was visually detected but urine is less than 90° degrees or greater than 100°F), a second sample is required from the client who must remain at the collection facility under observation by the collection staff and is allowed to drink up to 40 ounces of water until a second sample is provided. In most cases, the second sample will test positive while the first sample will test negative, clearly indicating that the first sample was substituted. Drug court probation terms must include a provision that the clients are required to remain and provide another sample if the collection staff suspect any tampering with or falsification of a sample.

Training of Collection Personnel

The training of collection personnel in detecting substitution or adulteration attempts is an important aspect of being an effective collector. Training cannot anticipate all of the creative scams used by clients. Training must teach collectors to be intuitive about mannerisms, posture, and unusual behaviors of the clients that will help them detect and prevent such attempts. Training must also clearly explain the need for direct observation and overcome any embarrassment or squeamishness about scrutinizing the genitalia of the clients while they provide a specimen.

It is important to train collection staff on what to do when confronted with bribes or belligerent behavior. Role playing, standard operating procedures, and careful instructions can overcome this problem. Also important is a dedicated phone in the collection area to call the police if necessary.

Because the testing process is critical to success of the drug court, appropriate sanctions must be implemented for disruptions to the process. Clients who attempt to adulterate or falsify the samples should have significant sanctions imposed immediately. This response will send a clear message to the offending client as well as to the rest of the drug court participants. Clients who assault, threaten, or attempt to bribe testing personnel are probably not amenable to further participation in the drug court, and consideration should be given to immediate expulsion whenever such an offense is proven.

Accuracy and Reliability

The accuracy and reliability of the testing results is a significant component of the process. However, the manner in which accuracy and reliability are achieved must be balanced with the cost of the process in order to keep costs low and affordable for the clients. Urine samples are first tested using a laboratory double immunoassay (EMIT) process in which the results are tested for all drugs of abuse. Then, if the sample is determined to be positive for one or more drugs, the original index sample is tested again for only those drugs in order to confirm the first positive result.

A secondary testing method such as gas chromatography–mass spectrometry or thin-layer chromatography testing is not completed at this point in the process in order to avoid the costs of extra, and often unnecessary, processing. When the clients appear in court, they are asked if they have been clean and sober since their last appearance before the judge. At this point, they are faced with the choice of telling the truth or telling a lie. Because the behavior of not being truthful is swiftly punished, the clients learn early in the program that they are rewarded for their truthfulness. If they have relapsed or abused substances between court visits, they often admit such behavior to the judge, thereby confirming the positive result established in the double EMIT testing process, and no further confirmation testing is necessary.

Reporting Results to the Client

There are advantages and disadvantages to reporting the results to the clients prior to their appearing in court. The drug court team must decide which approach to use.

Withholding Results to Promote Honesty

Test results must be reported to the court in a timely manner, usually within 1 day of the test. Results should also be reported to the treatment provider as soon as possible. Not informing the client of the results has the advantage of forcing the client to wrestle with the question of whether to be honest with the counselors and the judge.

Addiction causes such intense cravings that those in the early stages of attempting recovery will experience powerful incentives to continue drug use. The drive to use is insurmountable in many individuals, who succumb and use drugs despite their determination not to. In a moment of exposure to the drug, they deceive themselves by numerous stratagems such as, "I just need to use this once, and then never again," "My wife made me so mad, I need to use just this time to settle me down," "Once this bag is gone I will never buy another," or "I probably won't have to test for the next few days because I just tested this morning." Because the physiologic reward of drug use is intense, the benefit of dishonesty is reinforced with every use episode. Unless this cycle is arrested, the client will never cease drug use.

After drug use, clients experience guilt, shame, and an immediate desire to escape the consequences through flight, falsification, or dishonesty. The conflict between continuing in the program and facing adverse consequences or escaping the consequences through being dishonest comes to a head when they appear before the judge at the next status hearing.

Many participants will feel a strong bonding with the judge. This is particularly true of those who have experience before judges who have imposed punishments such as jail or prison. For the first time a judge has offered them help instead of punishment, an escape from the criminal justice system instead of internment within it. They feel a sense of gratitude to the judge and a desire to please him or her. For many, the judge assumes a parent-like role that engenders respect, affection, and a desire to please through compliance with drug court rules and abstinence from drug use.

After a drug use episode, the participant is faced with the decision whether to be honest and admit the use, thereby risking displeasure and disappointment from the judge or denying the use and hoping that the test results will not reflect it. Their rationality is clouded by fear and the effects of drug use, and they may "hope against hope" that the test will somehow not be positive, even while knowing that the potential for such a result is minuscule.

When the results of the drug and alcohol testing are not revealed to the clients before their court appearance, and when the judge asks the clients if they have been clean and sober since their last court appearance, only the judge, the probation officers, and the counseling providers are aware of the actual results. One approach is to ask them at the beginning of the status review whether they have been drug free since their last appearance; for example, "Hi Joe, have you been clean and sober since I saw you last?"

In that moment, the participant who has not been clean and sober will have to decide whether to admit the use or deny it. In such a setting it is not unusual to observe the struggle for several seconds before a response. It is particularly obvious to those knowing the test results.

At times, the clients will admit to a relapse in court when the testing results show a clean urine sample from their last test. Because many of the drugs of abuse metabolize out of their systems in 2 or 3 days, the random testing cycle may have tested them 4 or 5 days after that use, and the drugs will not be present in their urine sample. Under these circumstances, the judge should recognize and reward the honesty and apply appropriate sanctions but not inform the client of the clean test result. Treating the use episode with increased treatment rather than with punishment will enhance the benefits of honesty and engender continued honesty in the client, thus promoting future abstinence.

For those clients who tell the judge that they have been clean and sober since their last appearance in court when the double EMIT testing process has tested positive, the judge should tell them of the results and ask them to explain. At this point, many of the clients will simply admit that they "used" and lied to the judge. In rare cases, clients, after being told their test was positive, will deny that they used and will steadfastly maintain that they have been clean and sober since their last appearance. The judge then has an option of placing the clients in jail for a sanction or referring them back to the testing agency where a "put your money where your mouth is" process is implemented.

An effective strategy is to incarcerate the clients for a day or two, then bring them back to court and again inquire if they know how the drugs got into their system. Experience has shown that almost all of the time they will admit to use, whereupon they should be considered for reinstatement. This experience has a strong impact in reinforcing the need for honesty. It is more likely that in future opportunities for drug use the client will either resist the temptation to use or be honest about it.

The chief disadvantage of this procedure is that counselors who are aware of positive test results will not be able to confront the clients immediately after the results are known and may lose an opportunity to deal with the use episode rapidly. They may be placed in the uncomfortable position of obliquely attempting to elicit an admission to the use rather than openly discussing it. Counseling sessions under these conditions will have an artificial feel.

Informing the Client

Notifying the client of a positive test result allows the counselor to directly and immediately deal with the use episode. Appropriate treatment assignments can be given and denial broken in a timely manner.

It is still possible for the client to deny the use to both the counselor and the judge. Frequently, the client will deny use to the counselor but admit the use to the judge rather than risk sanctions for dishonesty. In such cases, the judge should carefully explain the need for honesty to the treatment staff as well as the court, for the benefit of the client. This is an opportunity for the judge to explain that unless the client develops a habit of being honest in all circumstances, the client will quickly return to drug use when involvement with the court ceases, and all the work and effort of getting clean will be lost. If the client continues to deny use to the judge, the same options are available as explained in the previous section.

Referral for Confirmatory Testing

Clients who adamantly deny drug use despite a positive test are offered an opportunity to appeal or contest the positive result by depositing the costs of a GC-MS test with the testing agency. The clients are told that if the test results from the double EMIT testing are confirmed at another independent laboratory by GC-MS testing methodology, then they have paid for the costs of that testing and the confirmed positive result will be reported back to the court. They are also told that if their results from the GC-MS testing come back negative, then this result will be reported back to the court and will reverse the original testing result, and they will be refunded the cost of the GC-MS testing. In other words, if they are confirmed dirty, they paid for it. If they are determined to be negative, then they will get their money back because the screen was inaccurate.

This becomes another decision point for the clients at which they must decide to waste their money if they know they have used or continue on with the appeal process knowing that they have not used. They also have the option of continuing with the appeal knowing that they have used and irrationally hoping for a negative confirmation. In most cases, the clients return back to court without depositing the money and admit to the judge that they used and lied. In some cases, the appeal process continues, and the original index sample is retrieved from frozen storage, packaged with an appropriate chain of custody, and sent to an independent laboratory for confirmation testing by GC-MS. Over 99% of the time, the result comes back confirmed, the court is notified, and the client suffers the consequences. In extremely rare circumstances, the original index sample will not be confirmed by GC-MS (typically borderline positives close to the cut-off level), and the clients are refunded their deposit with no sanctions by the court. It is imperative that confirmatory testing not be done at a higher cut-off level than the screening, or negative confirmations will be frequent. The GC-MS confirmations are accurate and must be arranged at a cut-off level equivalent to or lower than the screening cut-off level.

The double EMIT laboratory testing process combined with the "put your money where your mouth is" program has proven over the past 9 years to be effective in keeping the costs of the random drug testing program affordable for the clients, and, at the same time, it has proven to be extremely accurate and reliable as a tool in court. This process has also been effective in holding the clients accountable for their behaviors and has been beneficial in helping the clients learn to tell the truth.

Organization of Drug Testing Programs

This section reviews the key elements in the organization of the drug court drug testing program. These elements are:

1. Agreement with the court.
2. Drug testing locations.
3. Drug testing site design.
4. Forms and paperwork.
5. Laboratory management.
6. Result reporting.

Agreement with the Court

The nature of the agreements between the drug testing provider and the courts depends on the circumstances of the payment. In programs in which clients pay their own way, simple agreements between the provider and the probation department or courts may be sufficient. Such an agreement may spell out how many tests will be done, how the collections are conducted, and how the specimen will be tested.

In programs in which the court, probation department, or grants pay for the drug testing, formal performance contracts may be necessary. These agreements mainly concern accountability for money; however, they spell out the same points as the agreements: collection frequency, collection protocols, and testing methodologies.

Drug Testing Locations

The selection of the location is driven by geography and client density. Obviously, the collection point should be placed in a central area where most clients live and work. Other factors include expense, safety, availability of public transportation, accessibility for people with disabilities, and impact on the neighborhood.

Drug Testing Site Design

The testing site must be designed for easy accessibility and smooth flow. There must be a small waiting area, a check-in area for observing identification, a point for collection of hair or breath samples, and a toilet arrangement for observed, same-sex urine donations. It is also helpful to have the laboratory on the site to expedite the reporting of results. Although privacy is a concern, an open area with lots of collection personnel (except for the toilet) may prevent threats or bribe attempts on the collection staff. Installation of a urinal that does not retain water in the bottom will eliminate the potential for scooping water and make collection easier for men.

Forms and Paperwork

A one-page form should be designed to use for each test. The form is used to record the client identification, which tests were done, the results of witnessing, and the test results.

The form also serves as a chain-of-custody document for the laboratory and for positive specimens that need to be frozen. The original is kept on file at the testing provider, and copies are sent to the court, probation officers, and counselors.

Laboratory Management

Laboratories on the testing site provide rapid results and obviate the necessity of having to transport the samples and maintain a chain of custody while doing so. Regardless of the system used, basic laboratory procedures include the following:

1. Site security (the technician must come into eye contact with the donor to avoid attempts at intimidation and bribes).
2. Maintenance of the chain of custody and identification of the specimen.
3. Careful maintenance of equipment.
4. Appropriate training of the technicians.
5. Careful protective technique to avoid blood-borne exposures.
6. Proper reporting of results.
7. Secure storage of frozen specimens when the results are positive.
8. Appropriate disposal of gloves, specimens, cups, and so forth.

Result Reporting

The results of each test, negative or positive, must be reported to the court, probation officers, and counselors. All tests results should reach their destinations within 24 hours. Special results may be transmitted immediately to the court and probation officers in cases of:

1. Uncooperative or belligerent behavior.
2. Attempts at a bribe.
3. Evidence of improper identification (forgery or impersonation).
4. Evidence of adulteration, substitution, or tampering with the sample.

Conclusions

For drug testing to be effective in modifying drug-using behavior, it must have accuracy, reproducibility, and integrity. A system must be devised that anticipates forgeries, impersonation, substitution, adulteration, and tampering and guards against them. Truly random drug testing is a potent tool to promote abstinence and recovery and to bring clients to the realization that they cannot beat the system.

16
Drug Testing Scams

Richard L. McIntire and James E. Lessenger

A variety of scams are employed by drug court clients to circumvent the drug collection process and avoid detection of their drug use. There are five main ways in which clients attempt to avoid detection in drug testing (1):

1. Adulteration.
2. Tampering.
3. Substitution.
4. Impostors.
5. Bribes and threats.

We review these methods in this chapter.

The advantage of drug testing through the drug court collection process, in contrast to those of the U.S. Department of Transportation or industrial testing programs, is that the courts can:

1. Witness all tests with same-sex collectors.
2. Compel the physical examination of the client if the screening tests are outside the parameters of an acceptable test.
3. Perform on-site breath testing for alcohol and on-site monitoring for temperature and pH.
4. Standardize the collection and laboratory processes.
5. Generate reports to the court.

The Tulare County testing experience is presented in Table 16.1 (1). Although the numbers of persons who were caught tampering with their drug sample was relatively low (0.001%) when compared to the actual number of urine drug collections performed, the fact that they were caught confirms the integrity of the system.

Nobody is under the delusion that every cheater is caught, but the data demonstrate the numbers and types of scams being tried by clients. In addition, the Tulare County program couples the urine drug tests with a breathalyzer test. When the client presents to the check-in desk, he or she must submit to an alcohol breathalyzer to check for recent alcohol use. The two-step system increases the number of drugs tested and the accuracy.

TABLE 16.1. Scams and their extent (N = 171).

Scam	Number	Percent
Bottle of urine inside vagina	61	35.7
Temperature out of range and no device recovered	16	9.4
Impostor	12	7.0
Attempted bribe	11	6.5
Bottle of urine in female outside vagina	11	6.5
Bottle of urine, male	9	5.4
Rubber penis (includes rubber condom)	8	4.7
Client became abusive and walked out	8	4.7
Whizzinator™ without heater	8	4.7
Rubber balloon	5	2.9
Tampon soaked in bleach	4	2.4
Douche bag taped to the small of the back with a rubber tube	4	2.4
Blew a passive alcohol test and refused the rest of the process	2	1.1
Toothpaste tube with rubber tube attached	2	1.1
Whizzinator™ with heater	2	1.1
Synthetic urine substituted	2	1.1
No device or bottle found		
Turkey baster in vagina	2	1.1
Syringe with urine	2	1.1
Rubber grape	2	1.1
Totals	171	100.0

Source: Lessenger and McIntire (1).

Most of the scams detected were tried by women. It is theorized that this is because it is relatively tempting for women to attempt to secrete bottles of substitute urine in their vaginas in the belief that it will be difficult for a witness to detect.

In some situations, especially if the client was belligerent, the urine test was not requested after the scam was discovered. In those cases, the scam was discovered before the specimen was produced. In addition, some clients refused to go through with a drug test after their scam was discovered. After the scam was discovered, and if the specimen was obtained, the initial urine was typically sent into the laboratory anyway; 71.3% of the original specimens were negative and 4% tested positive for the presence of drugs. When the second witnessed urine was collected from the same clients, 5.0% were negative and 61% were positive.

The key to detecting collection scams (2) is an organization that:

1. Hires honest, reliable employees.
2. Trains its employees to maintain a chain of custody and witness the collections.
3. Maintains a physical plant that expedites witnessed collections.
4. Is aggressive in demanding identification, removal of outer clothing, hand washing, and inspections when screens are positive.

It is important to subject the specimen to a series of simple tests to make sure they are freshly produced, human specimens. These tests are for:

1. Color.
2. Odor.
3. pH (acidity and alkalinity).
4. Specific gravity.
5. Temperature.

Many clients committing a collection scam can be caught by using these screening tests on their urine samples. However, in a number of instances, no device was discovered, which suggests that they catheterized themselves and introduced some other person's urine.

Collection Scams by Category

Adulteration

Adulteration is the introduction of a substance into the donor's urine in an attempt to turn a positive test negative. A good example of this is the use of bleach-soaked tampons, referred to in Table 16.1. Most adulterants are household chemicals such as bleach, ammonia, baking soda, and the like. A more common method of introducing an adulterant into the urine sample is by caking the substance on their hands or under their fingernails. The screening tests quickly pick up these substances, and requiring the donors to wash their hands in the presence of the collector eliminates most of this. Other, more subtle, methods are the introduction of large amounts of a medication such as ibuprofen that can sometimes block or overwhelm some older and unsophisticated testing systems (Figure 16.1) (3,4).

Tampering

Tampering is the removal of the lid of the bottle and replacement of the urine with another person's urine or another substance. Tampering can be prevented by using security tape and placing the sample in a secure location, such as a locked refrigerator, until it is tested (4,5).

Substitution

Substitution (4,5) is the replacement of a person's urine with:

1. Another person's (presumably clean) urine.
2. A solution with the chemical constituents of urine.
3. Animal urine.
4. Water, bleach, ammonia, chlorine, or any other household chemical.

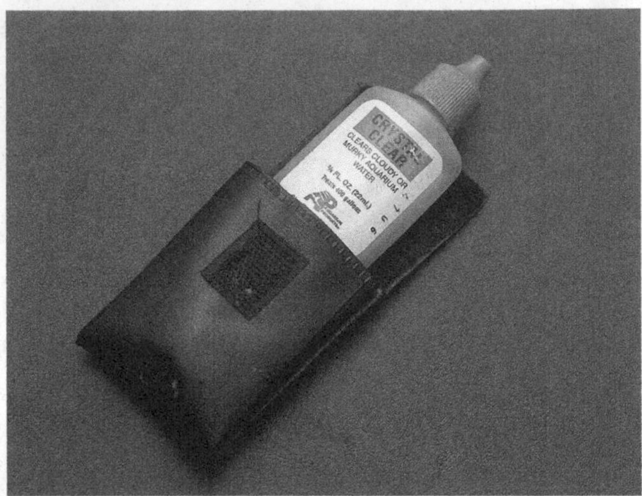

FIGURE 16.1. Adulterants to be added to the donor's urine.

There are several different methods of substitution. For males these include:

1. Artificial bladders and penises, with or without heaters (Figure 16.2).
2. Containers of fluid, either with or without heaters, secreted in pockets, the rectum, or underwear (Figure 16.3).
3. Contraptions such as douche bags, balloons, syringes, or other apparatus strapped to the back or thighs and with a tube running to the penis where it is either glued or taped (Figure 16.4).

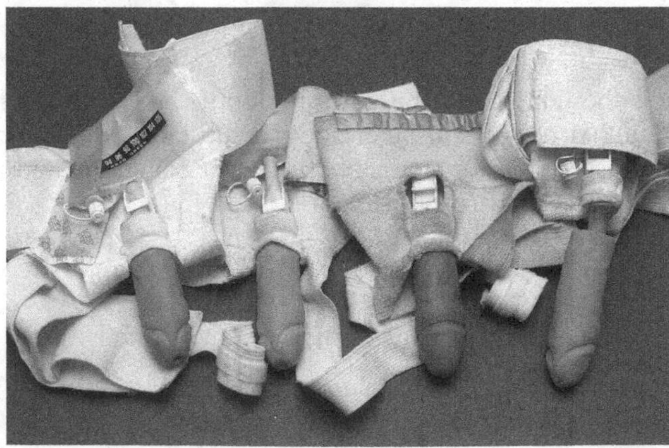

FIGURE 16.2. Artificial penises and bladders come in multiple skin tones and sizes, with and without heaters. These objects include the now-famous Whizzinator^{TM}.

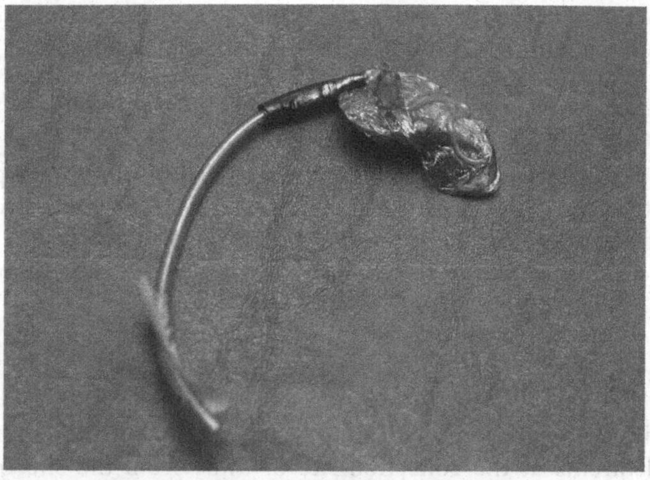

FIGURE 16.3. This condom with a tube taped to it was taped to the donor's penis. The specimen was too cold and the pH was abnormal. A second specimen tested positive.

Women typically secret bottles of substitute urine or fluid in their vaginas, underwear, or clothing. They may also strap or tape containers to their backs or thighs and run a tube between their legs (Figure 16.5). Their fingernails should be observed for sharpening into a point, used to prick the cover of a bottle inserted into the vagina. The donor must be required to keep her hands away from her pubic area prior to beginning urination. It

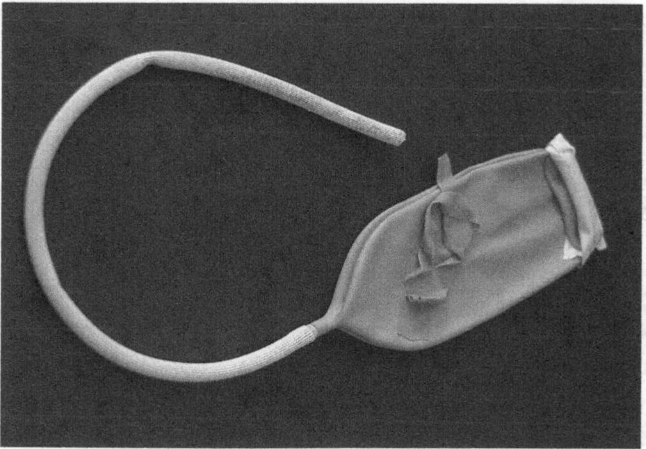

FIGURE 16.4. This douche bag was attached with straps to the back and to the penis with superglue.

is imperative that collectors watch the urine flow directly from the body. Close inspection will detect the openings of tubes and containers.

Impostors

Clients may entice friends or relatives through rewards of friendship, drugs, or money to pose as the client for donating a drug test sample. Ironically, some of those impostors may themselves be positive for drugs. Careful attention to identification of the donors is critical in the prevention of this scam.

Bribes and Threats

The most insidious problem with drug test collections is the potential for bribes and threats at the collection site or away from the site or at the laboratory. Many clients are desperate and looking at years in prison if they fail the test, so the pressure is present to attempt to bribe collection site personnel with drugs or money to allow a substitution of their urine. Desperation and the presence of drugs in their bloodstream, especially methamphetamines, can motivate donors to threats of violence against collection personnel and their families. These problems can be mitigated with:

1. Careful selection of collection staff.
2. Training of collection staff.
3. Well-lit facilities with barriers such as counters (Figure 16.6).
4. Immediate notification to appropriate authorities of threats or bribe attempts.

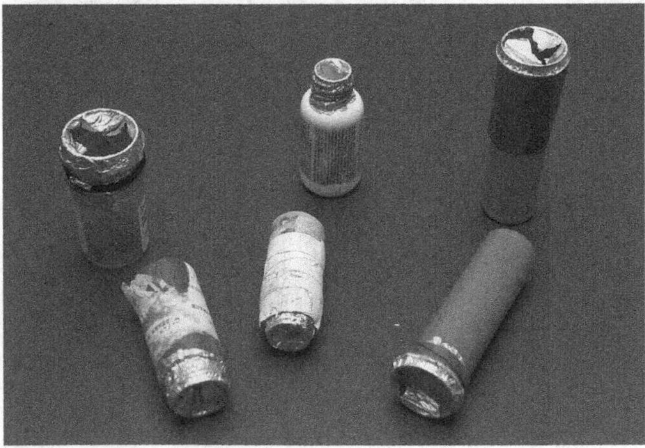

FIGURE 16.5. Containers secreted in the vaginas of donors. Fingernails will break the aluminum foil lids.

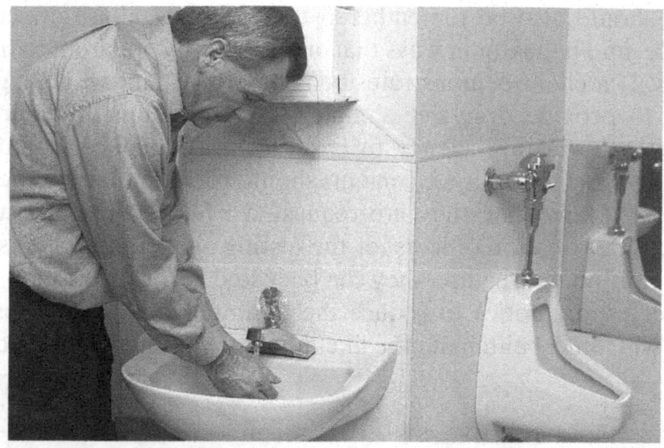

FIGURE 16.6. The facility should be well-lit and have barriers such as counters and with plenty of personnel so that nobody is left alone. This person is washing his hands before donating a specimen.

5. Ensuring the anonymity of the collection personnel and laboratory sites.
6. Monitoring the laboratory results and looking for trends that might suggest a falsification of the data.
7. Planting a decoy client who will attempt to bribe or threaten collection personnel to ensure that proper procedures are followed.

Conclusions

Maintenance of the integrity of the drug testing system is the key to the integrity of the entire drug court program. If clients think or know they can get away with scams to beat the drug tests, then they can get the idea that they can scam the judge, the counselors, and the probation officers. Eventually, that attitude will lead them to state prison.

This chapter has presented a collection of scams detected in a methodical manner. Clients can be very creative in trying to avoid facing the reality that they have a serious problem and that they are the cause of that problem. Therefore, more scams will be discovered every day, and drug court personnel must be vigilant to the creation of unique ways to beat the system.

It is important to note that, despite the best efforts of testing personnel, it is likely that some clients will succeed at defeating some tests. In a well-run testing program, these instances will be infrequent. Recognizing this, it should be remembered that drug court participants will be tested hundreds of times, usually over a 1- to 3-year period. It is highly unlikely that they will be successful in continuing their drug use undetected over a long period. It should also be remembered that drugs of abuse affect speech, appearance, and behavior in ways that are frequently apparent to treatment counselors. If a client demonstrates behavior consistent with drug use but continues to provide drug-free samples, the treatment providers should consult with the testing agency to ensure extra vigilance in looking for scams. Drug court terms or agreements should provide that the clients must submit to tests any time they are requested by the court, the treatment providers, the probation officers, or the testing agencies. If clients are suspected of continued drug use, they can be tested at more frequent intervals or with very short notice to reduce the potential for falsified tests. Such measures will almost eliminate the likelihood of continued undetected drug use.

References

1. Lessenger JE, McIntire R. Unpublished data. March 31, 2006.
2. Kerns DL, Stopperan WI. Keys to a successful program. Occup Health Saf 2000;69(10):230, 232–234.
3. Schwarzhoff R, Cody JT. The effects of adulterating agents on FPIA analysis of urine for drugs of abuse. J Anal Toxicol 1993;17(1):14–17.
4. Mikkelsen SL, Ash KO. Adulterants causing false negatives in illicit drug testing. Clin Chem 1998;34(11):2333–2336.
5. DuPont RL. Medicines and drug testing in the workplace. J Psychoactive Drugs 1990;22(4):451–459.

17
Analysis of Drug Testing Results

Olga A. Katz, Nikita B. Katz, Steven Mandel,
and James E. Lessenger

All scientific assays are potentially prone to errors, especially false-negative and false-positive results, which necessitates careful analysis of results. This chapter is a basic guide for the interpretation of the results of drug tests in the setting of a drug court.

The Patterns of Use Shift: Effects on Prediction Values of Drug Testing

A part of the interpretation of the results of a drug test is the issue of how widespread a specific type of abuse may be. The National Institute on Drug Abuses "NIDA 5" drug tests are often criticized as having fallen behind modern trends of drug use. The NIDA 5 tests (1) include measurements of the following:

1. Cannabinoids (from marijuana, hashish).
2. Cocaine.
3. Amphetamines.
4. Opiates (heroin, opium, codeine, morphine).
5. Phencyclidine.

These tests do not include synthetic opiates, such as oxycodone, oxymorphone, hydrocodone, and hydromorphone—compounds that are often abused. Also excluded from the NIDA 5 panel are benzodiazepines (Valium®/diazepam, Xanax®/alprazolam, Klonopin®/clonazepam, Restoril®/temazepam) and barbiturates, although tests for these are usually available and are both sensitive and specific (2–4).

For example, the confirmation test, usually gas chromatography–mass spectrometry (GC-MS), can tell the difference between methamphetamine and 3,4-methylenedioxyethamphetamine (MDMA, ecstasy). In the absence of detectable amounts of methamphetamine in the sample, the laboratory will either report the sample as negative or report it as positive for MDMA. What the laboratory reports to the client depends on whether MDMA was included in the panel as something to be tested for (3,4).

Gamma-hydroxybutyrate, meperidine (Demerol), fentanyl, propoxyphene, methadone, and ketamine are also easily measured, whereas hallucinogens other than cannabis and phencyclidine, such as mushrooms (psilocybin), lysergic acid diethylamide, and peyote (mescaline), are rarely tested for, most likely because each additional test leads to an overall increase in drug-testing expenditures (3–5). Although tests such as GC-MS have specificity and sensitivity close to 99%, if the tests are done for drugs that are abused less commonly, the positive prediction value of these exceptional test modalities deteriorates.

In other words, by not adjusting the testing patterns to correspond with the changing patterns of illicit drug use, employers, drug enforcement, and medical professionals cause erosion of statistical reliability of drug testing. Any drug court testing program must have the latitude and plasticity to alter the testing panel to detect the current drugs on the market.

False-Positive Results: The Drug-User Lore, Myths, and Urban Legends

Claims of false-positive results often come to the attention of a drug court. Although cases of false-positive results due to legitimate behaviors, equipment malfunction, and human error exist, it is important to consider that the confirmatory testing of the standard modalities, such as urine, blood, saliva/oral fluid, and hair, with GC-MS (or paired EMIT testing to save money) is remarkably reliable.

Ibuprofen

Prior to the development of confirmatory tests, occasional false-positive results would be observed in patients taking high quantities of ibuprofen (Advil™, Aleve™) because the antibody to the tetrahydrocannabinol used in the 1980s was not sufficiently specific. This is no longer an issue, as the newly developed antibodies do not cross-react with ibuprofen (5).

Lidocaine and Novocaine

Another urban legend, traceable to an Internet discussion group, states that dental anesthetics such as lidocaine (also an antiarrhythmia drug) and novocaine may cause false-positive results on a cocaine test. This is an example of lexicologic error. Although both drugs rhyme with cocaine, neither is structurally similar to the illicit drug, and the cross-reactivity is no more than a myth (6).

Over-the-Counter Steroid Supplements

The over-the-counter steroid supplement dehydroepiandrosterone is easily and inexpensively distinguishable from the illicit anabolic/androgenic steroids by the high-performance liquid chromatography technique developed in 2001 by a group of Japanese scientists (6).

Ritalin®/Methylphenidate

While the prescription drug Ritalin®/methylphenidate may be by itself an abused substance, it is not the case that its presence in the client will cause a false-positive result of the amphetamine screen. Methylphenidate is sufficiently structurally different from amphetamines not to cross-react with the antibody employed in the immunoassay tests. A GC-MS assay identifies methylphenidate decisively and should be considered in all questionable outcomes of the initial test (7).

Poppy Seeds

The issue of poppy seed consumption and its link with false-positive results on opioid screens is often misunderstood. Commercially available poppy seeds have been shown to contain 2 to 294 μg of morphine and 0.4 to 57 μg of codeine per gram of seed. It is not uncommon for people to consume significant amounts of poppy seeds in the form of the traditional Jewish pastry hamantashen, each of which contains up to 5 tablespoonfuls of poppy seeds. Following poppy seed ingestion, morphine concentrations in the urine generally peak within 3 to 8 hours and may be positive for as long as 48 to 60 hours postingestion. Morphine levels in urine of poppy seed eaters may climb as high as 2,797 ng/mL, and codeine levels up to 214 ng/mL have been identified in specimens of individuals who have consumed large amounts of poppy seed. Utilizing a 300 ng/mL limit of detection cut-off point with the opiate immunoassays will readily detect the presence of opiates in these specimens. Raising the detection limit to 2,000 ng/mL (also cited as 2 mcg/mL or 2 μg/mL) will reduce the false-positive results drastically. In the drug court setting, a successful strategy is to notify participants at the outset that they will be responsible for the cost of confirming all samples that detect opiates as the result of ingesting poppy seeds. The cost of the GC-MS confirmation will usually be sufficient to deter the consumption of poppy seed products during participation in the drug court.

Obtaining the limit of detection information from the testing laboratory is necessary to completely evaluate a test result. However, most modern kits and GC-MS can distinguish between morphine (poppy seeds) and 6-monoacetylmorphine (heroin) (8–10).

Urine Substitution and Adulteration of Samples

The small but determined industry that specializes in detection avoidance has produced several ingenious, a large number of questionable, and an even larger number of patently false chemical remedies, substitution devices, and drug test–defeating schemes. Most of these schemes target urinalysis as the most commonly performed testing modality that is somewhat open to tampering. However, certain schemes target other collection methods and testing modalities.

Endogenous Dilution of the Urine

Endogenous schemes attempt to use or circumvent the body's natural metabolism in order to make the illicit substance undetectable. Common approaches include the use of diuretics with names that include Ultimate Blend, Detoxify Carbo Clean, Precleanse, and Naturally Klean Herbal Tea. A mixture of mild diuretics is also sold: dandelion, burdock, red clover, chamomile, slippery elm, hibiscus, and rose hips. These substances, combined with ingestion of large amounts of water, dilute the specimen. More targeted and potent herbal remedies include St. John's wort, a known inducer of higher activity of liver enzymes that, among other things, metabolize benzodiazepine drugs such as alprazolam (Xanax®). Over-the-counter and prescription medications are used to either mask an illicit substance or facilitate more rapid turnover of an illicit substance in the body of the patient. Several hundred over-the-counter medications, like St. John's wort, can induce the liver enzymes (11,12).

The water washout may be easily detected by the fact that the urine sample is of very low specific gravity and contains unnaturally small amounts of the natural biomarkers such as creatinine. If the specific gravity is below 1.003 and the levels of the biomarker creatinine are below 20 mg/dL, the specimen should be considered to be dilute (13).

Creatinine is a product of muscle contraction and is excreted at a relatively constant rate in urine. Because creatinine is released into body fluids at a constant rate, its level in urine may be used as an indication of body hydration. The normal range for creatinine in urine is 20 to 400 mg/dL. A creatinine level of less than 20 mg/dL suggests overhydration of urine by excessive drinking or intentionally diluting the specimen with an adulterant such as water (14).

Specific gravity assesses the amount of solid substances dissolved in the urine. As increasing amounts of substances are added to urine, the specific gravity increases. Specific gravity measures the density of urine relative to the density of water. Normal range is from 1.003 to 1.030. The greater the specific gravity, the more concentrated the urine. A urine specific gravity of 1.000 is essentially water (13).

The more sophisticated herbal and medication approaches are much harder to detect and defeat. However, they do have a drawback: they have never been proven to work reliably.

Exogenous Dilution of the Urine

There is a multitude of what may be called *exogenous* schemes that involve tampering with the sample or substituting human, animal, or synthetic urine. Substitution methods vary from concealed containers (including the now infamous prosthetic penis device, the Whizzinator, and the lesser known intravaginal container device, often a condom, filled with "clean" urine) to injections into the bladder via needle or catheter, both of which may lead to severe urinary tract infections.

Clean urine may be provided by a donor, may be derived from animals, or may be reconstituted from dry urine sold by outfits on the Internet. Donor urine may not match gender-specific biomarkers, but these are rarely tested. Animal urine will not contain the human-specific biomarker IgG, but this is also rarely tested. Dry urine may undergo chemical degradation both before and after the reconstitution with water and also is likely to be identifiable because of the differences in temperature and pH. Under normal situations fresh urine would display a temperature between 90° and 100°F on the temperature strip, if read within 4 minutes of the collection. Specimens with a temperature out of range may indicate a substituted or adulterated sample (3).

Tampering with the Urine

Tampering with the urine sample is common and relatively well researched. Some of the adulterants include the following (13):

1. Water: detected by the low specific gravity and low levels of creatinine in the adulterated sample.
2. Oxidants: hydrogen peroxide, pyridinium chlorochromate, bleaches.
3. Nitrites used to induce chemical deactivation of the metabolites of tetrahydrocannabinol.
4. Chemicals that denature enzymes and antibodies used in immunoassays (glutaraldehyde, formaldehyde).
5. Chemicals that change the acidity/alkalinity of the urine, thus interfering with most assays (acids, alkali, including Drano, muriatic acid, lemon juice, and bleach).

Several commercial products, usually in the form of test strips, are available for detection of sample adulteration or tampering. A commonly used test strip detects the following:

1. The urine pH: acidity, characterized by pH lower than 4 or alkalinity, with pH higher than 9, leads to sample rejection.
2. Creatinine: with cut-off point for detection <5 mg/dL, while the range for normal urine is between 20 to 400 mg/dL.
3. Nitrates and glutaraldehyde: the presence of related substances may be expected in patients with uncontrolled diabetes.
4. Urinary tract infections.
5. Oxidants.

The usefulness of the test strip is reduced for individuals who follow high-protein, "Atkins-style" diets. Oxidants are normally not present in the urine; however, high amounts of ascorbic acid (vitamin C) in urine following the ingestion of very high amounts of the vitamin (5 to 10 g) may mask the presence of hydrogen peroxide and other oxidants. Although no test for urine adulteration is completely specific, the commercially available tests are generally considered to be reliable (12).

Using Visine™ to Block Marijuana and Cocaine

A point of significant scientific interest is the use of Visine™ eye drops and other products that contain the preservative benzalkonium chloride. Benzalkonium chloride may interfere with detection of tetrahydrocannabinol and cocaine. However, specific tests for this substance are available, and, most important, the adulterated sample loses its ability to foam, allowing for easy detection of tampering without the use of any equipment (13).

Secondhand Marijuana Smoke

Several well-done studies have been conducted by placing volunteers in a closed space, sometimes in actual automobiles, and exposing them to secondhand marijuana smoke. On occasion, very slight amounts of tetrahydrocannabinol were detected, but they were well below the cut-off limits used by commercial laboratory testing kits. Exposures necessary to produce these slightly elevated levels were extremely heavy to the point of causing bronchitis and many times longer than the typical automobile ride (14).

Vicks™ Inhalers

Vicks™ inhalers contain l-methamphetamine, which can cross-react with d-methamphetamine, the drug of abuse often called *meth* or *crank*. When drug testing began in the 1980s there were problems with testing kits testing positive for both forms. Current test kits report only the *d* or "dextro" form of methamphetamines, which is the addictive and abused form. If there is a concern that a false-positive result is due to cross-reactivity, a separate test can be performed to confirm that the specimen is the d form (15).

Legal Use of Medications

The issue of legally prescribed medications that may cause a positive drug test for drugs of abuse is critical in all testing venues. Although issues such as medical marijuana should not appear in drug court, the appropriate use of opiates in the treatment of acute trauma is a problem that appears constantly. Occasionally, amphetamines such as Adderal™ are legitimately prescribed to adults for attention deficit hyperactivity disorder, and methamphetamines are legitimately prescribed for narcolepsy.

Steps that can be taken to ensure that prescription medications are appropriate and are causing a false-positive test include the following:

1. Confirmation that the patient is taking the medications under a physician's care and prescription.
2. Confirmation, using a *Physician's Desk Reference*, that the medications in the container match the medications listed on the label.
3. Counting medications and comparing them to the issue date of the medication on the container to see if they are being overutilized.
4. Use of a medical review officer or medical-legal examination to determine if the medication is being used appropriately.

Steps in the Analysis of a Test Result for Drug Court

The use of a trained physician as a medical review officer is typically too expensive and cumbersome for most drug courts. To make drug testing work in drug courts, testing must not only be reliable but economical as well.

Steps that a judge, probation officer, or counselor can take to ensure the integrity of a testing result are based on the U.S. Department of Transportation testing program for truck drivers and upon private programs conducted for industry. These steps include the following:

1. *Ensure*: the standards of collection security are established and followed, including proper identification, specimen security, and chain of custody.
2. *Confirm*: proper laboratory testing techniques are followed.
3. *Review*: reporting documents to make sure they are in order.
4. *Establish*: the client is not taking any prescription or over-the-counter medications that may account for the positive drug test.
5. *Reject*: grandiose excuses told by clients as a pretext for a positive test.

Conclusions

Although no scientific method is without flaws and most are susceptible to both intentional and unintentional errors, the field of drug testing, especially with the introduction of the newer, more sensitive, and specific modalities, remains essentially reliable. The challenges to interpretation of the results are also numerous but not insurmountable. Proper application of the laws of logic and the principles of causality provides an unshakeable foundation for interpretation of the results of scientific investigation, particularly as it applies to drug testing.

References

1. Shults T. Medical Review Officer Handbook, 8th ed. Triangle Park: Quadrangle Research LLC; 2002.
2. Baselt RC. Disposition of Toxic Drugs and Chemicals in Man, 6th ed. Foster City, CA: Biomedical Publications; 2002.
3. Tsai SC, ElSohly MA, Dubrovsky T, Twarowska B, Towt J, Salamonde SJ. Determination of five abused drugs in nitrite-adulterated urine by immunoassays and gas chromatography–mass spectrometry. J Anal Toxicol 1998;22(6): 474–480.
4. Lotsch J. Pharmacokinetic-pharmacodynamic modeling of opioids. J Pain Symptom Manage 2005;29(5 Suppl):S90–S103.
5. Cody JT. Specimen adulteration in drug urinalysis. Forensic Sci Rev 1990;2: 63–68.
6. Maeda Y, Kamimura R, Higashi S, Namba K, Tanaka E, Iwamura T, Setoguchi T. A simple, accurate, and sensitive assay method of dehydroepiandrosterone sulfate: application for quantitative determination in human breast cyst and duct fluids. Steroids 2002;67(5):333–338.
7. Manzi S, Law T, Shannon MW. Methylphenidate produces a false-positive urine amphetamine screen. Pediatr Emerg Care 2002;18(5):401.
8. Hayes LW, Krasselt WG, Mueggler PA. Concentrations of morphine and codeine in serum and urine after ingestion of poppy seeds. Clin Chem 1987; 33:806–808.
9. Pelders MG, Ross JJ. Poppy seeds: differences in morphine and codeine content and variation in inter- and intra-individual excretion. J Forensic Sci 1996; 41(2):209–212.
10. ElSohly HN, ElSohly MA, Stanford DF. Poppy seed ingestion and opiate urinalysis: a closer look. J Anal Toxicol 1990;14:308–310.
11. Markowitz JS, Donovan JL, DeVane CL, Taylor RM, Ruan Y, Wang JS, et al. Effect of St. John's wort on drug metabolism by induction of cytochrome P450 3A4 enzyme. JAMA 2003;290:1500–1504.
12. Mikkelsen SL, Ash KO. Adulterants causing false negatives in illicit drug testing. Clin Chem 1988;34(11):2333–2336.
13. Jones AW, Karlsson L. Relation between blood- and urine-amphetamine concentrations in impaired drivers as influenced by urinary pH and creatinine. Hum Exp Toxicol 2005;24:615–622.
14. Law B. Mason PA, Moffat AC, King LJ, Marks V. Passive inhalation of cannabis smoke. J Pharm Pharmacol 1984;36:578–581.
15. Fitzgerald RL, Ramos JM Jr, Bogema SC, Poklis A. Resolution of methamphetamine stereoisomers in urine drug testing: Urinary excretion of R(–)-methamphetamine following use of nasal inhalers. J Anal Toxicol 1988;12: 255–259.

18
Juvenile Drug Courts

Cheryl L. Asmus and Denise E. Colombini

Juvenile drug courts are founded on the same philosophical and empirical premises as adult drug courts: A therapeutic approach to alcohol or drug abuse and dependence is more effective than a punitive one. This chapter describes the principles, organization, operation, and evaluation of a juvenile drug court, using the Colorado Eighth Judicial District Juvenile Drug Court as an example.

Offenses and Eligibility

Juvenile drug courts serve eligible males and females aged 10 to 18 years who are charged with petty misdemeanor and felony offenses. Juvenile drug courts are not designed to serve clients who are merely experimenting with alcohol or other drugs. Dispositions include diversion, deferred prosecution, and postadjudication. Juvenile drug courts do not accept violent offenders, sex offenders, or offenders involved in selling drugs for profit. Clients must be able to comply with juvenile drug court terms and conditions. The program does not discriminate based on race, creed, or religion. Parent participation is an essential part of the program; a parent or guardian must agree to participate regularly in the program.

Each court sets the parameters for the level of offender it accepts into its program. The date of the offense determines acceptance into the court. A youth is acceptable if the offense is committed while the youth is 17 years of age or younger. In the event that a youth turns 18 while in the program, the case remains in juvenile drug court until that youth successfully completes the program or is terminated without completion. Should the juvenile commit additional crimes after the age of 18 years, those charges will be handled in the adult court system.

The local district attorney's office commonly approves the juvenile's legal eligibility. Juveniles must admit to the underlying offenses. A qualifying offense is usually drug related, including possession of drug paraphernalia, alcohol, and other drugs. Some courts do not include alcohol in juvenile drug court. Juveniles with drug-related criminal offenses such as theft can also be accepted. For instance, a youth who steals money from his parents to purchase marijuana may be appropriate for juvenile drug court. In some cases, juvenile drug court may accept a juvenile who is known to have a substance abuse problem although the charge is not directly or indirectly drug related. The juvenile drug court may also accept a probation client facing revocation for drug-related violations.

Entrance into the Program

A juvenile's legal status varies from court to court. There are both presentence and postsentence programs. Generally, the district attorney is the gatekeeper. In this role, the district attorney determines which type of disposition is offered. A presentence case may be diverted or placed on deferred adjudication status. In a diversion case, no formal charges are filed. Therefore, there is no official court record of the case. If the youth successfully completes the drug court diversion program, no charges are filed. The court can offer the youth a deferred adjudication or deferred prosecution in exchange for successful completion of the juvenile drug court program. When a juvenile successfully completes juvenile drug court, the case is formally closed without prejudice.

Post-plea cases can either be adjudicated to be delinquent or placed on a stayed mittimus. This gives the youth the opportunity to address substance use issues while remaining in the community instead of being committed to youth corrections.

Based on a set of criteria, the *Diagnostic and Statistical Manual of Mental Disorders*, 4th ed, describes two general types of substance abuse disorders: substance abuse and substance dependence. Juvenile drug courts use these criteria to identify youth with substance abuse or substance dependence diagnoses and to screen out experimenters. Assessments are administered upon client referral and may include a substance abuse evaluation, mental status form, mental health evaluation, and psychosocial history (1–3).

Principles of the Juvenile Drug Court System

A juvenile drug court provides youth with positive social relationships and a system that cares for them as individuals. It typically adheres to the principles outlined below, depending on the resources of the jurisdiction and community (4,5). The combination of these principles provides youth and their families with a rich arsenal of rehabilitation tools based on evidence-based prevention and intervention in alcohol and drug use.

Drug Court Team

Establishment of a drug court team is critical and should include, at a minimum, a judge, prosecutor, defense attorney, treatment provider, evaluator, and school representative who work collaboratively to meet the needs of the juvenile and his or her family. When youth are involved in positive social relationships with peers and a variety of adults, such as parents and teachers, they are more likely to have good self-esteem, think and act in socially responsible ways, and have good problem-solving skills (6,7). A juvenile drug court provides positive and frequent contact and relationships with adult mentors. Clients get to know a judge, defense attorney, case manager, and treatment provider. In a juvenile drug court system, youths can be cocooned by their family, community, court, and schools. In addition, the system integrates these entities to provide a seamless structure for communication and information. Clients have the rich experience of observing their peers' setbacks and successes at the various levels in drug court.

Intervention

Intervention by the court as soon as possible following the juvenile's initial contact with the justice system is the key to success, along with continuous judicial supervision of the juvenile through frequent status hearings. Immediate reinforcement is critical to either increase or decrease any behavior. Too often, youths are arrested or charged with a crime and no consequences occur for several weeks or months depending on the caseload of a justice system. By the time the juvenile has consequences for a particular action, he may not associate the delinquent behavior with the punishment. The juvenile drug court reduces the amount of time between an act and reinforcement. This occurs through a rapid mechanism to get the youth into the court and in front of a judge, into treatment, and assessed for critical mental health issues.

Court-Supervised Substance Abuse Treatment

Development of a court-supervised program of substance abuse treatment and other core services is necessary to address the multifaceted issues that the juvenile and his family face. Issues may include the juvenile's substance use, family, educational needs, and behavioral problems as they affect his ability to lead a drug-free life.

Accountability

Treatment and other services must be coordinated to provide accountability and integrity. Optimal conditions for positive youth development exist when there is meaningful communication among the different settings of the adolescent's life. Juvenile drug courts provide frequent and clear links among the youth, his family, the school, and other community entities. Lack of these important links among home, school, and community is associated with problem behavior (8–10).

Monitoring

The juvenile's progress in the program is monitored through frequent random urinalysis, continuous supervision, and proactive case management. Extended interventions of longer than 6 months for individuals with alcohol and other drug use disorders have been found to result in better long-term outcomes than shorter treatment protocols (11). Juvenile drug courts typically are 6 to 18 months in length. Ongoing assessment of a client's treatment plan is necessary to ensure it meets changing needs. As the youth progresses through the program, his or her attitudes, skills, and behavior need to be constantly assessed to ensure that the most effective treatment and response by the staff are employed.

The amount of supervision necessary is dependent on the risk level of the abuser. Those at high risk respond better when they are closely and frequently monitored by a judge so that consequences can be consistently delivered for treatment noncompliance. A judge and courtroom may be the only and most effective method to instill the accountability and behavior modification necessary to end the cycle of drug and alcohol abuse (12,13).

Ongoing Interaction

There is immediate judicial response to the progress of all participating juveniles or their noncompliance with the court's program conditions. Juvenile drug court provides a mechanism to see the youth on a weekly basis so that any behavior, positive or negative, can be reinforced immediately, thus strengthening the association of the two in the youth's mind.

Juvenile Focused

The judge is concerned about juveniles and their families, sensitive to cultural and other factors unique to all participants, and interested and trained in adolescent development and behavior, substance abuse, and pharmacology. Youths need several types of caring support from adults in their lives. Caring is a protective factor for children and youth. It helps humans develop social competence, identity, confidence, and a sense of purpose and future. It can also be empowering. The caring that juveniles experience in a juvenile drug court helps them to gain a sense of independence, control, and mastery and to understand and analyze the communities and environments in which they live. The caring of the juvenile drug court team promotes positive development by providing the youth with clear expectations and resources to help them succeed in all areas of their lives, jobs, school, relationships, community, and health (8,14).

Strengths-Based Philosophy

The program philosophy capitalizes on the strengths of each juvenile and his or her family (4). A strengths perspective is both a philosophy and practice that identifies, builds, reinforces, and enhances the positive qualities, attributes, and aspirations of youth through the use of counseling and intervention techniques. It is in contrast to identifying the negative qualities, attributes, and aspirations of youth in trouble or at risk and concentrating on those through counseling or other intervention techniques. Applying the research findings of the strengths-based approach for youth and families in the juvenile justice system provides 15 areas of competencies that practitioners can follow as they work this perspective into juvenile drug courts (15,16).

Continued Assessments

There is a comprehensive assessment of the juvenile at intake, with follow-up assessments conducted periodically thereafter. Information obtained during the intake and assessment is integrated into subsequent decisions in the case.

Between 60% and 70% of youths in the juvenile justice system suffer from mood, anxiety, substance abuse, or thought disorders. This prevalence rate is approximately two to three times higher than that of U.S. youth in general. Juvenile drug courts use reliable screening assessment instruments at intake and periodically thereafter to ensure that the treatment is immediate and appropriate (17–19).

Family Oriented

Focus is kept on the functioning of the family and its effects on the juvenile throughout his participation in the program. Whether a family is functionally healthy or unhealthy, the family knows the youth better than anyone. The family is also the environment in which the youth lives, and family counseling has been found to reduce recidivism. The extent of the family's involvement in the child's school has a direct impact on the success of that child academically. The same holds true for juveniles in the criminal justice system: Family involvement is directly correlated with reduced recidivism. Youths who grow up in families witnessing violence and family conflict often exhibit poor school performance, poor mental health, and increased juvenile delinquency. They exhibit the same violence and conflict in their own families as adults. However, a family can also provide positive influences and protective mechanisms through supportive relationships with their child, positive disciplinary methods, supervision, and communication. Juvenile drug courts insist on family involvement for a youth to be part of the programs, and most also mandate family counseling or therapy (20–23).

Parents must be present and involved consistently in all aspects of the youth in the program. It is clear how important it is for parents to know what is going on with the youth so that they can be in touch and have a shared perception of standards for behavior with their child. This ensures that neither the parent nor the adolescent will be confused about expectations facilitating the youth as they go through the program.

Appropriately Trained Officials

Officials involved in the program are trained in adolescent developmental issues and the effect these issues have on drug use and withdrawal (5). It is imperative to develop and maintain a trained and interdisciplinary, nonadversarial team. Although members come to the team with a role they must maintain, they must also be willing to listen and accept another member's opinion without bringing forward any turf issues, keeping the overall goals of the program at the forefront. To do this, all members need to understand and be trained in the philosophies and principles of the juvenile drug court system (24,25).

Case Studies Illustrating Benefit of Teamwork

The following two case studies are examples of successful outcomes resulting from effective interdisciplinary teamwork in the juvenile drug court system and serious work by the juvenile clients.

Case Study 18.1

Joey was an 18-year-old white male diagnosed with substance dependence. His substance of choice was prescription drugs, and he had exhausted treatment ranging from group to residential treatment. Drug court was a last chance for Joey. Joey entered the program and took it seriously. He attended outpatient treatment and 12 Step meetings. He made monumental changes in his life. After 10 months in juvenile drug court, Joey was sober and chaired 12 Step meetings, had a job at a grocery store deli, completed his Graduate Equivalency Degree (GED), and enrolled in college. Two months before juvenile drug court graduation, Joey surprised the court with an unusual request. He asked to stay in the program a little longer, until after he completed his first full semester at college, because he needed the support of the juvenile drug court.

Case Study 18.2

Cody had been in the system before and did not have a good reputation with the court. During his intake, it was explained to Cody and his parents that juvenile drug court was different from the traditional court system because it is a strengths-based program. Although they were somewhat apprehensive, they agreed to participate in the program. Cody struggled to meet all the requirements. In turn, the court responded with sanctions when he broke the rules. Things were spiraling downward when the director received a call from Cody's mother. She was angry that her son was being treated in a punitive fashion while the court overlooked his positive accomplishments. She reminded the director that she had agreed to participate in juvenile drug court because it was a strengths-based program rather than a traditional court program. She said that she knew her son and that this punitive approach would not work for him. She said that he would respond well to positive recognition. She was right. After the counselor had a gentle discussion with the magistrate, the court tried another approach with Cody. Although Cody was still sanctioned for noncompliance, the court changed its tone and focused on the positive things that he had accomplished. This turned things around for him. He responded positively to the strengths-based approach. He got his GED and ultimately successfully completed the program.

Program Goals

Each juvenile drug court is designed to fulfill the needs of the community that it serves. The programs generally accomplish the following:

1. Reduce the number of juveniles who are using alcohol or other drugs as measured by drug court clients who achieve successful program completion with no additional alcohol or other drug use.
2. Reduce the number of juveniles who are using alcohol or other drugs and committing delinquent acts (clients complete the program with no further filings with the judicial system).
3. Empower parents and actively involve them in the drug court program.
4. Assist juveniles to actively resume, participate in, and complete school.
5. Facilitate cooperation and interaction among schools, the community, and juvenile agencies.

Adversity in life, whether physical or psychological, has at least four potential outcomes:

1. To continue a downward slide, compounding the effects and eventually succumbing to them.

2. To survive the event, but somehow become weakened by it, never really returning to the physical or psychological state prior to the event.
3. To return to the preadversity level of functioning.
4. To surpass the condition before the adversity, to not just survive but to thrive.

O'Leary and Ickovics (1) first discussed this concept to argue that some people can actually emerge from an adverse experience as better people, perhaps with qualities they did not have before.

This principle is often seen in physical well-being. For example, a child with the mumps will emerge with antibodies that ward off further infections of the virus. A person who experiences a heart attack may change his lifestyle and become healthier. Some people can and do thrive physically after an adverse event happens. For over a decade, youth development researchers and practitioners have studied this principle as it relates to psychological thriving for young people who are at-risk or have already experienced an adverse event (2,3).

Youth who find themselves in the juvenile justice system because of their alcohol and drug abuse have experienced an adverse life event. The juvenile drug court system looks at this adverse event as an opportunity to become a part of this person's life at this crucial time and work toward the fourth possible outcome of this adversity: thriving.

The Juvenile Drug Court Organization

The organization of the program consists of four components: (1) setting goals, (2) establishing the structure, (3) establishing the programs, and (4) managing the data and measuring the outcomes.

Setting Goals

The first activity of a juvenile drug court is to establish the goals and the mission and strategies to achieve those goals. They provide a foundation to measure where the program is and where it should be headed.

Establishing a Structure

Advisory Board

Most juvenile drug courts initiate an advisory board. The advisory board may consist of a judge, probation officer, district attorney, chief public defender, law enforcement representative, mental health representative, and evaluator. The board meets frequently in the planning stage of the court and then less frequently as the court is implemented and the problems have been resolved.

The Drug Court Team

The juvenile drug court team may consist of the presiding judge, the director or coordinator, the district attorney, the public defender, case managers, and treatment providers. The team meets on a regular basis to develop, monitor, or change policies and procedures to ensure the integrity of the program. The team reviews juvenile cases prior to each court session.

The Judge

The judge oversees the program and staff and runs each court session, including chairing the team staffing. The judge sentences the juvenile, conducts review hearings concerning compliance issues, imposes sanctions and rewards, and has ongoing interaction with each participant.

Drug court is held on a set docket at a set time and date so that everybody knows when to be there and there are no excuses for failing to come. Participants appear initially every week to 2 weeks. Court appearances may be more or less frequent, based on a juvenile's progress. During court proceedings, the judge provides positive reinforcement to juveniles who are in compliance with program requirements or imposes sanctions for noncompliance. Case managers report participants' progress regarding treatment, school, employment, and home issues to the judge.

The Program Director

The director or coordinator is responsible for all program and interteam communication; case manager monitoring; treatment provider monitoring; team training; policy and procedure development, maintenance, and implementation; hiring; presentation of new cases to the team; facilitation and communication with agencies outside of drug court; sustainability of the program; data monitoring for program implementation and evaluation; budget management; and administrative duties.

The District Attorney

The district attorney serves as the gatekeeper for the program in many jurisdictions, assesses whether cases meet the criteria, and determines if juveniles are appropriate for the juvenile drug court program. If the juvenile is found appropriate, the district attorney gives sentencing recommendations to the court and refers the juvenile to the program.

The Public Defender

The public defender represents some juveniles and serves as a team member, acts as a consultant, advocates for the legal rights of juveniles, and monitors sanctions imposed by the court to ensure they are within the legal and philosophical parameters of the program.

The Social Services Representative

The social services representative provides knowledge of community resources and in some cases can supply funding for alcohol and other drug treatment.

Case Managers

Case managers may supervise diversion agencies, social service agencies, private probation, or probation services. The term *case manager* is used to describe the staff member who supervises a case, whether that person is a mental health worker, a probation officer, or has no function other than supervising the case. Many juvenile drug courts use interns from local colleges or universities to assist with caseloads and monitoring. Case managers have dual roles as they serve to monitor youth and to advocate for the youth when appropriate. They are the essential link among the court, the youth, and the family.

Treatment Providers

Treatment providers are also commonly part of a drug court team and attend all staff meetings. Some programs have treatment in-house, and the case managers coordinate and monitor the juveniles with the treatment provider. The case manager also keeps track of the juvenile's progress and compliance with the assigned treatment by constant communication with the treatment providers whether they are in-house or community providers.

Parents

Parents or guardians must attend court with the juvenile for each scheduled appearance. Parents must keep the team, through the case manager, informed of any setbacks or progress of the juvenile in the family home. For most programs, family counseling is also a requirement. Parents also may be required to complete a parental survey at intake, at graduation, and 6 to 12 months postgraduation for evaluation purposes and to help engage the parent with the activities of the program. Juveniles are required to comply with a curfew. The parents and the team establish the curfew jointly, and the parents are responsible for reporting any violation to the case manager as soon as possible.

Establishing the Programs

Once a basic juvenile drug court structure is established, layers of on-site programming are added, ultimately creating a unique community among participants and a distinct culture within the existing justice system. The creation of this culture allows the varying members of a team to maintain their professional roles yet embrace the goals of a juvenile drug court.

Examples of on-site programs include on-site treatment, education, the arts, planned physical activities, parent involvement, and gender-specific programming. These program enhancements provide a positive impact on individuals within the program by affording access to these services and create a sense of community among the participants.

Managing the Data and Measuring the Outcomes

All programs need some way to manage the data and measure the outcomes of their work. These usually require the development and implementation of a simple, but complete, monitoring and evaluation database to keep track of clients and their behavior while entering and going through the program. The data are important for ongoing monitoring and weekly staff decision making and to measure the success of the program for improvement and continued funding.

Juvenile Drug Court Operations

Screening and Assessment

Once a juvenile is determined to be eligible for juvenile drug court by the team, the juvenile and his parents accept or decline the terms of participation. All juveniles who decide to take part in the program must complete the screening and intake evaluation with a trained provider. Often the alcohol and drug screen information is acquired before the drug court staff meeting in which the juvenile is discussed

Court

Juvenile drug court dockets are typically held weekly. Before court, the team meets and discusses each juvenile one at a time. The team then goes to the courtroom and gives their input as participants appear before the judge. The hearing of one client typically lasts no more than 5 minutes.

Levels and Phases

Although various programs are organized differently, the Colorado programs place new clients in one of two levels, according to the extent and severity of their crimes and the nature of their difficulties.

Within Level I there are two stages (Table 18.1). In stage one (first month), the juvenile appears in court weekly for the first month or biweekly

TABLE 18.1. Levels and stages of the juvenile drug court.

Level	Stages	Criteria	Number of visits	Average number of visits	Average length in months
I				23	6.3
	1	First month	Weekly		
	2	Second month to graduation	Monthly		
II				45	8.6
	1	First month or until urine drug screens are negative	Weekly		
	2	Second month or after drug screens are negative	Weekly to monthly depending on compliance in the program		

if he or she had a clean baseline drug screen. In stage two (second month until completion or termination), the juvenile appears in court at least monthly. Court appearances increase or decrease in frequency as determined by the team based on the juvenile's compliance with the program requirements. Even though some youth have very high compliance levels right from the beginning, most programs will still require that the youth be alcohol and drug free and law abiding for at least 4 months. The following conditions could determine a Level I placement:

1. A first time petty offense or misdemeanor.
2. A less serious offense (juveniles who are cited into court rather than being held in custody).
3. Diversion by a district attorney's office before filing of formal charges.

Level II juveniles attend weekly court reviews for the first month and thereafter until drug screens are negative. Frequency of appearances increases or decreases as determined by the team based on the juvenile's compliance with the program requirements. The Level II program typically lasts 6 months to 1 year or more. The following conditions could determine Level II placement:

1. Multiple offenses, misdemeanor offense, or low-level felony offense.
2. Deferred or suspended adjudication.
3. Condition of probation.

On occasion, a juvenile may move from Level I to Level II. Conditions that can precipitate this move could be an additional charge while in the program or an inability to remain alcohol or drug free during the program.

Length of the Program

The average length of time in a juvenile drug court program for Level I clients is given in Table 18.1. Typically, the juvenile must have a minimum of 4 months of sobriety and negative drug screens to be considered for graduation. If a juvenile enters the lower level program with a negative baseline alcohol and drug screen, the program can be completed in less time. In the Level II program, the juvenile must typically have a minimum of 4 months of sobriety and negative drug screens to be considered for graduation. In addition to abstaining from alcohol and drugs, the juvenile must remain law abiding while in the program. The juvenile must also be compliant with the other requirements of the program, such as attending meetings with case managers, attending and participating in treatment, appearing in court as scheduled, meeting school or work requirements, complying with a mandated curfew, maintaining a daily journal, and being available for possible home visits. Noncompliance with any of these requirements or others stated in court or in a contract could lengthen the time the juvenile spends in the program.

Treatment

At intake, juveniles complete an alcohol and drug evaluation performed by a certified provider. The juvenile and the parents must comply with the evaluation recommendations as required by the team. Typically, the juvenile will attend individual treatment for thc first 1 to 2 months up to five times per week, with a two times per week minimum. For the third month, individual treatment continues. For the fourth month and thereafter until termination, the participant attends support groups, relapse prevention training, family therapy, and other treatment as necessary based on the team recommendations. These include anger management, intensive outpatient therapy, group therapy, detoxification, inpatient therapy, mental health counseling, psychological evaluation, and psychiatric consultation.

Most clients participate in aftercare and are referred to community programs. A relapse prevention plan is in place within 2 weeks of entry in the aftercare program and is followed after the juvenile graduates to the community program.

School and Work Contracts

Juveniles must be either enrolled in school, actively pursuing a GED, or gainfully employed as approved by the team. If enrolled in school, the juveniles will work up to their ability without attendance or discipline problems. The case manager maintains regular contact with school staff. Changes in employment or school status are first reviewed with the case manager, who presents it to the team for a decision.

Alcohol and Drug Screening

For the first month of participation, each juvenile submits to a minimum of two drug screens per week. After the first month, the frequency is determined on an individual basis by the drug court team. Drug screens may be increased or decreased at the discretion of the team. Breath analysis is requested as appropriate. Clients are responsible for the costs of the drug screens unless other arrangements are made. A missed, altered, or diluted drug screen is considered a positive drug screen. Clients are told to refrain from eating poppy seeds while in the program. Secondhand marijuana smoke is not considered a legitimate excuse for a positive test.

Sanctions and Incentives

The juvenile drug court team imposes graduated sanctions for noncompliance with program requirements and rules. It also implements rewards or incentives for progress and success demonstrated by the juvenile. The case manager learns the interests and motivations of each juvenile and suggests sanctions and incentives that are meaningful and motivating. The judge makes the final decision with regard to the frequency and implementation of sanctions and incentives. Relapse is considered on a case-by-case basis.

Graduation or Expulsion

Clients who meet the program requirements are eligible to graduate, and their initial charge is typically dropped. Both the client and parents are given a postprogram survey to complete. In addition, they are given a debriefing form that explains the program they just completed. It also gives them a contact name and number should they require any information or assistance with regard to the program in the future. The client participates in an exit interview geared toward letting the juvenile know that the task of staying law abiding and drug free is an ongoing process and that there is support available should he or she need it.

Expulsion from the program occurs for the following reasons:

1. The drug court is no longer helping the juvenile.
2. The juvenile has received maximum benefit from the program and has exhausted the resources.
3. The juvenile has demonstrated continuous noncompliance with the program requirements.

The team understands that relapse happens. However, if the implementation of appropriate sanctions or increased treatment is still not effective, the juvenile will more than likely face expulsion from the program. If the juvenile continuously misses scheduled appointments for treatment or with the case management, in addition to other breaches in the contract, the team will typically decide to expel the juvenile. When a juvenile is expelled from the program, the initial charges that were deferred while the juvenile was participating in juvenile drug court are brought against the juvenile.

Case Study 18.3

A negative termination can still have a positive impact. Adam is a 15-year-old white male who lived with his mother. He was accepted into the program after a failed diversion opportunity because of alcohol-related charges. His drug of choice was alcohol, and he drank to dangerous levels that resulted in visits to the emergency room. Adam and his mother had a conflicted relationship that spilled over into the courtroom. At times, his mother was at odds with the magistrate and the program. After several serious drinking episodes while in juvenile drug court, Adam's treatment and enhancement activities were increased. His time was structured; he was placed on electronic home monitoring. After failing as an outpatient, he was placed in a residential treatment facility. Following discharge, he did well for a brief period but had another incident of drinking, and again a high level of structure was put in place. Finally, Adam got drunk and took his mother's car without her consent and caused an automobile accident. He received new charges and was negatively discharged from juvenile drug court.

Adam was committed to the Department of Youth Corrections several months after his discharge from juvenile drug court. The program staff received a call from his mother. She let them know that Adam was doing well in treatment. She thanked them for working with her son and told them that she supports the juvenile drug court program. She informed them that she sits on a local community interfaith board, and she invited juvenile drug court personnel to come and speak to her board members. She also invited juvenile drug court personnel to submit an application for a small grant to help fund items needed for the program.

Barriers to Success

Many communities already have efforts and initiatives in place to reduce juvenile delinquency and drug use. Funding can be competitive and scarce. Initially, juvenile drug courts may encounter resistance to change from the existing system. Criminal justice professionals may be reluctant to support a therapeutic approach for serious offenders, and communities may fear that they are soft on crime. Traditional treatment providers and correctional systems may feel threatened by the reallocation of funds.

On a local level, families have limited resources to pay for juvenile drug court treatment costs. Parents have limited insurance coverage and may have exhausted their benefits. They are often frustrated by the juvenile's delinquent behavior and want the juvenile to be responsible for program participation. The majority of participants are high school students and, if employed, have part-time, low-wage jobs. As a result, juveniles have a limited ability or no ability to pay for treatment.

The following solutions were offered at several drug court training workshops held across the country in 2005 (4):

1. Develop a long-term, systemic strategy and create partnerships that will generate ongoing support.
2. Maximize positive media coverage.
3. Become more efficient at using existing resources.
4. Draft legislation that will create a consistent framework for drug court operations.
5. Create additional community partnerships.
6. Explore creative funding such as receiving restitution payments.
7. Advocate for incorporation of drug court into the state judicial system.
8. Promote community awareness of drug court by inviting the press and local dignitaries to graduation ceremonies.

Funding for general operating costs is also an obstacle. Federal grants and other funding will only cover part of the costs and are not a long-term solution. Drug court planners need to focus on developing a sustainable funding stream that goes beyond initial start-up funds or one-time grants and that can support a larger program. They need to become part of the system. This can only be done by providing the system and other funding resources with positive outcomes of the juvenile drug court program. People and organizations need to know if they are spending their money wisely.

As drug courts grow in size, new obstacles arise. Courts may revert to more traditional procedures and lose the practices specific to drug courts. Also, changes may occur in the participant population. For example, when methamphetamine became easily available, it quickly became the drug of choice and changed almost every demographic.

Evaluation of The Eighth Judicial Juvenile Drug Court, 2002

In the early years, the juvenile drug court in the Eighth Judicial District of Colorado did not have a mature program with a stable evaluation base. Instead, it consisted of evolving interventions where results were not only hard to describe but were even difficult to name. Questions we had to consider included the following:

1. What should be measured?
2. What is the true independent variable?
3. Can we be sure that the results are due to the intervention?

4. How do we best capture the subtle interactions between the agency and the clients?
5. What are the indicators we should use? Who are the stakeholders or audience?

A major difficulty was determining the variables that influenced any observed change. Otherwise stated: Did the program actually contribute to the improvements in a youth? What about the program made the change possible? Many parts of a program that exist throughout one particular year are not the same from one month to the next. Perhaps there was a staff or provider change. Even the juvenile drug court as a comprehensive collaboration agency might add a program such as family therapy or eliminate a program as funding cycles began and ended. Many outcomes that were worth studying had many causes, including social conditions that affect individuals and families.

Evaluation is the systematic attempt to make sense of the outcomes of comprehensive services for stakeholder audiences and policy groups. Specifically, the purpose of the implementation evaluation is to develop a system for data compilation that is coordinated, comprehensive, reliable, valid, easy to use, and addresses the program goals.

Analysis Method: The Logic Model

The logic model was used as the conceptual framework to design the evaluation of the program. Based on the Bennett hierarchy of program effectiveness, the logic model describes what the program is and will do and the sequence of events that links program investments to results. It classifies activities as inputs, outputs, outcomes, and impacts. The framework was used to examine the implementation phase of the juvenile drug court. It provided a model to document the inputs, outputs, and outcomes of the program and staff. In addition it assisted in the design of the next phase of evaluation for the enhancement grant. The model provides a common vocabulary with which to conduct program planning and evolution and focuses on quality and continuous improvement in the juvenile drug court (26).

Based on the logic model as the framework to collect the information for the evaluation, program inputs included executive committee, members, staff, volunteers, mission and goal statements, and partners. In addition, specific output information was collected on type of program, program goals, program description, duration, and how the program was funded. Program target population characteristics were also collected and included age, ethnicity, gender, education, income, program levels, and employment status.

Results of the Analysis

A total of 386 juveniles were presented to the team for consideration of participation in drug court from 1999 to 2002. Of these 386, 97 were denied by the team, 38 declined, and 251 became drug court participants. Four were still in the program, and four withdrew after being accepted.

Of the 251 participants, 167 (67%) graduated successfully from the program and 84 (33%) did not graduate. Of the graduates, 87 were in Level I and 80 were in Level II. Of those who did not graduate, 42 were in Level I and 42 were in Level II. For 15 participants there is no record of whether they graduated or not.

The program accepted juveniles aged 10 through 18 years with petty, misdemeanor, and felony charges. The juveniles were mostly male (79%), aged 16 or 17 years (46 percent), and white (85%).

The charges most commonly filed were possession of marijuana (32%), drug paraphernalia (16%), or alcohol (11%). The most common charge the juveniles faced at intake was a petty offense (49%), felonies (26%), and misdemeanors (25%).

Most participants at intake were in school (76%). The juveniles who had dropped out (9%) or were suspended (2%) at intake had to be in school to participate in the program. These juveniles resumed their work toward a high school diploma as a program requirement.

Using a sample of the population (only the participants who came into drug court in 2001, as the earlier years had too much incomplete data), the results show that 80% of the juveniles had some sort of co-occurring mental disorder on their intake evaluation. Juveniles diagnosed with depression (36%) and attention deficit disorder (31%) together made up over two thirds of the drug court population in the year 2001. Some of the juveniles reported a history of emotional (6%), psychological (8%), physical (5%), and sexual (3%) abuse. Most of the juveniles were employed while they were in the program (72%).

The results of the early evaluation of the program demonstrated that even though the juvenile drug court costs the criminal justice system and the general public less than half that of the typical criminal justice program, it still has a 67% success rate (percentage who graduated from the program). In addition, over 100 juveniles in this community have remained out of the criminal justice system and gained the skills and knowledge to lead satisfying and law-abiding lives. Almost all have either remained in school or acquired their degree. Almost all have positively impacted their relationship with their families.

Campus Drug Courts

There is one campus drug court in operation in the United States, although several are in the organization stage. The campus drug court at Colorado State University was an experiment to see if a drug court of this type would work on a university campus and has become a prototype for future programs.

In the 1999–2000 academic year, the Center for Drug and Alcohol Education, in collaboration with the University Counseling Center at Colorado State University, conducted a pilot program utilizing a small group format to help students deal with issues related to substance abuse and to teach more adaptive socialization skills, harm reduction, and coping strategies. Although the approach showed promise, it lacked the structure and well-established knowledge-base already in operation through the community drug court (27).

In conjunction with the Colorado District Court judge and the juvenile and adult drug court coordinator, the author invited members of the Colorado State University Office of Judicial Affairs (OJA), Center for Drug and Alcohol Education, Counseling Center, and Police Department to experience a juvenile drug court staffing and court session. Dr. Asmus acquired a grant achieving 3 years of support and $345,000 from the United States Department of Education for the first campus drug court adaptation.

Over the following 2 years, a dedicated effort was implemented to create and sustain the Drugs, Alcohol and You, IV (DAY IV) protocol.The reasoning behind the "DAY" name was that at the time, the campus student affairs office was apprehensive about having any type of court on campus. They already had a DAY I to III program that consisted of drug and alcohol education programming with counseling and assessment.

In its first 3 years of operation, the DAY IV program cost Colorado State University $233,000 and, through the retention of otherwise dismissed students, it has allowed the University to retain $1.8 million in tuition, fees, room and board, and Colorado Commission on Higher Education funding. As an example of its first few years, 231 students entered the program and 75% graduated from it.

In 2006, the National Judicial College sponsored and implemented the Back on TRAC (Treatment, Responsibility, and Accountability on Campus) National Initiative. The initiative offered competitive funding to colleges and universities seeking training and sponsorship from Colorado State University and the National Judicial College to replicate the campus drug court model piloted at Colorado State University. At the time of this writing, awards were pending for several universities and colleges.

Conclusions

In general, juvenile drug courts are the most effective means of stopping the revolving door of substance abuse and crime. Through accountability and application of treatment, they increase public safety and provide people with the tools that are needed to lead productive lives. Across the nation there are 406 juvenile drug courts fully operational in the United States and 101 juvenile, 86 family, and 5 combined drug courts that are in the planning stages. Still, only 4% to 8% of juveniles eligible for drug court are given the opportunity to participate because many communities do not have a juvenile drug court. The Eighth Judicial District Juvenile Drug Court was the first juvenile drug court in Colorado. In its first 2 years of operation, almost 200 youth were given the opportunity and the tools to create and maintain productive and successful lives.

References

1. O'Leary VE, Ickovics JR. Resilience and thriving in response to challenge: an opportunity for a paradigm shift in women's health. Womens Health 1995;1: 121–142.
2. Catalano RF, Hawkins JD, Berglund L, Pollard J, Arthur M. Prevention Science and Positive Youth Development: Competitive or Cooperative Frameworks? Seattle: University of Washington Press; 2000.
3. Scales P, Benson PL, Leffert N, Blyth D. Contribution of developmental assets to the prediction of thriving among adolescents. Appl Dev Sci 2000;4(1):27–46.
4. OJP Drug Court Clearinghouse and Technical Assistance Project. Juvenile and Family Drug Courts: An Overview. Washington, DC: American University; 1999.
5. Roberts M, Brophy J, Cooper C. The Juvenile Drug Court Movement, Fact Sheet. Washington, DC: U.S. Department of Justice, Office of Justice Programs, Office of Juvenile Justice and Delinquency Prevention; 1997.
6. Conrad D, Hedin D. School based community service: what we know from research and theory. Phi Delta Kappan 1991;72(10):743–749.
7. Lerner RM. America's Youth in Crisis: Challenges and Options for Programs and Policies. Thousand Oaks, CA: Sage Publications; 1999.
8. Bronfenbrenner U. The Ecology of Human Development: Experiments by Nature and Design. Boston: Harvard University Press; 1979.
9. Booth A, Dunn J, eds. Family–School Links: How Do They Affect Educational Outcomes? Hillsdale, NJ: Lawrence Erlbaum Associates; 1996.
10. Dryfoos JG. Coalition for Community Schools: Evaluation of Community Schools. Findings to Date. Washington, DC: Coalition for Community Schools; 2006.
11. McKay JR. Is there a case for extended interventions for alcohol and drug use disorders? Addiction 2004;100(11):1594–1610.
12. Marlowe DB, Festinger DS, Lee PA, Dugosh KL, Benasutti KM. Matching judicial supervision to clients' risk status in drug court. Crime Delinquency 2006;52(1):52–76.
13. Harrell A, Roman J. Reducing drug use and crime among offenders: the impact of graduated sanctions. J Drug Issues 2001;31:207–232.
14. Pittman K, Cahill M. Youth and Caring: The Role of Youth Programs in the Development of Caring. Indianapolis, IN: Lilly Endowment; 1992.
15. Mackin J, Weller J, Tarte J, Nissen L. Breaking new ground in juvenile justice settings: Assessing for competencies in juvenile offenders. Journal of the National Council of Juvenile and Family Court Judges. 2005;56(2):25–37.
16. Nissen LB. Bringing strengths-based philosophy to life in juvenile justice settings: A primer for understanding the power of strengths in action. Reclaiming Children Youth 2006;15(1):40–46.

17. Teplin L, Abram K, McClelland G, Dulcan M, Mericle A. Psychiatric disorders in youth in juvenile detention. Arch Gen Psychiatry 2002;59:1133–1143.
18. Atkins D, Pumariega W, Rogers K. Mental health and incarcerated youth: I. Prevalence and nature of psychopathology. J Child Fam Stud 1999;8:193–204.
19. Costello E, Angold A, Burns H, Stangle D, Tweed D, Erkanli A, et al. The Great Smoky Mountains Study of Youth: goals, design, methods and the prevalence of DSM-III-R disorders. Arch Gen Psychiatry 1996;53:1129–1136.
20. Kumpfer K. Strengthening America's families: exemplary parenting and family strategies for delinquency prevention. Washington, DC: U.S. Department of Justice, Office of Juvenile Justice and Delinquency Prevention; 1999.
21. Dague B, Tolin C. Developing Parent Supports Within the Juvenile Justice Setting: One Community's Experience. Portland, OR: Portland State University; 1999.
22. Thornberry TP, Lizotte AJ, Krohn MD, Farnworth M, Jang SJ. Delinquent peers, beliefs, and delinquent behavior: a longitudinal test of interactional theory. Criminology 1994;94:47–83.
23. Kumpfer KL, Alvardo R. Effective Family Strengthening Interventions. Washington, DC: Office of Juvenile Justice and Delinquency Prevention; 1998.
24. Bureau of Justice Assistance. Juvenile Drug Courts: Strategies in Practice. Washington, DC: Bureau of Justice Assistance; 2003.
25. Institute of Medicine. Fostering Rapid Advances in Healthcare: Learning From Systems Demonstrations. Washington, DC: Institute of Medicine; 2002.
26. Taylor-Powell E, Hermann C. Collecting Evaluation Data: Surveys. Madison: University of Wisconsin-Extension; 2000.
27. Asmus CL. A campus drug court: Colorado State University. Natl Drug Court Inst Rev 2003;4(1):1–36.

19
Drug Court Organization and Operations

Glade F. Roper and James E. Lessenger

This chapter explains the typical organization of a drug court and the everyday operation of the program. Drug courts are a team effort in which various organizations that are not accustomed to working in concert must work together so that the clients can achieve sobriety, eliminate criminal behaviors, stay out of the criminal justice system, and become productive members of the community. The basic organization of a drug court is the bedrock of the program. Although the concept of drug court is flexible enough to be adapted to the needs and laws of any jurisdiction, the principles enumerated herein have been proven to work, and there is no need to reinvent the basics.

Organization of Drug Court

Judge

The judge sets the tenor and pace of the drug court organization and operation. He or she will provide leadership to the drug court and see that it is effectively implemented. This is not an easy task and requires dedication and commitment, characteristics possessed by most judges. No one personality type is required; indeed, many different types of judges have been successful in presiding over drug courts. Some drug court judges are inherently compassionate and understanding; others are more inclined to be authoritarian and strict. Both types can be successful, although they will deal with drug court defendants differently. The common attributes are a desire to improve the system rather than merely to grind through cases and a willingness to consider novel approaches and alliances.

Drug court judges are typically jurists who have volunteered for the task because they think they can make a positive impact on people's lives and on the worldwide drug problem. Many are dissatisfied with recycling drug defendants through the criminal justice system, only to see them return to their courts days, weeks, or months later. In some jurisdictions, judges have been assigned by presiding judges without volunteering. If they are conscientious and open minded, most will embrace the concept and willingly continue once they observe the efficacy of the program and begin to feel the sense of accomplishment from being part of a successful team that has a significant beneficial effect on people who were deteriorating rapidly and consistently.

Drug court judges need to understand the following basic features of the program and concepts of addiction before assuming their task:

1. The basic concepts and principles of drug courts, especially the difference between failure to comply with treatment and not responding to treatment when compliant.
2. The cycles of addiction and withdrawal.
3. The 12 steps of 12 Step fellowships.
4. The true power of their place in the process as a role model and leader.
5. The likelihood of relapse for many people, even those seriously engaged in recovery.

Because presiding over a drug court is different from other judicial assignments, an untrained judge will have difficulty stepping into the assignment on short notice and may disrupt the consistency of the drug court. It is beneficial to have a judge trained as a backup to substitute when the regular drug court judge is on vacation, in training, or ill. Another viable option, where it is legal, is to have an attorney who is willing to sit as a drug court judge pro tem, or on temporary assignment. Criminal defense attorneys who have seen the benefits of drug court for their clients are a ready source of pro tems, as are attorneys who have personal experience with recovery from addiction. While it is rare for a sitting judge to be a recovering drug addict or alcoholic, it is more common for members of the bar to be so. Attorneys who are recovering addicts or alcoholics make excellent advisors to the drug court judge and as *pro tem* jurists.

Court Officers

Court clerks, bailiffs, and other officials attached to drug court are permanently assigned to the judge, so they do not typically represent an increase in spending. However, it is helpful to have one clerk or a team of clerks assigned to drug court to handle the specialized paperwork. They get to know the clients, can recognize when something appears not to make sense, and can anticipate what the judge will do in most situations. Because of the number of status review hearings, clerks should work with the judge to develop shortened minute order forms that have standard boxes to check to minimize hand writing. Clerks and bailiffs see progress made by the participants and may become involved and supportive of the program.

It is important for a bailiff to understand that the operation and philosophy of a drug court are distinct from those of other courts. Although a defendant who appeared under the influence of drugs would immediately be incarcerated in most courtrooms, that may not be the outcome in a drug court. Unless bailiffs understand that the purpose of a drug court is to assist and nurture addicted people in the process of recovery, they will be at odds with many of the procedures. Judges may choose to come down from the bench to present awards, shake hands, and even give hugs to the participants. While this might be seen as a major breach of security in most courtrooms, it is common in drug courts. The bailiff also needs to be aware that the judge may allow participants to approach the bench to deliver written assignments or receive congratulations and rewards. The bailiff must be willing to consult with the judge and amend common security procedures to allow more informality without sacrificing the safety of the judge and other personnel.

Some programs hire program coordinators, case managers, and consultants to organize the various components of the program and to keep track of the clients as they advance through the phases. Computer programs are available on the Internet to track clients through the program and handle the load of forms and paperwork.

Some drug courts write complicated operations manuals that spell out every phase of treatment, sanctions, and recovery. Others have short memos that do the same or have no written protocols. A written organization manual can be helpful in making the program accessible, perpetual, and equally applicable to all clients in terms of sanctions and rewards. It is also helpful to make the manual available to the clients so that they know what is expected of them and the consequences of unacceptable behavior. The drug court should be organized as a permanent process, and written procedure manuals should detail the responsibilities of all personnel involved. With inevitable promotions, retirements, and other reassignments, it is likely that a constant flow of people will come in and out of the drug court positions. It is important to have written procedures to ensure consistency of operation.

Treatment Providers

Many effective treatment providers and case managers are recovering alcoholics or drug addicts who know and can anticipate attempts to circumvent program requirements such as falsifying test results or attendance at 12 Step meetings. It is also important that they have:

1. Written protocols.
2. Appropriate certification and state licensure, if required.
3. A method of accountability to the court.
4. Availability to the clients in terms of hours of operation and geographic location.

5. Adherence to the drug court requirements and protocols for treatment and reports.

For the court, it is critical that treatment providers be monitored carefully for appropriateness of care and the treatment of clients. Clients must be treated firmly and with respect. Complaints, especially of a sexual nature, must be immediately investigated and resolved.

Of special concern are faith-based treatment providers, many of whom have sincere desires to assist people. A desire to help, although necessary, is not sufficient, and many sincere people have done more harm to recovery than good. A drug court must ensure that its treatment providers are adequately trained and supervised to provide meaningful treatment. That is not to say that all effective counselors must have a PhD or masters degree, but they must have an understanding of basic treatment principles and have experience under qualified supervisors to make sure that they do not substitute personal desires for sound practices.

Committees

Committees generally fall into a formation committee and an operations committee, which may be an extension of the first.

Formation Committee

The establishment of a formation committee is critical to recruit the various participants to support the program. At first, the committee may meet weekly to plan and discuss various aspects of the program formation. People who should be invited to the committee must have policy-making authority and should include the following:

1. Interested judges.
2. A representative from the district attorney or county prosecutor (or similar title in various jurisdictions).
3. A representative from the public defender's office.
4. Representatives from the local criminal defense bar association.
5. Treatment providers.
6. Educators.
7. County or city government.
8. Law enforcement agencies.
9. Mothers Against Drunk Driving (MADD) or other organizations that advocate positions about substance abuse.
10. Interested people from the community, especially service clubs and other traditional segments of the community.
11. Representatives of 12 Step fellowships if the treatment will be based on the 12 Step model of recovery.

The most critical decision of the committee is whether to invest the time and energy into forming a drug court. The second is how it is going to be paid for. Once these two hurdles are overcome, there will be an idea of how much money is available from grants and other sources. The committee must determine what the program will require from the criminal justice system in terms of staffing, rewards, and sanctions and what commitment will be required from the clients.

Operations Committee

The operations committee oversees ongoing operation and makes necessary changes in the drug court. The best planned drug court will need to make changes as obstacles present themselves and conditions change. For example, the formation committee may set a target client population. Once that target is reached, the operations committee may want to increase the population as success is achieved and benefits are manifest. Alternatively, a problem might arise with a treatment provider, and it may become necessary to terminate or modify the contract with that provider. Clients who are in recovery can become extremely agitated and paranoid about any gap in the system, which can contribute to relapse. Disruption should be minimized as much as possible. Standing members of the committee may consist of the following:

1. The judges.
2. The case managers and program manager.
3. Representatives from the treatment providers.
4. A representative from the drug test provider.
5. The prosecutor.
6. The public defender.
7. Other representative of the defense bar.
8. Drug court alumni members.
9. Interested members of the public.

Other members of the community who may be important in the operation and improvement of the drug court include the following:

1. Members of the bar who are in recovery.
2. Physicians knowledgeable in addiction, withdrawal, recovery, and drug test result evaluation.
3. Psychologists.
4. Legal consultants.

Experts who have special knowledge and skill in treating and dealing with addicted people are an invaluable resource to the drug court. Physicians and psychologists may not wish to make the time commitment to serve on a standing committee but may be willing to assist when necessary and to consult when specific problems arise. Many are familiar with the deficits in the traditional criminal system and are willing to contribute their expertise when they understand the benefits of the drug court approach. It is a great benefit to the drug court when influential members of the community outside the court system support the drug court.

Drug Testing

Drug testing can be done by court officers, treatment providers, or a separate, independent contractor or company. Tests can be paid for by the client, through operation funds, or by a grant, although reliance on grant funding for testing is a sure recipe for conflict and struggle when the grant funds are exhausted. Whoever performs the testing must be aware of some simple facts:

1. The tests must be economical so that the client can pay for them or so they can be paid out without depleting grant or operation funds.
2. It is important to test for all commonly abused drugs and not just the client's drug of choice.
3. The specimen must be handled and destroyed as contaminated medical waste.
4. The results must be reproducible and reliable.
5. Chain-of-custody must be maintained.
6. Appropriate reports must be made to the treatment providers and court.
7. Testing must not overwhelm the clients. Testing sites and times must be convenient to the clients to meet the demands of employment and drug court requirements.
8. Testing schedules must be truly random and unpredictable.
9. Testing must be observed to prevent tampering or falsification.

Community Support

Support from nonprofit, service, and community organizations within the community is invaluable. They can provide:

1. Political support.
2. Money for graduation facility rentals and refreshments.
3. Money for incidentals such as clothing and makeup for the clients.
4. Contacts for client jobs.
5. Special job training and education programs.
6. Rewards and incentives.

Some drug courts have created 501(c)(3) nonprofit foundations that provide ongoing support for the drug courts. Most judges are ethically prohibited from soliciting funds but are free to speak about the operation and benefits of a drug court. After hearing such benefits, many civic groups and individuals inquire about what they can do to help. A judge may refer such individuals to a foundation board member who can then explain how donations can be made to the foundation. In most jurisdictions, board members and other drug court team members are not restrained from soliciting donations. Court personnel must be careful not to appear to represent the judge in soliciting donations. Prominent community members and business executives who are in recovery are ideally suited to sit on foundation boards (1).

Operation of the Drug Court

The day-to-day operation of the drug court is typically organized by a program coordinator or, if one is lacking, the judge and an operations committee. The operation of a program begins with the day the client is arrested (2).

Arrest

When arrested for a drug-related crime, detainees are either released on their own recognizance or incarcerated in the county jail, depending on the jurisdiction, crime, and circumstances of arrest. The arresting officer transmits a report to the prosecuting attorney's office, where a complaint is prepared and filed with the court.

Arraignment

At arraignment the defendants are formally charged, and a defense counsel is arranged if the defendant pleads not guilty. Either at the arraignment or at subsequent hearings, the defendant's eligibility for drug court is determined. Basic criteria may include the following:

1. The defendant has committed a drug-related crime, such as possession of drugs, possession of paraphernalia, intoxication with drugs, or sale of small amounts of drugs to support their personal drug use. In many jurisdictions, small theft offenses, such as shoplifting, that are clearly related to drug addiction are referred to the drug court.
2. The client has no history of violent crimes such as assault, spousal abuse, or child abuse.
3. The defendant has no history of sex offenses.
4. The defendant was not in possession of a deadly weapon.
5. The defendant is not a large-scale drug dealer.

Those defendants not selected for a probation interview are channeled into regular criminal justice processing.

Probation Interview

The defendants seeking admission into drug court typically interview with a probation officer or some other court officer charged with screening for eligibility and suitability. The officers typically ask a series of questions and complete an interview sheet. Most officers conduct numerous interviews, so the questions are intended to learn a lot about the defendant in a short period of time. For example, in the Tulare County program, probation officers initially asked a lot of questions about drug use. Yet when an analysis was done on the data, it was discovered there was no statistical benefit from knowing the answers. All that is asked now is the drug of choice and the route of choice. Conversely, questions about disability, military service, and psychiatric problems were added to ferret out evidence of mental illness (3).

Later in the program, it was found that the probation interview form essentially duplicated the initial treatment program assessments, so the program became less selective to allow more defendants to potentially benefit from the program. The probation intake form was shortened to include only that information deemed necessary to determine eligibility. The lengthy questionnaire was found to be a poor predictor of success, and the philosophy was changed to admit anyone meeting the eligibility criteria who expressed a willingness to participate, which moved the court closer to a comprehensive drug court system designed to treat a broad range of drug-using offenders (3). In jurisdictions with limited slots available, a more thorough suitability determination is employed. Such an arrangement will produce better outcome statistics for completion of the program but may exclude many potential participants.

The screening officer typically makes a decision to offer drug court based on the following:

1. The defendant's responses to the questions.
2. The defendant's criminal justice computer history report (rap sheet).
3. The circumstances of the arrest.
4. A subjective determination of probable success based on the defendant's demeanor.

If the officer determines the defendant is appropriate for drug court, the officer explains the costs (if any) of the program, the amount of work that is expected, and the other requirements such as drug testing, 12 Step fellowship meetings, counseling, and court appearances.

An effective strategy is to require prospective clients to sit through a day of drug court and see the effect of the sanctions and rewards before making the commitment to participate. At that time they also have an opportunity to talk with other clients and graduates and learn what the program is about from the client's point of view.

The defendant has the choice of accepting or rejecting the program. Most of those who reject drug court do so because they are unwilling or perceive themselves as unable to cease drug use. Many, however, have concerns about the pain of withdrawal, the costs of the program, or charges pending in other courts. Sometimes, the officer can answer those questions and the defendant will elect to go into the program despite perceived obstacles.

Defendants who decline drug court are returned to the criminal justice system where one of the following can occur:

1. They go to trial.
2. They plead guilty or arrange some form of plea bargain, or,
3. Their cases are occasionally dropped for various reasons, including lack of evidence.

Judgment

Once defendants accept drug court, they appear before the drug court judge and plead guilty to the crime or (more often) crimes. The defendants are then placed on probation; once they sign an agreement, they become clients of drug court. In some jurisdictions a plea may occur in another courtroom, but it is always the best practice to have the drug court judge pronounce sentence. The sooner defendants can become familiar with the drug court judge, the sooner they can begin to understand the nature of the drug court and to comprehend that they are there to receive help and support, not punishment.

Probation agreements vary by jurisdictions, but in general the client makes many significant commitments to the court, waiving several rights and making a number of promises. In addition, clients may sign agreements to allow their photographs to be used in graduation ceremonies or other agreements as required in the various jurisdictions. In jurisdictions where defense attorneys do not appear in court for regular status hearings, that should be made clear to the defendants at the inception and appropriate waivers signed. Waivers of confidentiality are also required by The Health Insurance and Portability Act (HIPAA) and 42 USC (4,5).

In the Tulare County drug court, photographs are taken at arrest, arraignment, or at sentencing to be used as a baseline for the client's progress and to compare to a graduation photograph at the graduation ceremony. Although a participant should not be forced to allow presentation of photographs, displaying the difference in appearance between starting and graduating from the drug court is a powerful message of success to the participants and the general public. Most graduates are proud to display the progress they have made.

Assignment of Treatment Providers

Case managers and treatment providers may be officers of the court or, more commonly, personnel of nonprofit or public treatment clinics. They may be assigned randomly, but consideration should be given to special treatment requirements, such as the following:

1. The location of the client's residence.
2. The client's transportation resources.

3. Possible conflicts of interest.
4. The client's detoxification and withdrawal needs.
5. Gender-specific groups.
6. Mental illness.
7. Language limitations.

The number of providers available, their affiliations, and their place in a rotation pool often dictates which one is selected for a given client. Often providers are assigned according to where the client lives. Another selection factor is the lack of a conflict of interest such as family members of the client being associated with the provider or other relatives being clients of the provider. Most important is whether the client needs an inpatient, residential, or outpatient facility for detoxification, withdrawal, and intensive therapy. Intravenous methamphetamine users are especially in need of inpatient facilities and seem to have the most problems in withdrawal. Unfortunately, inpatient and residential beds are scarce and expensive so the client may have to wait in jail until an inpatient or residential bed becomes available if he or she is unable to remain abstinent.

Recent research suggests that many people referred to drug courts may not be diagnosable as chemically dependant but may actually use or abuse drugs. Total abstinence may be a reasonable expectation for them, whereas total abstinence is an unrealistic expectation for truly addicted people. It may be unwise to mix the two groups, and consideration should be given to segregating participants according to the extent of their addiction (1).

The Drug Court Process

While it varies from one jurisdiction to another, the drug court process generally follows a pattern of three treatment phases and aftercare (Table 19.1).

TABLE 19.1. Outpatient phases and requirements of Tulare County Drug Court.

Phase	Minimum length	Court dates	Individual therapy	Recovery group	Education classes	12 Step meetings	Drug tests
I	2 Months	Weekly	Weekly	Weekly	Weekly	Four times a week	Twice a week
II	4 Months	Every other week	Every other week	Weekly	Weekly	Four times a week	One and a half weekly
III	6 Months	Monthly	Every other week	Monthly	Monthly	Four times a week	One and a half weekly
Graduation							
Aftercare	6 Months	Every third month		Twice a month		Four times a week	Weekly

During the process, clients must attend regular court hearings and are monitored by drug tests, probation officers, and treatment providers.

In addition, clients are expected to:

1. Attend individual and group counseling.
2. Engage in client life skills training.
3. Graduate from high school or obtain the equivalent unless they are mentally incapable of doing so.
4. Get a job, unless legitimately disabled.
5. Attend 12 Step fellowship programs.

In 12 Step–based programs, clients are required to attend self-help meetings, such as Narcotics Anonymous (NA) and Alcoholics Anonymous (AA). In certain jurisdictions, courts have held that NA and AA meetings are religious in nature and cannot be required for defendants who object to attending them (6). Such rulings have questionable applicability since in most areas AA and NA have made it clear that they are open to persons of all beliefs and that they can designate anything to be their "higher power." Many people who have no religious inclinations are able to embrace the principles of AA and NA and effectively apply them to their recovery. It is beneficial to include AA and NA leaders in drug court planning so that nonreligious participants may be welcomed to their fellowships and so that meetings are sufficiently tolerant to accommodate people of all persuasions. However, in areas where AA or NA has been adjudicated as religious in nature, drug court participants must be given access to an alternative, nonreligious 12 Step fellowship if they desire it.

The Court Day

The drug court team should convene before court opens to discuss client progress and appropriate responses. Some drug courts discuss every client; others find it necessary to discuss only those who have particular problems or who have made exceptional progress. Differing philosophies dictate how much influence each team member will have in the decision-making process. Some programs give equal weight to all team members who vote whenever there is a disagreement on what course should be followed. Others give extra weight to the treatment providers for treatment decisions and to the judge and attorneys for legal matters. A judge cannot abdicate his or her responsibility to administer the law, so in certain areas the judge will have the sole decision-making authority after consulting with the other team members. These occasions are rare, and in general a team that works together well will have very few conflicts. Judges, attorneys, coordinators, and probation officers should give great deference to the guidance of trained treatment providers on treatment issues. Treatment providers and coordinators will have much less experience and knowledge of legal matters and should defer to attorneys and the judge on those issues.

The court appearance of the client before the drug court judge is an essential part of the program. It is here that the feedback loop of behavior and consequences is completed and where sanctions are delivered for bad behavior and rewards given for appropriate behavior. Each client is called before the court and queried about his or her progress and compliance with the recovery program. In general, the team will have discussed any violation of treatment requirements or ongoing drug use, and the judge will implement the decision made by the team. It is not unusual for a surprise to occur during the status hearing. Reports are prepared in advance of the hearing and may not include all relevant information. In the event that something new or unforeseen arises in the course of the dialogue between the judge and the participant, or new information comes to the attention of a team member, he or she should request a recess or approach the bench to inform the judge of the new information. Judges readily accept such information to avoid imposing an improper sanction or rewarding a participant who is out of compliance.

Court Schedule

Clients are attempting to comply with the requirements of a job, education, and treatment, so a court schedule that interferes with these requirements is counterproductive. In Tulare County, the court is held on one day and in one courtroom so that the clients do not get confused while they are detoxifying from drugs. Six hourly times are offered to attempt to accommodate work and school schedules as much as possible. Participants who are employed full-time or attending school are given priority in scheduling, and the remaining participants are divided among the calendars to even out the day.

Documents for Court

During the court hearing, the judge has the legal file and any other files on charges or crimes that may have filtered through the system. Present are representatives of the treatment providers who give a report orally and in writing on the client's progress. The court also has a copy of the client's drug testing record to test the veracity of the client's statements. Lying is not tolerated and is considered a violation of treatment rules; drug use is considered a symptom of withdrawal. Decisions are made from the bench after consultation with the drug court team and a record generated for the legal file. Bench warrants and remands for incarceration hearings are also executed if the client absconds or fails the program.

Proof of Compliance

Accountability is key to the success of the program; therefore, at each court hearing the clients are required to submit proof of attendance at 12 Step fellowship meetings. Some jurisdictions require the meeting organizer to send a form to the court; in Tulare County the client must ask the secretary of the meeting to initial a card with the date. The client then brings the card into the court.

Reports for education, counseling, and other programs are provided by the case managers or treatment providers. The courts may require the client to bring in proof of attendance in a high school continuation program, college classes, or vocational training schools.

The Court Interview and the Implementation of Sanctions and Awards

The clients are called up before the court and queried by the judge about their progress for the previous week or weeks. If sanctions are needed, they are immediately implemented. Implementing sanctions immediately in front of other clients and those thinking of joining drug court makes a powerful statement about the consequences of their actions (Table 19.2).

When certain significant rewards are presented, the judge may choose to walk to the floor, hand clients their rewards, and shake their hands. Such a gesture communicates acceptance and constitutes a reward for achievement. An effective strategy is to have clients make a short speech about what recovery means to them and how their lives have changed with sobriety. The speeches are often emotional, very powerful, and therapeutic for the client (Table 19.3).

Courtroom Decorum

Each drug court will have to decide how formal the courtroom will be during drug court reviews. Some judges find it appropriate to hold more informal hearings than they have in other court proceedings. They allow clapping for significant milestones, refer to the defendants by first name, and may come off the bench to shake hands or hug the defendants when they achieve certain levels. The theory in such lessening of courtroom strictures is that a drug court differs from other court proceedings and is a place to help, rather than punish, the defendants.

Other judges run their drug courts just like other criminal proceedings with strict formality. No approach has been proven more effective than the other, and it is suggested that judges experiment and follow the procedure they find most comfortable and shows the most success.

Because many participants have experienced sexual abuse as children and adults, they should never be required to hug anyone. Part of the recovery process requires participants who have been subjected to sexual abuse to draw appropriate boundaries, and judges should not initiate embraces. If a judge feels comfortable giving an appropriate embrace to a participant,

TABLE 19.2. Tulare county drug court minimum sanctions.

Violation	Sanction
1. Miss 12 Step meetings after being placed on star track	a. First time: sit in jury box next drug court day, make up meetings b. Second time: spend 1 night in jail, make up meetings c. Third time: spend 2 nights in jail, make up meetings d. Fourth time: spend 1 week in jail, make up meetings e. Fifth time: spend 2 weeks in jail, make up meetings f. Sixth time: spend 1 month in jail, move back a phase, make up meetings g. Seventh time: spend 2 months in jail, move back a phase, make up meetings
2. Miss test	a. First time: sit in jury box next drug court day b. Second time: spend 1 night in jail c. Third time: spend 2 nights in jail, may move back a phase d. Fourth time: spend 1 week in jail, consider moving back a phase e. Fifth time: spend 2 weeks in jail, consider moving back to Phase 1 f. Sixth time: spend 1 month in jail, consider termination g. Seventh time: spend 2 months in jail, consider termination
3. Miss counseling	Pay for missed session, extension of 1 week to move to next phase
4. Adulterate test	a. First time: spend 30 days in jail after next drug court day, possible termination from drug court b. Second time: termination from drug court
5. Falsify signature	a. First time: spend 14 days in jail after next drug court day b. Second time: termination from the drug court
6. Miss aftercare meeting	Extend aftercare 1 month
7. Take unauthorized medication	Clean date adjusted, write essay about importance of not taking unauthorized medications
8. Miss test in aftercare	a. First time: pay for hair test b. Second time: pay for hair test, move back to Phase 3
9. Fail to attend graduation ceremony	Spend 1 week in jail

Note: These standard sanctions are the minimum that will be imposed for the listed violations of the drug court program. Additional or increased sanctions may be imposed at the discretion of the judge after consultation with the drug court team. In the absence of compelling circumstances, all sanctions will be imposed at the next court date to connect the behavior with the sanction as much as possible. Once someone has established a record of not attending meetings, a little "star" or asterisk is placed in the file next to the running total of how many meetings they owe, and they are on the "star track," meaning that they then start getting sanctioned for every meeting they miss.

he or she should do so only when the participant initiates it and it should be brief and clearly platonic in nature.

In any event, participants should dress appropriately for court appearances, should always refer to the judge as "Your Honor," and comply with

Table 19.3. Rewards.

Type	Phase	Action	Reward
Standard	I	Completion	Key ring with drug court logo and message, "Recovery is a process that lasts a lifetime because sooner or later you have to plant your feet"
		180 days clean and sober	Small handcuffs, given with the advice, "These are to remind you that you don't have to wear the big ones anymore"
	II	Completion	Coffee mug with drug court logo depicting a car on a road and a sign pointing to freedom and the message: Half way there
	III	Completion, at graduation ceremony.	T-shirt with drug court logo depicting closed and open handcuffs, and a certificate signed by the judge and probation officer.
	Aftercare	Completion	Embossed gold seal to place on the graduation certificate
Variable, given as needed or available		10 days clean and sober	Small bottle of shampoo, soap, or conditioner collected from a hotel
		30 days clean and sober	Souvenir pen or pencil from some interesting place
		60 days clean and sober	Small clock or similar item
		One year clean and sober	Squeeze ball donated by NCAA
		Graduating from high school or getting or improving employment	Covered clipboard, carry bag, calculator, or similar item

Note: Additional ad hoc rewards are given any time someone donates something appropriate and a participant needs some encouragement for his or her performance.

other rules such as remaining quiet, listening in court, and not chewing gum. Part of the process of changing from outlaws to law-abiding citizens involves appreciation for civic rules and learning to behave appropriately.

Graduation

Many drug court clients have never completed anything important in their lives and think of themselves as losers and outcasts. Most feel isolated and are under the impression that they are unique in their experience. Some never graduated from high school. The graduation ceremony at the end of the third phase is designed to make them feel accomplished and accepted into society as rehabilitated. The ceremony may be held in an auditorium, often with more solemnity than a college graduation. The judge presides with bailiffs and other court officials in attendance. Local politicians and representatives of the legal, medical, and law enforcement communities attend. Popular personalities might be invited to speak; for example, in Tulare County, David Crosby, Larry Hagman, Todd Bridges, Mackenzie Phillips, Art Linkletter, and Joe Walsh have spoken to the graduates and handed out diplomas. Each graduate is handed a diploma by the probation officers and congratulated by the dignitaries.

Part of the program is a slide presentation that shows contrasting arrest and graduation photographs of the clients. There are also videos of some of the clients speaking, expressing appreciation for those who have supported them on the road to recovery, and citing the benefits of sobriety. Some express appreciation to the police officers who arrested them and interdicted their declines. Refreshments are typically served after the graduation and may be provided by service clubs such as Rotary or a drug court foundation.

Graduation gives the clients a sense of accomplishment and instills the concept that they can complete a difficult task. The ceremony puts them on public notice that continued drug-using behavior would not only be a failure on their part but a grave source of disappointment to the judge and the members of the audience. This social expectation can be a stronger deterrent to drug use than the threat of incarceration.

Aftercare

The aftercare program consists of less frequent appearances before the court, continued attendance at 12 Step fellowship meetings, and attendance at alumni association meetings. Aftercare for clients reinforces habits created during the formal program and develops a new culture devoid of habits and friends that contributed to addiction. If after 6 months the clients have paid all fines and expenses, attendance has been perfect, and there has been no new crime or positive drug test, the charges can be dismissed. In addition, depending on the circumstances, crime, and jurisdiction, fines can be decreased, other charges dismissed, convictions overturned, and records expunged.

If at any time during the aftercare program clients are arrested on drug charges, they are sent to jail for a period determined by the judge after consultation with the other team members. On release, they may be reevaluated for drug court. If they decline the program or commit another offence, they are incarcerated in jail or state prison under standard sentencing practices.

Confidentiality Issues

Confidentiality issues have become complex and uncertain. The United States Code (42 USC 290dd-2) authorizes the Secretary of Health and Human Services to promulgate regulations to protect the confidentiality of patients receiving any type of substance abuse treatment, counseling, or rehabilitation. These regulations are codified at 42 Code of Federal Regulations Part 160 and Subparts A and E of Part 164. In 1996, Congress passed HIPAA, which also required the Department of Health and Human Services to develop regulations to protect the privacy of anyone receiving health care. Both of these laws are complex and difficult to understand. They require specific waivers to be executed by drug court participants before information about their treatment can be communicated from treatment providers to others, and anyone receiving the information is probably bound not to further communicate that information to anyone else without a similar waiver. In addition, state laws govern communication of this information and may have more stringent requirements than federal law. Sample waiver forms have been included in the Appendix for illustration only; there is no guarantee that they meet the requirements of all federal and state laws and regulations, and they should not be relied on.

Very few court decisions have clarified the numerous questions that arise from the interaction of drug courts with HIPAA and 42 CFR. For example, because drug court status review hearings are done in open court, may treatment reports and issues be openly discussed? One court opinion indicates that they may, but there could be varying opinions from other jurisdictions (7). It is mandatory that all drug courts seek legal advice from knowledgeable attorneys who can review all waiver forms and ensure that they meet the requirements of current state and federal laws.

References

1. Tauber J, Huddleston CW. Development and Implementation of Drug Court Systems. Washington, DC: National Drug Court Institute; 1999.
2. Lessenger JE, Roper GF. Drug courts: a primer for the family physician. J Am Board Fam Pract 2002;15(4):298–303.
3. Lessenger JE, Lessenger LH, Lessenger EW. An Outcome Analysis of Drug Court in Tulare County, California. Visalia: Tulare County Superior Court; 2000.
4. Health Insurance Portability and Accountability Act, 45 CFR Part 160 and Subparts A and E of Part 164.
5. 42 USC 290dd and 42 CFR Chapter 1, Part 2.
6. *Warner v. Orange County Department of Probation*, 115 F.3d 1068 (2d Cir. 1997).
7. *State of Florida v. Noelle L. Bush*, Case No. 48-02-CF-6371-0, Circuit Court for the Ninth Judicial Circuit, Orange County, Florida (2002).

20
The Legal Basis for Drug Courts

Glade F. Roper

During the 1950s, rehabilitation was the primary goal of the criminal justice system (1). In the 1970s, the effectiveness of rehabilitative programs began to be questioned. By the 1980s, support for rehabilitation had eroded, and the focus shifted from rehabilitation of criminals to punishing and taking them off the street through incarceration (2). In 1990, an assistant warden of a California prison facility told the author that all hope of rehabilitation in the prisons had been abandoned and that the sole purpose of the Department of Corrections was to warehouse the inmates.

Not only did the focus on warehousing inmates prove to be a very expensive policy but judges around the country began to see the same drug offenders repeatedly, and with increasing frequency, as early release programs were instated to alleviate prison and jail overcrowding. As studies showed that an increasing number of offenders for all crimes were under the influence of drugs at the time of arrest, judges began to search for alternative ways to sentence defendants that would not only be less costly than incarceration but would also address the cause of the crime. Research showed that treating addicted offenders would reduce their tendency to commit crimes and that coerced addiction treatment was at least as effective as voluntary treatment (2–4). Judges and prosecutors in Dade County, Florida, developed the first drug court to reduce drug crime recidivism and reserve scarce penal facilities for more serious and violent offenders. Other drug courts soon followed around the country.

Because drug courts were formed by judges and prosecutors working with probation officers, treatment providers, and law enforcement officials, there were no statutes authorizing their development. The legal basis for their structure was either the inherent ability of judges to impose probation in postconviction drug court models or the authority of prosecutors to dismiss charges in preconviction models.

In every state jurisdiction, judges have the discretion to impose probation for most crimes. The purposes of probation are to deter further criminal behavior, punish the offender, help provide reparation to crime victims and their communities, and provide offenders with opportunities for rehabilitation (5,6). In general, a judge may impose any terms of probation that are rationally related to the crime and the purposes of probation (7). Although this is not unfettered discretion, a judge has broad discretion to impose conditions of probation that are reasonably calculated to control the conduct of the defendant (8). It is this latitude that allows judges to impose drug court requirements as terms of probation that regulate what the defendants must do in the drug court. Judges must collaborate with all members of the drug court team and have agreement from each on the probation terms to be imposed for the drug court to function smoothly.

In pre-plea drug courts, it is the decision of the prosecutor to offer to dismiss charges after successful completion of the treatment program that constitutes the legal basis for the drug court. The prosecutor's decision to institute criminal charges is the broadest and least regulated power in American criminal law. The judicial deference shown to prosecutors generally is most noticeable with respect to the charging function. This is not to say that the prosecutor's discretion is unbounded. Various legal, political, experiential, and ethical considerations inform and guide the charging decision (9). Thus, the prosecutor has wide latitude in deciding what charges to file. Certainly in a pre-plea drug court setting, this latitude would have little meaning unless there is an express agreement between the court, the defense bar, and other drug court team members about who will be admitted into the program.

Having observed the success of drug courts, some state legislatures have adopted statutes authorizing drug courts and regulating how they are to be operated. For example, Virginia adopted a detailed statute called the *Drug Treatment Court Act* explaining exactly how drug courts are to be operated and establishing state and local advisory committees to oversee them (10). Drug courts in existence prior to the effective date of the act, March 1, 2004, are exempt from the provisions of the act. Similarly, Idaho and Illinois specifically authorize drug courts and mental health courts and regulate how they are to be created and operated (11,12). It is probable that many states that do not yet have legislation governing drug courts will adopt such legislation in the future as drug courts become more widely established.

Other statutes have provided funds to operate drug courts, although not expressly authorizing them or closely regulating them. For example, the California Drug Court Partnership Act of 1998 (13) provided funds to counties wishing to implement or enhance their existing drug courts through a grant process (14). No county was required to have a drug court nor were counties with drug courts required to apply for a grant. Grantees were required to comply with standards set forth in the act and to report on the outcomes of their programs. In this way, they were regulated on how their drug courts were operated.

Drug courts have become an integral part of the overall drug control strategy of some states. In Florida, a main section of the state's Drug Control Strategy is entitled "Drug Courts—An Integral Part of Stopping

Drug Abuse." It incorporates 10 components of drug court adopted by the Florida Supreme Court Treatment-Based Drug Court Committee and cites the findings that drug court programs reduce the annual cost for participants from $19,000 for incarceration to $1,800 for drug court. The strategy strongly advocates the need to expand drug courts into all parts of Florida not adequately served at the present time (15).

The federal government has played a major role in establishing drug courts through funding mechanisms. Title V of the Violent Crime Control and Law Enforcement Act of 1994 authorized awards of federal grants for drug courts. Since 1995, the Office of Justice Programs has awarded grants for planning and implementation of new drug courts and enhancement of existing ones. These grants required the funded drug courts to have early and continuing judicial supervision, mandatory periodic drug testing, addiction and substance abuse treatment, integrated administration of services, and graduated sanctions. The grants also required that violent offenders be excluded and that upon unsuccessful completion, participants be prosecuted and punished (16). While not expressly mandating or authorizing drug courts, congressional appropriations have been one of the chief motivations for state courts to create them.

Interestingly, even though Congress has provided millions of dollars to fund the creation, operation, and expansion of drug courts, it has not authorized federal courts to operate drug courts. In a *New York Times* opinion article, Senior Judge Donald P. Lay of the United States Court of Appeals for the Eighth Circuit explained that mandatory minimum sentences, enacted by Congress, have contributed to the rising costs of imprisonment and crowding in federal prisons. Judge Lay argued that 54% of the federal prison population are drug felons and, unlike the states, the federal criminal justice system offers no alternatives for nonviolent offenders charged with drug-related crimes. Lay wrote that, given the success of drug courts in the states, the federal government should study how to modify its sentencing to incorporate elements of the drug court model and to assess the effectiveness of community-based alternatives to imprisonment for nonviolent federal drug felons (17).

References

1. American Correctional Association. Manual of Correctional Standards. College Park, MD: American Correctional Association, Committee for the Revision of the 1954 Manual; 1959.
2. Gebelein RS. The Rebirth of Rehabilitation: Promise and Perils of Drug Courts. Sentencing and Corrections: Issues for the 21st Century, No. 6. Washington, DC: U.S. Department of Justice, Office of Justice Programs, National Institute of Justice; 2000.
3. Farabee D, Prendergast M, Anglin MD. Effectiveness of Coerced Treatment of Drug-Abusing Offenders. Federal Probation 1998;62(1):3–10.

4. Marlow DB. Effective Strategies for Intervening With Drug Abusing Offenders. Villanova Law Rev 2002:14:989–1025.
5. Minnesota Statutes 2005 609.02 Subd. 15.
6. *Commonwealth v. Pike*, 428 Mass. 393, 403 (1998).
7. *Commonwealth v. LaPointe*, 435 Mass. 455 (2001).
8. *Commonwealth v. Williams*, 60 Mass. App. Ct. 331 (2004).
9. Gershman BL. A Moral Standard for the Prosecutor's Exercise of the Charging Discretion. Fordham Urban Law J 1993;20:513–530.
10. Virginia Statutes 18.2-254.1. Drug Treatment Court Act.
11. Idaho Statutes Title 19 Section 19-5606.
12. Illinois Statutes 730 ILCS 166 and 705 ILCS 410.
13. California Health and Safety Code, Section 11970.
14. Drug Court Partnership Act of 1998, Chapter 1007, Statutes of 1998 Final Report. Sacramento, CA: The California Department of Alcohol and Drug Programs and the Judicial Council of California, Administrative Office of the Courts; 2002.
15. Florida Drug Control Strategy 1999–2005. Tallahassee, FL: Office of Drug Control, Executive Office of the Governor, State of Florida; 2005.
16. Turner S, Longshore D, Wenzel S, et al. A National Evaluation of 14 Drug Courts. Santa Monica, CA: RAND Corporation, 2001. Available at: http://www.ncjrs.gov/pdffiles1/nij/grants/191200.pdf.
17. Lay DP. New York Times. November 18, 2004.

21
Drug Court Funding Options

Glade F. Roper, Dennis A. Reilly, Dee S. Owens,
and James E. Lessenger

Although the success of drug courts has been remarkable, the cost of implementing them is always a challenge. Placing offenders in treatment programs saves the cost of incarceration, but the treatment, usually a fraction of the cost of jail or prison, must be financed. For example, in California it costs approximately $26,000 to incarcerate one person for 1 year in the state prison system, while the cost of a year in a county jail varies between $12,500 and $40,000. Effective treatment for a year can cost as little as $3,000. Testing and supervision are critical elements of drug court, and each incurs a significant cost (1–8).

Drug court funding varies according to the activity within the system being used by the client. Sources of funding include general revenue funds, grants, contracts, insurance, and private pay by the clients themselves. For a given client and drug court system, multiple funding sources may be used.

Drug court activities that require funding include the following:

1. Court operations.
2. Probation department operations.
3. Medical treatment.
4. Dental treatment.
5. Counseling.
6. Education.
7. Drug testing.
8. Client life training.
9. Tattoo removal.
10. Research.
11. Miscellaneous needs such as food at the graduation and gifts and rewards for graduates.

Funding Sources

Funding for drug court operations and for the clients' progress through the program can come from several sources. In reality, a mix of various funding tools is used in a modern drug court setting. The composition of the mix depends on the country, state, or province and on the local political commitment to the program (Table 21.1). Sources of funding include the following:

1. General and special revenue funds.
2. Interagency cooperation.
3. Nonprofit organizations.
4. Community-based service and philanthropic organizations.
5. Grants.

Table 21.1. List of funding tools.

Drug court activity	Funding Source
Court operations	General revenue funds Special revenue funds
Probation department operations	General revenue funds Special revenue funds Fines Client paid Grants
Medical and dental testing and treatment	Client paid Insurance Grants Donations
Counseling	Client paid Insurance Grants Contracts
Education	Client paid Scholarships Grants
Drug testing	Client paid Grants Donations Contracts
Client life training	Client paid Grants Contracts
Tattoo removal	Client paid Insurance Donations Grants
Research	Grants Donations
Miscellaneous, gifts, handouts, diplomas, refreshments	Donations Service clubs Client paid

6. Fundraising.
7. Insurance.
8. Client-paid fees.

General and Special Revenue Funds

State agencies with common missions can join together to support drug courts. State agencies can fund grants that can be used to support drug court program components. State agencies may fund a portion of a service program once it has been shown to be effective, such as drug testing, inpatient detoxification, training programs, or dental work. State commissions formed to reduce crime, improve highway safety, or increase access to treatment may be tapped for drug court or service program funding. State agencies can fund drug court services through pretrial or probation supervision fees or conviction surcharges imposed on offenders convicted of drug offenses. Education and prevention programs mandated for at-risk offenders are often sources of funding for services, utilizing lower level offender's program fees to support higher level offender treatment and supervision costs.

One key for drug courts to obtain local resources is to develop strong personal relationships with local government officials and to present an effective case for the need for drug courts by demonstrating the economic benefit to the local community. Local funding application processes are relatively simple and have minimal reporting requirements. Not all funds obtained through city or county governments originate as local dollars. Local officials may control many federal funds. Good examples of locally controlled federal funds are the community development block grants.

Municipalities and counties have been able to support drug court models by reallocating other state or federal funds or creating new funding streams. Cities, municipalities, and counties have supported drug court programs by redirecting money from taxes, fines, and forfeitures or reapplying funding from prevention and health programs or from offender programs such as traffic safety. Other possible funding sources on the local level include abandoned property funds, abandoned trust funds, punitive damage awards, and nondispersed class action funds. Federal transportation funding or special treatment funding such as the recent Access to Recovery treatment voucher program may expand resources for drug courts.

Interagency Cooperation

Drug courts, especially newly formed ones, can finance themselves better by focusing on interagency cooperation than by trying to pay for resources in a drug court budget that are already available through other agencies. Other agency services, such as medical care, dental care, child care, and counseling, may already be provided to people in recovery, and the drug court can easily tap into those resources without establishing a separate line item in its own budget.

Nonprofit Organizations

Nonprofit organizations that can provide money include organizations dedicated to a specific court, philanthropic organizations, and faith-based organizations. Nonprofit organizations can assist the drug court in developing relationships and identifying potential funding sources. Drug courts have established nonprofit organizations under IRS tax code 501(c)(3) to seek funding for supportive services from foundations and other nonprofit organizations and to promote public awareness. Forming a nonprofit corporation permits judges and attorneys to distance themselves from development activities and reduce the risk of real or perceived conflicts of interest.

If drug courts do not want to start a new nonprofit corporation, they can partner effectively with existing nonprofit corporations such as the United Way that can set up an account for funds to be passed through to the program. Local United Way organizations convene representatives of human service providers, clients, and community leaders to evaluate the needs of the community. Drug courts can address these meetings to raise awareness of their mission and improve access to services.

Community-Based Service and Philanthropic Organizations

Drug courts have received financial support from local corporations, faith-based organizations, foundations, and service clubs. These organizations may have mission statements and community outreach goals that can be fulfilled by supporting a drug court. Community service clubs have been instrumental in building meaningful incentive systems and community service opportunities to support critical components of drug court such as tattoo removal, employment training, and graduation ceremonies. Corporations may provide matching funds for fundraisers or donate incentives to recognize client and community achievements. Citizen's councils, community antidrug coalitions, and prevention groups facilitate access to services. The existence of foundation and other support systems boosts a court's ability to demonstrate sustainability to funding agencies. Partner organizations can also assist drug court practitioners to focus resources and to create broad-based support.

Community partnerships improve the court's chances of accessing funds that were not attainable as a judicial entity. By combining social service eligibility factors with criminal justice involvement, the increased risk factors of the drug court population can help to establish a case for increased grant, foundation, and state agency funding. Conversely, by partnering with the court, community treatment providers can gain access to funding that has traditionally been the province of the courts.

Building accountable service systems with community partners increases opportunities for funding. A fiscal management team for the drug court can be developed utilizing members of the program steering committee or pro bono professionals. Funding sources recognize that time-limited grants to assist in planning or to provide seed money for operations must be evaluated and awarded based on the sustainability of the project. Community partners that share the burden of sustaining new programs and services provide some assurance that services will not terminate upon the completion of grant funding.

Partnerships provide opportunities to enhance existing projects and create opportunities to fulfill grant requirements or reach capacity in existing grant-funded programs. Pilot projects and clinical trials can lay the foundation for future grant funding. Community coalitions attract funding to improve their coordination efforts and improve the delivery of services. Drug courts create effective service strategies when developed and operated by multidisciplinary teams that create a stable environment for the drug court. Criminal justice agencies often provide staff, financial resources, or in-kind services to the drug court, knowing that the offenders would be the responsibility of their agency in the absence of a drug court. The relationship with prosecution and law enforcement agencies is critical to community credibility of a program. Beyond political support, building relationships with probation and law enforcement can assist in client supervision through home visits, drug and alcohol testing, and street intelligence.

Grants

Drug courts, service providers, treatment providers, and individual clients may apply for grants to fund part or all of a component program of drug court or a client's treatment. Sources of grants include the following:

1. Government agencies.
2. Nonprofit organizations.
3. Service and philanthropic organizations.
4. Corporations.
5. Interested individuals.

There are many classes that can give drug court development staff the grant proposal writing tools needed to write an effective proposal for grant applications. What is often more difficult is developing relationships with the community providers to execute a plan and to sustain the plan in the future once the grant funds have run their course. The grant writers must:

1. Formulate a service delivery plan that meets the needs of the target population and describe how the program will specifically achieve measurable goals.
2. Highlight the innovative aspects of the program and prepare a clear budget that directly relates to program activities.

3. Clearly outline responsibilities and time frames, including a resource management plan.
4. Identify an experienced evaluator and conduct ongoing research so they may change court operations quickly if problems become apparent.
5. Agree to a realistic sustainability plan and provide some assurances regarding their long-term commitment.

Fundraising

Drug courts have also considered fundraising to provide for operating costs, treatment, and supportive services. To make fundraising a viable and significant part of a financial support strategy, courts may need to formalize and develop an infrastructure for fundraising. Fund drives are labor intensive and only achieve financial success if the efforts and commitment of volunteers are maintained. Financial support is often required to get a campaign started. Insufficient up-front funding can lead to failure of what otherwise might be a successful campaign. Experienced consultants can be hired initially to ensure that a solid fundraising plan is established. This resource may be obtained *pro bono* from community partners who wish to support the drug court. Talking with key community leaders can assist in determining the feasibility of a campaign.

It is important to recognize that in most jurisdictions judges are prohibited by law and ethical rules from participating in fundraising activities. In such jurisdictions, fundraisers must be clear that they are not acting on behalf of the judge or the court. Failure to do so will lead to disciplinary action being taken against the judge.

Insurance

A large number of clients may qualify for some kind of insurance. Sources of insurance may be social programs such as Medicare and Medicaid or private insurance programs. Insurance may pay for at least part of the following services:

1. Drug and alcohol detoxification.
2. Medical testing and treatment.
3. Dental treatment.
4. Inpatient detoxification.
5. Counseling.
6. Psychotherapy.
7. Drug and alcohol rehabilitation therapy.
8. Medications to support abstinence and to treat medical illnesses.
9. Tattoo removal.

Client-Paid Fees

The cost of starting a drug court can be considerable, and courts commonly apply for state or federal grants to cover these costs. The United States Department of Justice has awarded numerous competitive grants, providing up to $300,000 for start-up, implementation, or enhancement for the first 3 years of operation of a drug court. Some state agencies have provided grants to assist in implementing or enhancing drug court operations. For example, in 1995, Oklahoma started the first state-operated drug court in the nation, blending both state and federal funding and incorporating standards into statute.

Once the grants expire, many drug courts are threatened with closure because replacement funds are not available. Some programs have closed when grant funds ran out. Other courts wanting to create a drug court were unable to qualify for a grant or lacked the resources to write a competitive application.

The experience of Tulare County, California, demonstrates the benefits of funding a drug court through client-paid fees. It was the opinion of the judges that no additional judicial resources would be required to start a drug court, since the defendants would either be involved in the drug court or proceed through the routine criminal process. If the drug court option induced only a few defendants to plead guilty without proceeding to jury trials, a large amount of court time and money would be saved. Probation officers assigned to each division of the court were willing to take on the additional burden of administering the program. The major obstacle was funding for drug treatment. Although the county alcohol and drug program administrators expressed support for the concept, they indicated they had no funds to contribute toward treatment.

Despite the existence of several alcohol-rehabilitation programs, there was little knowledge of treatment for nonalcohol drug addiction in the county. The owner of the local program for driving under the influence of alcohol offenders proposed that participants be sent to this program, with modifications, and that they pay the cost of their treatment. At first this seemed unrealistic, as most people in the county with untreated addiction were thought to be destitute. The argument was made that if addicts are paying up to $200 per day for drugs, they could afford to pay $50 per week for treatment. The difficulty with this argument was that they were stealing, prostituting themselves, or selling drugs to finance their own drug use, all of which the court wanted to eradicate. However, another treatment provider, himself in recovery, indicated that such behaviors are inconsistent with the process of recovery and that addicts would not steal, sell drugs, or prostitute to pay for recovery. A judge from a neighboring county with experience in a drug court laughed out loud when presented with that idea, saying, "Addicts are not going to waste their money from stealing or prostitution on treatment!"

Many offenders had jobs and could be expected to use income for treatment that in the past had been used to buy drugs. It was discovered later in a retrospective study that approximately 70% of the drug court clients had jobs at the time of their arrest and continued to work while in the program, many in state jobs (9).

With no other resources to draw on, the court was faced with the harsh choice of either starting the program by having participants pay for their own treatment or not having a drug court at all. Given those options, it seemed preferable to experiment with client-funded treatment rather than abandoning the concept entirely. With misgivings, the drug court began.

Potential participants were identified by the judges and referred to the probation officer for an interview in which the program was explained and background information about the defendant obtained. If the probation officer determined the defendant was interested in changing his or her life and embracing recovery, and could pay the cost of treatment, the defendant was offered drug court. Formal terms of probation were signed that constituted an agreement to comply with the drug court requirements. The defendant was referred to the drug court judge and sentenced into the drug court.

Because participants pay their own cost of treatment, each additional participant adds only a small incremental burden on the system, principally in court time needed to review their cases. Larger populations increase the efficiency of the program because of economies of scale. For example, larger numbers help keep the cost of testing low, as fixed costs for the testing agency are spread among more clients. The treatment providers are able to add more counselors as needed to accommodate greater client bases. By early 2004, over 500 people were participating in the program.

The approach in Tulare County has been that if the drug court is to have a significant impact on the drug problem, as many people as possible should be directed into treatment. A system was developed whereby prosecutors, using agreed on criteria, screened every offender and completed a form indicating whether the offender was eligible to participate in the program. If eligible, the program was offered at the first pre-trial conference, encouraging an early settlement of the case and avoiding additional court hearings.

The concept that people can and will pay for the cost of their addiction treatment has flourished and enabled hundreds of people every year to avoid jail, embrace recovery, and return to a normal lifestyle. To this point, there is no evidence that any participant has committed theft, drug sales, or prostitution to pay for treatment.

Disadvantages of the Client-Funded Approach

Publicly funded drug courts can better supervise participants. These courts are frequently able to hire coordinators and case managers who contact the participants frequently and make home visits to ensure compliance. These courts also enjoy the full participation of prosecutors and defense attorneys who add valuable perspectives to the drug court team. The self-funded approach requires that treatment providers do much of the case management along with the probation officer. In jurisdictions where a probation officer is not available for dedication to the drug court, treatment providers do all case management functions.

The greatest disadvantage of the self-funded approach is that many defendants who would otherwise be eligible to participate and desirous of doing so are excluded because they cannot bear the cost of treatment. Many participants in the Tulare County Drug Court are initially unable to personally pay for treatment but have relatives or other supporters who are willing to advance the cost of treatment for some period of time, feeling it is money well spent because of the high level of supervision by the court. Many family members who have abandoned hope for their addicted relatives are willing to pay the cost of treatment for several months because they know that if the participants do not comply with requirements they will be immediately corrected. The court expects this outside support to end within a few months of entry into the drug court because participants are required to obtain employment and become self-supporting.

Lack of funding prevents ongoing study of outcomes and substantiation of success for policymakers who might otherwise be willing to contribute public funds for drug courts. This is partly offset by the annual graduation ceremony that celebrates the return to society of those who have graduated during the past year. At the ceremony, photographs of the participants at arrest are compared with a current photograph, graphically and powerfully showing the changes made by participation in the drug court. Publicity from these graduations has made it clear to policymakers that the drug court is a valuable asset to the criminal justice programs of the county.

Treatment is necessarily no-frills and basic to keep it as inexpensive as possible. All counselors are state certified and licensed, but many need more training. This is mitigated by the availability of local community colleges that offer human services degrees with an emphasis on addiction treatment and by involvement in state continuing education programs. The counseling provided to the program is worth far more than the cost paid by the drug court participants.

The lack of public funding also means that the drug court team is responsible for payment of ongoing training. For example, involvement in the National Association of Drug Court Professionals requires substantial annual dues, and the cost of attending its annual training conference is considerable. This expense can be offset somewhat by state associations that also provide training and by other training opportunities. One example is the National Rural Institute on Alcohol and Drug Abuse at the University of Wisconsin, which offers annual training for drug courts subsidized by the Office of National Drug Control Policy and the United States Department of Justice. Participants can receive scholarships to attend this training, including the full cost of travel, lodging, and tuition.

Advantages of the Client-Funded Approach

The self-funded approach offers many advantages, chief among them is freedom from constant worry about where the next funding will come from. The economic downturn following the September 11, 2001, tragedy in New York caused some drug courts to close for lack of funding. Other drug court coordinators have had to spend hours searching and applying for grants, which diverts them from their intended purpose of coordinating the drug court. Under the self-funded approach, economic downturns resulting in government budget cuts will not affect the operation of the program.

Free of bureaucratic interference, the drug court team can consider local needs for particular circumstances. The court can adapt quickly to changes in local drug use trends and resources. There are no time-consuming reports and forms that must be submitted to grant providers or individuals whose political agenda does not include drug court.

The most significant advantage of the self-funded approach is that it allows any jurisdiction, no matter how poorly funded, to have a drug court. There is no need to locate a grant writer to write a proposal and then wait for funding cycles. People in large metropolitan areas frequently have advantages over rural areas when applying for grants because they are familiar with the grant application processes and have better access to grant information. Furthermore, once an implementation grant is awarded, immediate attention must be directed toward ongoing applications for continuation grants or soliciting funds from other sources. All this is avoided if those who need the services and derive the most benefit—the addicted people—fund the program.

The public is highly supportive of the self-funded approach, seeing drug court as not just another government program that uses taxpayer dollars squeezed from already strapped budgets. The drug court judge and other team members can proudly speak about the efficacy of the program, all without additional cost to the taxpayers. Service clubs and other civic groups are very supportive when they hear that those who violated the law in the first place are paying their own cost of treatment. The study by the California Judicial Council and the California Department of Alcohol and Drug Programs completed in March 2002 showed that California drug courts saved taxpayers over $43,400,000 or more than $200,000 for every 100 participants. These savings are enhanced when the cost of treatment is borne by the participants (7).

Many services such as medical care, employment training, vocational and educational counseling, housing, parenting classes, and child care can be provided from existing government programs. Alert team members can arrange liaisons with such programs to give special attention to drug court participants. For example, the adult school and adult literacy programs in Tulare County found that drug court participants are highly motivated to succeed because, barring disability, completion of their education is a requirement of participation in the drug court. If they do not follow through on commitments to these programs, they face expulsion from the program and incarceration. With appropriate waivers, periodic reports can inform the judge of progress, and any necessary corrective measures can be applied to put the participants back on the right track.

Finally, experience has shown what is intuitive: People value something according to their investment to obtain it. The Tulare County Drug Court emphasizes to the graduates that they can be proud of the fact that they paid for their treatment and are responsible for their own success in achieving recovery. Graduates leave with an unprecedented feeling of pride in their accomplishments. Many graduates have never done anything deserving of positive public recognition. One man in his 30s stood silently for more than a minute, looking at his certificate after graduating, then looked up with tears in his eyes and said, "This is the first thing I have ever accomplished."

Most participants have lengthy criminal records and suffer feelings of worthlessness upon entry into the drug court. This lack of self-esteem contributes to the cycle of helplessness and hopelessness that spirals into ongoing and increasing drug use. Instilling a sense of pride of accomplishment, which is bolstered by paying for treatment, is a key element in future sobriety. Graduates leave knowing that their sobriety came dearly purchased, and they guard it closely.

References

1. Hora PF, Schma WG, Rosenthal JTA. Therapeutic jurisprudence and the drug treatment court movement: revolutionizing the criminal justice system's response to drug abuse and crime in America. Notre Dame Law Rev 1999;74(2):439–537.
2. Bureau of Justice Statistics, Office of Justice Programs. Recidivism of Prisoners Released in 1983. Washington, DC: U.S. Department of Justice; 1989.
3. Langan PA, Levin DJ. Recidivism of Prisoners Released in 1994. Washington, DC: U.S. Department of Justice, Office of Justice Programs, Bureau of Justice Statistics; 2002.
4. Miller NS. History and review of contemporary addiction treatment. Alcohol Treat Q 1995;12(2):1–22.
5. Belenko, S. Research on Drug Courts: A Critical Review, 2001 Update. New York: The National Center on Addition and Substance Abuse at Columbia University; 2001.
6. Lessenger JE, Roper GF. Drug courts: a primer for the family physician. J Am Board Fam Pract 2002;15(4):298–303.

7. California Department of Alcohol and Drug Programs and the Judicial Council of California, Administrative office of the Courts. Drug Court Partnership Act of 1998, Chapter 1007, Statutes of 1998, Final Report, 2002.
8. California Department of Corrections, California Department of Justice, Justice Statistics Center. Incarceration Rates for Drug-related Crimes, 1970–2002.
9. Lessenger JE, Lessenger LH, Lessenger EW. An Outcome Analysis of Drug Court in Tulare County, California. Porterville, California, unpublished report, 1999.

22 Strategies for Administering Rewards and Sanctions

Douglas B. Marlowe

In the social and psychological sciences, few findings have been so reliably demonstrated that they may qualify as laws of human behavior. The principles of operant conditioning or contingency management are one such set of laws. These principles have been proven time and again in a multitude of diverse settings to the point that they are no longer the subject of scientific dispute. The techniques for effective implementation of operant conditioning are reviewed in this chapter. If one's goal is to improve adaptive functioning and reduce antisocial behavior on the part of offenders, then it is essential to closely monitor their behavior and impose certain and immediate sanctions for infractions and rewards for achievements (1). Failing to punish misconduct inevitably makes behavior worse, and failing to reward accomplishments makes those accomplishments less likely to recur.

The criminal justice system is, in essence, a contingency management intervention designed to reduce crime and rehabilitate offenders. Unfortunately, rewards and sanctions are rarely applied by criminal justice professionals in a systematic manner that can maximize effects. Consequences are often applied in the absence of certainty or predictability and after unacceptably long delays (2). As a result, outcomes tend to be lackluster at best.

Drug courts represent an effort to apply rewards and sanctions for offenders more systematically and in accordance with effective principles of behavior modification (1,3,4). Few drug court practitioners are behavioral scientists by background or training or have a sophisticated grasp of the principles of operant conditioning. Regardless, the founders of drug courts had an intuitive sense of how to influence behavior and were successful in translating that anecdotal knowledge into workable, best-practice standards for the courts. In so doing, they borrowed concepts not only from operant conditioning but also from sociologic and criminologic theories that view perceptions of rewards and sanctions as influencing offenders' conduct. This chapter reviews these principles and how they can be most effectively applied in drug court programs.

Techniques of Operant Conditioning

The basic techniques of operant conditioning are shown in Figure 22.1. There are four ways to influence the behavior of offenders through the application of sanctions or rewards:

1. *Give a reward for good behavior (positive reinforcement)*. Praising a drug offender or giving token gifts for attending counseling sessions are examples of positive reinforcement.

2. *Give a sanction for bad behavior (punishment)*. Giving an offender a writing assignment or jail detention for using drugs are examples of punishment.

3. *Take away a reward or something of value for bad behavior (response cost)*. Imposing a monetary fine or revoking an offender's driver's license for driving under the influence are examples of response cost. Response cost is similar to punishment in that they both cause distress to the individual and are designed to reduce unwanted behaviors. For response cost, the sanction involves losing something of value such as money or driving privileges (5).

4. *Take away a sanction for good behavior (negative reinforcement)*. Drug courts often structure their incentives in the negative. That is, participants are commonly rewarded with reductions in treatment or supervisory obligations or with the elimination of a criminal record or avoidance of incarceration. Negative reinforcement is similar to positive reinforcement in that they are both desired by the individual and are both designed to increase wanted behaviors. Negative reinforcement involves relief from unpleasant circumstances, whereas positive reinforcement involves giving a new, prospective reward (6,7).

Overreliance on any one operant conditioning technique is unlikely to produce lasting gains. The most effective approach is to employ a combination of strategies that elicits synergistic effects by simultaneously squelching undesired behaviors and reinforcing desired behaviors (1). For this reason,

	REWARD	SANCTION
GIVE	Punishment	Punishment
TAKE	Response Cost	Negative Reinforcement

FIGURE 22.1. Basic techniques of operant conditioning or contingency management.

drug courts were designed to utilize all four of the operant conditioning techniques (8). Punishment and response cost are used to reduce bad behaviors, such as drug use and crime, and positive reinforcement and negative reinforcement are used to increase good behaviors, such as counseling attendance, employment, and fulfillment of familial responsibilities.

Parameters of Operant Conditioning

Regardless of which operant conditioning technique one employs, several critical parameters will directly influence the success of the intervention. If these parameters are applied weakly or incorrectly, effectiveness will be greatly diminished. These parameters include the following:

1. Certainty.
2. Celerity.
3. Magnitude.
4. Fairness.

Certainty

The single most important factor influencing the success of any behavioral intervention is certainty (4,9,10). This is expressed as a ratio of infractions to sanctions or as a ratio of achievements to rewards. For example, if drug court clients are sanctioned every time they fail to attend a treatment session, then the ratio of infractions to sanctions would be 1 : 1; this is called a "fixed ratio-1" or "FR-1" schedule. If they are sanctioned for every two missed sessions, this would be an FR-2 schedule, and so forth. The scientific evidence is unambiguous that the smaller the ratio, the more powerful the effects for initiating a new behavior or stopping an old behavior (5,11,12).

Unfortunately, certainty is often conspicuously absent in the criminal justice system. Offenders typically engage in repetitive instances of drug use or crime before being detected by law enforcement authorities (13). Once they have been arrested, the prosecution might not file charges because of insufficient evidence, resources, or interest. If the case does go to trial, the state bears the heavy evidentiary burden of proving guilt beyond a reasonable doubt. This makes the odds of imposing a criminal sanction in a given case decidedly small. Finally, convicted drug-possession offenders are typically sentenced to probation in the community for their first offenses. Because probation officers often have high caseloads and insufficient resources, it may be exceedingly difficult for them to monitor probationers effectively or to impose sanctions for violations of probation (10,14). Taking all of these factors into consideration, one should assume that the ratio of infractions to sanctions would ordinarily be too small to exert a meaningful influence on behavior.

Drug courts make it possible to increase the certainty of rewards and sanctions in several ways. First, drug courts ordinarily require clients to deliver frequent urine specimens in direct observation of clinical staff members on a random basis during the first several months of the program (8). In addition, clients are usually required to attend weekly appointments with a clinical case manager and appear at regular status hearings in court (8). The judge receives routine progress reports from the case manager concerning such matters as drug screen results and counseling attendance, and treatment providers or case managers may appear in court to give live testimony concerning clients' progress in the program. This greatly diminishes the likelihood that accomplishments or infractions will go undetected in the program or that clients will slip through the cracks and elude deserved sanctions or be denied deserved rewards.

Relaxing these measures reduces the certainty of detection, which in turn will reduce the effectiveness of the program. For example, a drug court that fails to conduct random drug testing at least weekly is unlikely to reliably detect drug use. This will have the effect of increasing the ratio of infractions to sanctions; for example, it might shift a client from an FR-1 schedule to an FR-10 schedule, because drug use might only be detected every tenth time it occurred. Such a weak schedule is unlikely to produce beneficial outcomes.

After clients have demonstrated an extended period of continuous abstinence, it might be appropriate to offer them an incentive by decreasing the frequency of urine testing. This would be an example of negative reinforcement, in which the burden of having to provide urine specimens is reduced as a reward for abstinence. However, starting out with a sparse schedule of urine monitoring reflects poor clinical practice and poor behavior modification.

A related issue concerns the practice of giving clients a second chance. Assume, for example, that a client delivers a dirty urine specimen, but the judge elects not to administer a sanction because the judge was in a good mood that day. This would have the effect of increasing the ratio of infractions to sanctions. For example, it might shift the client from an FR-1 schedule to an FR-2 schedule. This course of action, no matter how well intended, would be likely to reduce the efficacy of the program. Consider a different example in which the client used drugs but then felt guilty about it, spontaneously acknowledged the drug use to his or her counselor, and sought further treatment to avoid a continued relapse. In this example, it would be quite appropriate to withhold the sanction as an incentive for the client's being truthful and seeking treatment of his or her own volition. This is an example of negative reinforcement, in which the sanction is withheld as a reward for honesty and help-seeking behavior. Second chances can be appropriate but only when they have been earned. Mistakes do happen, and clients need to learn how to deal with the aftermath of their mistakes.

If a client behaves in a mature and responsible manner following a relapse, then the mature behavior may be seen as canceling out the impending sanction for drug use.

Celerity

The second most critical parameter of operant conditioning is celerity, which means rapidity or immediacy (4). The unfortunate reality is that the effects of sanctions and rewards begin to degrade within only hours or days after an offender has engaged in a target behavior (10,11). Worse still, this decline is not necessarily linear but can be exponential (7). For example, a delay of 10 days may not be merely twice as weak as 5 days; it may be 25 times as weak (i.e., 5^2).

A partial explanation for this precipitous decline in efficacy is that there is interference from new behaviors. Assume that an offender uses drugs on Monday but then is abstinent and compliant with treatment for the remainder of the week. If that same individual is sanctioned on Friday for the instance of drug use that occurred on Monday, it should be evident that the desirable behaviors transpiring on Tuesday through Thursday are actually closer in time to the sanction than the drug use. This explains why the effects of sanctions decline exponentially. New behaviors occur more recently in time, and operant conditioning works, in part, by proximity in time. In this example, the effects of the sanction could be, paradoxically, to punish the good behaviors that occurred most recently. This, of course, would be ineffective or counterproductive.

Celerity, too, is often conspicuously absent in the criminal justice system. The constitutional requirements of procedural due process make it virtually impossible for a finding of guilt or a criminal sentence to be imposed in less than 6 months, usually considerably longer. Even after conviction and sentencing, there are delays in punishing probation violations. In Philadelphia, for example, it takes roughly 4 to 6 months from the filing of a violation of probation petition to the date of a court hearing. Given such inordinate delays, the effects of sanctions should be expected to be minimal. In contrast, status hearings in drug courts are typically held in front of the judge on a weekly, biweekly, or monthly basis (8). This enables the court to impose sanctions and rewards on offenders in a more time-efficient, and thus more effective, manner.

A program of experimental research recently confirmed that holding status hearings more frequently can enhance the effectiveness of drug court programs (15–17). In these studies, improved outcomes were achieved by holding status hearings on a biweekly basis for high-risk drug offenders who had the most serious drug-use histories and antisocial predispositions. These incorrigible individuals were the ones who were most likely to engage in new instances of drug use or rule infractions and who had the poorest prognosis for treatment. When they were monitored closely by the court, allowing sanctions and rewards to be applied more readily, abstinence rates and graduation rates increased considerably.

Magnitude

The issue of magnitude is more complicated than most people realize. There is a common misconception that sanctions and rewards are most effective at high magnitudes, which could explain the penchant of some authorities to impose long and arduous prison sentences for drug possession offenses. In fact, evidence reveals that sanctions tend to be least effective at the lowest and highest magnitudes and most effective in the moderate range. This inverted U-shaped function is shown in Figure 22.2. The figure does not present actual research data but rather illustrates the essential relationship between the magnitude of sanctions and client outcomes.

Sanctions that are too weak in magnitude can precipitate habituation, in which the individual becomes accustomed to being sanctioned (1). The problem with habituation is not only that low-magnitude sanctions may fall below an effective threshold but also that they can make it less likely for higher magnitude sanctions to work in the future because they can raise the client's tolerance for sanctioning. This may account for the "been there, done that" attitude that many drug offenders exhibit in response to threats of punishment. Over time, they become hardened to the threats; therefore,

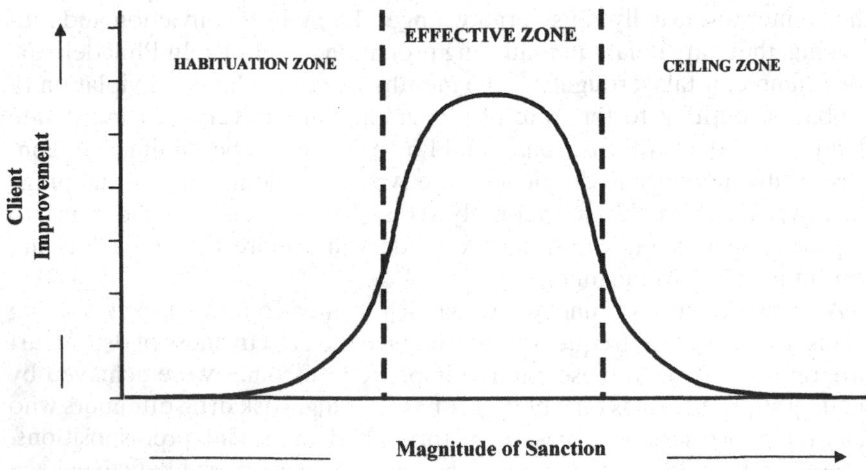

FIGURE 22.2. Relationship between the magnitude of sanctions and client outcomes.

they may be apt to push the limits to the point of no return, to the point of imprisonment, overdose, or drug-related death.

At the other extreme, sanctions that are too high in magnitude can lead to ceiling effects in which further escalation of punishment is impracticable (1). Once an offender has been imprisoned, for example, the authorities have used up their armamentarium of sanctions and the offender knows the authorities have exhausted their options. At this point, future efforts to improve the offender's behavior could be futile.

More important, high-magnitude sanctions are apt to precipitate a host of iatrogenic reactions or negative side effects, such as avoidance and escape responses, learned helplessness, and antitherapeutic feelings of anger and despondency (18,19). As will be discussed later, individuals who are exposed to high-magnitude sanctions often do everything in their power to avoid the sanctions, such as absconding from the program, lying, or tainting their urine specimens. As a result, staff members spend much of their time trying to overcome clients' resistances rather than conducting therapy. In addition, clients who receive severe sanctions may become depressed, angry, or despondent, which can interfere with the therapeutic alliance and the counseling process.

Unfortunately, the criminal justice system tends to operate at the lowest and highest magnitudes of sanctions. For example, offenders often receive a slap on the wrist, such as a reprimand or brief probation sentence, for their first crime (13). This may stem from a well-intentioned desire to be lenient with youthful offenders or a lack of correctional resources for first- or second-time offenders. Regardless, it presents a formidable risk of habituation. Subsequently, after multiple crimes, the only remaining sanction at the authorities' disposal may be imprisonment, which is the paradigm of a ceiling effect.

For this reason, drug courts were crafted to provide a wider and more creative range of intermediate-magnitude sanctions and rewards, which can be ratcheted upward or downward in response to clients' behaviors (8). The sanctions and rewards are administered on an escalating or graduated gradient, in which the magnitude increases progressively in response to each successive infraction or accomplishment in the program (8). This can enable a drug court to navigate between habituation and ceiling effects by altering the magnitude of punishment in response to successive infractions. It also permits the criminal justice system to offer a substantially richer and more effective range of rewards than is ordinarily available to offender populations.

The success of any given drug court will depend largely on its ability to apply a meaningful range of intermediate sanctions and rewards. Those programs that are too lenient will be apt to elicit habituation and make outcomes stagnant, whereas those that are too harsh will be apt to elicit resentment, avoidance, and ceiling effects. Those programs that are just right will tend to have the best results.

Fairness

Certainty, celerity, and magnitude refer to how rewards and sanctions are actually administered. However, perceptions of rewards and sanctions are also very important. One issue relates to the concept of *procedural justice.* Evidence from cognitive psychology reveals that individuals are more likely to perceive a decision as being correct and appropriate if they believe that fair procedures were employed in reaching that decision (20). In fact, the perceived fairness of the procedures exerts a greater influence over participants' reactions than the outcome of the decision. Specifically, clients will be most likely to accept an adverse judgment if they feel they had a fair opportunity to voice their side of the story, were treated in an equivalent manner to similar people in similar circumstances, and were accorded respect and dignity throughout the process (21). When any one of these factors is absent, behavior not only fails to improve, it may get worse and offenders may sabotage their treatment goals (22).

This does not mean that clients should always get what they want or that all clients should always be treated in the same manner for the same behaviors. The important point is that clients should be given a fair chance to explain their side of the story and should be offered a clear rationale for how and why a decision was reached. If staff members have difficulty articulating a reasonable explanation for why one client is being handled differently from others, then perhaps the team should rethink its responses. On the other hand, there will often be very good reasons for treating some clients differently. For example, research suggests that rewards and sanctions may need to be modified for certain high-risk offender populations, such as psychopaths, juveniles, or the dually diagnosed. For these types of clients, a "foolish consistency" can be counterproductive. This may require a drug court program to create separately stratified tracks for different types of clients or at least to have a convincing script at hand for explaining why rewards and sanctions are applied differently to different individuals.

Most important, it is never appropriate to be condescending or discourteous. Even the most severe sanctions, such as jail detention or termination, should be delivered in a dispassionate and even-handed manner, with no suggestion that the judge or other staff enjoy meting out punishment. Just as a good parent interacts with his or her child, it should be clear that the sanction is for the client's bad conduct and not because the client is a bad person or intrinsically deserves to be punished.

Complications of Operant Conditioning

Learned Helplessness

Clients in drug court may become angry or despondent if they are sanctioned for failing to comply with excessive or unrealistic demands. This process is called learned helplessness (23). Under such circumstances, behavior fails to improve, and clients may sabotage their own treatment goals (22).

The major factors that precipitate this iatrogenic reaction are an absence of predictability or controllability. Predictability refers to a client's ability to anticipate the precise behaviors that will elicit a sanction or reward. For example, if a client is told that he or she will be sanctioned for failing to be mature, this might seem unfair if the client is unable to predict the specific behaviors the judge would interpret as reflecting immaturity that deserved a sanction. This could cause the client to become resentful or despondent or to give up. Controllability refers to the ability to engage in a desired behavior or refrain from an undesired behavior. If, for example, a client is sanctioned for failing to obtain a GED, this could precipitate despondence if the client suffered from an undiagnosed learning disability that prevented him or her from understanding the study materials or completing the educational exercises. Under such circumstances, punishment would be unlikely to further educational aims and would be likely to interfere with other treatment goals.

Related to the factor of controllability is the issue of ratio burden. Drug courts often place multiple demands on clients that can be difficult to fulfill simultaneously. Clients may be required to attend counseling sessions, appear at court hearings, deliver urine specimens, remain abstinent, and complete vocational training; they may be sanctioned for failing to comply with any one of these directives. Under such circumstances, the sheer burden of response requirements could be so daunting as to trigger a learned helplessness response.

One way to forestall learned helplessness is to clearly specify in advance the concrete behaviors that can trigger a sanction or reward. At the point of entry into the program, clients should be clearly informed of the program's rules, the behaviors that may trigger sanctions or rewards, the types of sanctions and rewards that can be imposed, the criteria for graduation or termination from the program, and the consequences that may ensue from graduation or failure. Ideally, this information should be recorded in a written manual and may also be the subject of an oral colloquy between the judge and client that is memorialized in a stenographic record. Such procedures help to ensure that each client understands the rights given up and the risks assumed by entering the program. This serves to increase clients' perceptions of fairness and predictability, which will make clients more ready to accept negative sanctions that need to be imposed.

A second way to forestall learned helplessness is to separate proximal from distal behavioral goals. This process is known as shaping. Proximal goals are those behaviors that clients are readily capable of engaging in and that are necessary for long-term objectives to be attained. Examples of proximal behaviors include attendance at counseling sessions, attendance at court hearings, and delivery of urine specimens. Distal behaviors are those that are ultimately desired but may take clients some time to accomplish. Examples might include drug abstinence, gainful employment, and improved parenting skills.

This does not mean distal behaviors should be ignored during the early phases of drug court. As discussed earlier, the most important parameters of contingency management are certainty, celerity, and fairness. Therefore, staff should always respond to every infraction and every accomplishment in a quick and even-handed manner. However, the magnitude of the response should vary according to whether the behavior is a proximal or distal goal (24,25). During the early phases of the program, relatively higher magnitude sanctions and rewards should be imposed for proximal behaviors and relatively lower magnitude sanctions and rewards imposed for distal behaviors. For example, clients might receive verbal reprimands or writing assignments for providing drug-positive urine samples but might receive community service or brief jail detention for failing to show up for counseling sessions or failing to provide urine specimens. As the client progresses through later phases, the emphasis should shift to distal goals, and high-magnitude sanctions might be applied for positive urine screens as well. The goal is to navigate between habituation and ceiling effects by immediately and substantially reinforcing proximal, pro-treatment behaviors while reserving a larger range of responses for distal behaviors that could take some time to accomplish.

Of course, behaviors that present an immediate threat to public safety or program integrity, such as criminality or driving under the influence, are necessarily regarded as proximal because they cannot be permitted to continue. Offenders who fail to refrain from these behaviors might be considered poor candidates for drug court and might best be confined and treated in a correctional halfway house, residential facility, or prison or jail setting.

The Carrot Versus the Stick

There is a serious concern that some drug courts may place an inordinate emphasis on squelching undesired behaviors to the detriment of reinforcing desired behaviors (1,3). Although drug courts can be quite effective at reducing crime and drug use while clients are under the supervision of the judge, these effects cannot be expected to endure unless the clients contacted alternative rewards and sanctions in their natural social environments that maintained the effects over time (26). For instance, clients who find a job, develop hobbies, or improve their family relationships will be more likely to be continuously rewarded (e.g., with praise, social prestige, or wages) for prosocial behaviors and punished (e.g., by being ostracized from peers or fired from a job) for drug-related behaviors. In contrast, those clients who simply return to their previous habitats will most likely find themselves back in an environment that rewards drug use at the expense of prosocial attainments. The community reinforcement approach is a counseling strategy that capitalizes on natural systems of rewards and sanctions in clients' social environments to compete with the drug-using lifestyle (27).

To maintain treatment effects over time, it is essential that drug courts not merely punish crime and drug use but also reward productive activities that are incompatible with crime and drug use. This represents one of the greatest challenges facing drug courts because law professionals have not traditionally defined their role in this manner. Judges and prosecutors are trained to adjudicate controversies and reduce recidivism. Only recently have the courts recognized therapeutic jurisprudence as a legitimate legal philosophy, in which improving the psychological health of citizens is viewed as an appropriate function of the judiciary (28). A critical task facing the drug court field is to educate law practitioners about the importance of using more positive reinforcement in their work and selecting behavioral goals for their clients that are consistent with the principles of the community reinforcement approach.

Sanctions have been associated with a host of negative side effects that can make outcomes worse rather than better. For example, sanctions have been associated with avoidance responses, learned helplessness, anger, despondency, and ceiling effects. Positive reinforcements have also been associated with negative side effects; however, these side effects are of considerably lesser consequence than those associated with punishment. For example, some clients may become complacent or entitled if they come to expect something for nothing. That is, if clients are continuously rewarded for mediocre or substandard performance, this will not only fail to improve their performance but can also lead them to feel resentful or despondent if expectations for acceptable performance are subsequently increased (5). If later it becomes harder to earn rewards, the clients may perceive this as having rewards taken away from them. This is the very definition of response cost and can be experienced as a form of punishment. Although this is a legitimate concern, these unwanted effects can be easily avoided by increasing one's performance demands for clients over time. If expectations for appropriate behavior are continuously heightened, there should be little concern that clients' conduct will fail to improve.

Artificial extrinsic rewards can undermine clients' intrinsic motivation for change (29). However, this finding relates to detrimental effects on individuals who were already intrinsically motivated. Intrinsic motivation is often conspicuously absent among drug abusers and criminal offenders (30,31). If participants are not motivated to begin with, then it is difficult to envision how their motivation could possibly be interfered with. For unmotivated individuals, it is not only acceptable to use extrinsic rewards to start them on a course toward abstinence, but it may be necessary to do so. After they have experienced a sustained interval of sobriety, then clients will begin to experience the natural rewards that come with abstinence. For example, they will start feeling physically and emotionally healthier, may regain the respect of family members or friends, and may become employable. Then, and perhaps only then, will they begin to develop the intrinsic motivation that is necessary to maintain abstinence over the long haul.

Perhaps the most enduring objection to rewards is one of equity. Citizens are not ordinarily given tangible incentives for abstaining from drugs and crime. Therefore, it may seem inequitable to reward some people for doing what is minimally expected of most others, particularly when those being rewarded are among the less desirable elements of society, such as drug addicts and criminal offenders. Because this objection is based on sentiment and is not related to the actual effects of the intervention, it cannot be empirically disputed or confirmed. It is an unavoidable policy objection that can make it difficult for drug court professionals to conduct their work most effectively. The best recourse is to explain to stakeholders why positive reinforcement is necessary and why it may be among the most effective and cost-effective strategies to employ with drug offenders. Perhaps data can answer some of the objections raised against the use of positive rewards with offenders.

Special Populations

Rewards and sanctions may require modifications for use with certain populations of offenders characterized by higher levels of criminogenic risk or needs.

The Risk Principle

A substantial body of evidence demonstrates that intensive interventions are best suited for high-risk offenders who have more severe antisocial propensities or drug use histories but may be ineffective or contraindicated for low-risk offenders (32,33). Low-risk offenders are less likely to be on a fixed antisocial trajectory and are more likely to adjust course readily following a run-in with the law; therefore, intensive treatment and supervision may offer little incremental benefit for these individuals at a substantial cost (34). High-risk offenders, on the other hand, are likely to require intensive interventions to dislodge their entrenched, negative behavioral patterns. The greatest risk factors for failure in correctional rehabilitation include being younger, being male, having an earlier onset of crime or drug use, having multiple prior arrests, meeting criteria for antisocial personality disorder or psychopathy, or having previously failed in drug abuse treatment or a criminal diversion program (35,36).

Research suggests that certain high-risk offenders may respond differently to sanctions and rewards than other individuals. For example, psychopathic offenders, those with antisocial personality disorder, and youthful offenders tend to discount the probability of receiving a serious sanction in the long term in favor of earning an immediate reward (37). They are also more likely to opt for smaller short-term rewards than to forestall gratification in favor of larger rewards to be earned some time in the future (38). This apparent hypersensitivity to rewards, imperviousness to sanctions, and impulsivity could reflect executive-control deficits stemming from damage or immaturity to their prefrontal cortex (39). Alternatively, it could reflect the vagaries of their learning histories. By virtue of their recidivist proclivities, antisocial offenders may be more likely to have habituated to or reached a ceiling effect on sanctions. This could make them seem unresponsive to sanctions because of their maladaptive experiences with punishment in the past.

Etiology aside, evidence is convincing that structured behavioral interventions are ideally suited for high-risk offenders. Studies have shown that drug abuse clients who had a comorbid diagnosis of antisocial personality disorder performed as well as, or better, than non–antisocial personality disorder clients in voucher-based contingency management interventions that employed a good dosage of positive reinforcement (40–42). In fact, it would appear that the higher the risk level in a given population, the less margin of error there is for applying contingency management interventions effectively (43). Greater exactitude may be required in certainty, celerity, and procedural justice to achieve comparable gains for high-risk offenders as for other clients.

Substance Abuse Versus Substance Dependence

One critically important issue that has received insufficient attention in the drug court literature is the question of whether a client is a substance abuser as opposed to substance dependent. It is unwarranted to assume that simply because an individual has been arrested for a drug-related offense that he or she must be an addict or in denial about being an addict. In fact, research indicates that roughly 30% to 40% of drug offenders do not have a diagnosable or clinically significant substance use disorder (34,44). In some studies, nearly one half of misdemeanor drug court clients and one third of felony drug court clients produced subthreshold drug composite scores on the Addiction Severity Index, similar to a community sample of non–substance-abusing individuals (16,45–47). In another study, approximately one third of misdemeanor drug court clients provided a virtually unbroken string of drug-negative urine specimens over nearly a 4-month period following entry into drug court (48). If these individuals could readily abstain from drug use over such an extended interval of time, there is arguably little clinical justification for labeling their use as compulsive.

Of course, depending on the characteristics of the community in which a drug court is situated, as well as inclusion criteria for the program, the percentage of nonaddicted individuals could be higher or lower than in published studies. Regardless, it should be assumed that at least a substantial minority of individuals in drug court are not addicted. This has important implications for administering sanctions and rewards.

There are three critical symptoms for determining whether an individual is addicted to or dependent on drugs or alcohol:

1. Introduction of the substance precipitates a binge pattern. For example, the individual intends to have just one beer, but drinking that beer triggers a several-hour bender.
2. The individual experiences intense cravings or compulsions for the substance that are extremely difficult to resist and that steadily build in intensity during prolonged intervals of abstinence.
3. The individual suffers serious withdrawal symptoms when levels of the substance decline in the bloodstream.

For clients exhibiting one or more of these hallmark features of addiction, abstinence should generally be considered a distal goal. By definition, substance use is compulsive for these individuals; therefore, they should be expected to require a good deal of time and several instances of relapse before attaining sustained abstinence. If a drug court team were to impose high-magnitude sanctions on these individuals for drug use early in treatment, the odds are high that the team would hit a ceiling effect quite soon and the client would fail out of the program. This could have the paradoxical effect of making the most drug-dependent individuals ill-fated for success in drug court programs. Instead, high-magnitude sanctions should be reserved during the early phases of the program for treatment-related behaviors, such as attending counseling, appearing at status hearings, and submitting urine specimens. Positive urine screens should still be met with certain and swift sanctions; however, the magnitude of the sanctions should be relatively low, thus permitting ample opportunities to increase the sanctions over time.

In contrast, for clients who are not addicted to drugs or alcohol, abstinence should be considered a proximal goal. Because substance use is not compulsive for these individuals, they are capable of stopping their usage quickly or immediately. Applying low-magnitude sanctions for substance use would essentially give them a free run to continue their use for some time. This could lead to habituation effects, which would make outcomes worse. Instead, higher magnitude sanctions should be applied for drug use from the outset so as to put a rapid end to this misbehavior.

This practice may require some drug courts to develop separately stratified tracks for clients who are drug dependent as opposed to abusers. Separate tracks could avoid perceptions of unfairness when some clients are treated more leniently than others. Of course, for rural drug courts or those with low censuses, separate tracks might not be practical. Staff in these programs will need to explain to clients why they are being treated differently from other clients based on their clinical needs. Having a prepared script at hand to provide this explanation could reduce perceptions of unfairness.

Research on Sanctions and Rewards in Drug Court

Several descriptive and experimental studies have examined the application of sanctions and rewards in drug court programs.

Research on Sanctions

One experimental study in the District of Columbia (49) randomly assigned drug-abusing arrestees in a pretrial supervision program to one of three conditions:

1. Participants assigned to the standard condition received the typical regimen of pretrial services, which included infrequent court appearances, infrequent urine testing, and nonmandatory referrals to treatment services.
2. Participants assigned to the sanctions condition provided urine specimens on a random weekly basis and received progressively escalating sanctions for positive results, which included jail stays of up to 3 to 7 days.
3. Participants assigned to the treatment condition attended an intensive day-treatment program that provided clinical services, meals, and recreational activities several hours per week.

Contrary to expectations, the participants preferred the sanctions condition to day treatment (49). Only 40% of participants assigned to day treatment agreed to participate in treatment, whereas 66% of participants assigned to the sanctions condition agreed to comply with those requirements. Focus-group inquiries provided an explanation for this surprising finding. The participants reportedly objected to the substantial time burden and intrusiveness of day treatment, which far outweighed the minimally intrusive procedures employed in weekly urine collection (50).

Significantly, participants in both the treatment condition and sanctions condition had lower rates of drug use than those receiving standard pretrial services; however, participants in the sanctions condition had the best outcomes because they also had lower rearrest rates extending out to 1 year postentry (49). These results confirm that graduated sanctions, including the threat of brief jail detention, can be acceptable and effective for drug-abusing offenders.

Several researchers have conducted confidential focus groups with drug court participants to learn whether they perceived graduated sanctions to be a powerful motivator in treatment. The results confirmed that participants generally viewed the threat of sanctions to be a powerful inducement to succeed in the program but only when the sanctions were perceived as being imposed in accordance with the principles of procedural justice outlined earlier (51–53). Sanctions were viewed as detrimental to treatment goals when they were meted out in an arbitrary or inconsistent manner. In contrast, they were viewed as helpful when participants felt they had a chance to articulate their side of the story, believed they were treated equivalently to other clients, and felt they were accorded respect and dignity throughout the process.

Research on Rewards

No published study has investigated judicially administered rewards in a drug court. However, preliminary data from two ongoing studies suggest that enhancing tangible positive rewards may not improve outcomes for clients as a whole (54,55). These studies added payment vouchers or gift certificates as rewards for program compliance. Contrary to expectations, this procedure did not improve treatment outcomes. It appears that the powerful contingencies that were naturally in place in the drug courts (e.g., the threat of imprisonment for failure) produced such high rates of counseling attendance and drug abstinence (at least while the participants were enrolled) that augmenting tangible rewards did not yield incremental gains.

Planned interaction analyses conducted in one of the studies revealed positive effects of the enhanced rewards for high-risk participants who were younger or had a prior felony record (54). If these preliminary results are confirmed with a larger sample, this would suggest that increasing the density of tangible rewards can improve outcomes for the most incorrigible clients in drug courts.

Conclusions

At its core, the criminal justice system is a contingency management intervention designed to reduce crime and rehabilitate offenders. Traditionally, however, rewards and sanctions were rarely applied in a systematic manner that could produce meaningful or lasting effects. Dissatisfied with this state of affairs, a group of criminal court judges set aside dockets to provide closer supervision and greater accountability for drug-abusing offenders. Wittingly or unwittingly, these judges devised programs highly consonant with scientific principles of operant conditioning. Specifically, they

1. Introduced greater certainty, celerity, and fairness into the process of imposing criminal justice sanctions.
2. Combined various behavioral techniques to simultaneously squelch undesired conduct and increase desired conduct.
3. Crafted a range of intermediate-magnitude sanctions and rewards that could be ratcheted upward or downward in response to offender conduct.
4. Developed a phased program structure that separates proximal from distal goals and thus helps to reduce learned helplessness and ratio burden.
5. Introduced more positive reinforcement and therapeutic goals into the business of the courts.

As a result, outcomes from drug courts have substantially exceeded those typically achieved by other programs for drug-involved offender populations (2,56). Drug courts are far from perfect, and more research is needed to fine-tune the behavioral components of these programs. This will necessitate the development of collaborative partnerships between drug court practitioners and behavioral scientists and the forging of a planned research agenda that both permits rigorous scientific hypothesis testing and demonstrates relevance for criminal justice practice and drug policy.

References

1. Marlowe DB, Kirby KC. Effective use of sanctions in drug courts: lessons from behavioral research. Natl Drug Court Inst Rev 1999;2:1–31.
2. Marlowe DB. Effective strategies for intervening with drug abusing offenders. Villanova Law Rev 2002;47:989–1025.
3. Burdon WM, Roll JM, Prendergast ML, Rawson RA. Drug courts and contingency management. J Drug Issues 2001;31:73–90.
4. Harrell A, Roman J. Reducing drug use and crime among offenders: the impact of graduated sanctions. J Drug Issues 2001;31:207–232.
5. Martin G, Pear J. Behavior Modification: What It Is and How to Do It, 6th ed. Upper Saddle River, NJ: Prentice Hall; 1999.
6. Hineline PN. Negative reinforcement and avoidance. In Honig WK, Straddon JER, eds. Handbook of Operant Behavior. Englewood Cliffs, NJ: Prentice Hall 1976:364–414.
7. Sidman M. Avoidance behavior. In Honig WK, ed. Operant Behavior: Areas of Research and Application. New York: Appleton-Century-Crofts; 1966:448–498.
8. National Association of Drug Court Professionals. Defining Drug Courts: The Key Components. Washington, DC: Office of Justice Programs, U.S. Department of Justice; 1997.
9. Stitzer ML, McCaul ME. Criminal justice interventions with drug and alcohol abusers: the role of compulsory treatment. In Edwards EK, Braukmann CJ, eds. Behavioral Approaches to Crime and Delinquency. New York: Plenum; 1987: 225–233.
10. Taxman FS. Graduated sanctions: stepping into accountable systems and offenders. Prison J 1999;79:182–204.
11. Azrin NH, Holz WC. Punishment. In Honig WK, ed. Operant Behavior: Areas of Research and Application. New York: Appleton-Century-Crofts; 1966:388–447.
12. Van Houten R. Punishment: from the animal laboratory to the applied setting. In Axelrod S, Apsche J, eds. The Effects of Punishment on Human Behavior. New York: Academic Press; 1983:13–44.
13. Nurco DN, Hanlon TE, Kinlock TW. Recent research on the relationship between illicit drug use and crime. Behav Sci Law 1991;9:221–249.
14. Goldkamp JS. The drug court response: issues and implications for justice change. Albany Law Rev 2000;63:923–961.
15. Festinger DS, Marlowe DB, Lee PA, Kirby KC, Bovasso G, McLellan AT. Status hearings in drug court: when more is less and less is more. Drug Alcohol Depend 2002 68:151–157.

16. Marlowe DB, Festinger DS, Lee PA. The judge is a key component of drug court. Drug Court Rev 2004;4:1–34.
17. Marlowe DB, Festinger DS, Lee PA, Dugosh KL, Benasutti KM. Matching judicial supervision to clients' risk status in drug court. Crime Delinquency 2006;52:52–76.
18. Newsom C, Favell JE, Rincover A. The side effects of punishment. In Axelrod S, Apsche J, eds. The Effects of Punishment on Human Behavior. New York: Academic Press; 1983:285–316.
19. Sidman M. Coercion and its Fallout. Boston: Authors Cooperative; 1988.
20. Thibaut JW, Walker L. Procedural Justice: A Psychological Analysis. Hillsdale, NJ: Erlbaum; 1975.
21. Tyler TR. Psychological models of the justice motive: antecedents of distributive and procedural justice. J Pers Soc Psychol 1994;67:850–863.
22. Sherman LW. Defiance, deterrence, and irrelevance: a theory of the criminal justice sanction. J Res Crime Delinquency 1993;30:445–473.
23. Seligman MEP. Helplessness. San Francisco: W. H. Freeman; 1975.
24. Huddleston CW, Meyer W, Marlowe DB. Rethinking Court Responses to Client Behavior: Incentives and Sanctions—New Tools to Build a Better Drug Court. Alexandria, VA: National Drug Court Institute and Bureau of Justice Assistance; 2006.
25. Meyer WG. Developing Consensus on Sanction and Incentive Guidelines in the Drug Court. Alexandria, VA: National Drug Court Institute; 2002.
26. Higgins ST, Budney AJ, Bickel WK, Foerg FE, Donham R, Badger G. Incentives improve outcome in outpatient behavioral treatment of cocaine dependence. Arch Gen Psychiatry 1994;51:568–576.
27. Sisson RW, Azrin NH. The community reinforcement approach. In Hester RK, Miller WR, eds. Handbook of Alcoholism Treatment Approaches: Effective Alternatives. Elmsford, NY: Pergamon; 1989:242–258.
28. Hora PF, Schma WG, Rosenthal JTA. Therapeutic jurisprudence and the drug treatment court movement: Revolutionalizing the criminal justice system's response to drug abuse and crime in America. Notre Dame Law Rev 1999;74:439–538.
29. Deci EL, Koestner R, Ryan RM. A meta-analytic review of experiments examining the effects of extrinsic rewards on intrinsic motivation. Psychol Bull 1999;125:627–668.
30. Marlowe DB, Glass DJ, Merikle EP, Festinger DS, DeMatteo DS, Marczyk GR, et al. Efficacy of coercion in substance abuse treatment. In Tims FM, Leukefeld CG, Platt JJ, eds. Relapse and Recovery in Addictions. New Haven, CT: Yale University Press; 2001:208–227.
31. Satel SL. Drug Treatment: The Case for Coercion. Washington, DC: American Enterprise Institute; 1999.
32. Taxman FS, Marlowe DB. Risk, needs, responsivity: in action or inaction? Crime Delinquency 2006;52:3–6.
33. Andrews DA, Bonta J. The Psychology of Criminal Conduct, 2nd ed. Cincinnati: Anderson; 1998.
34. DeMatteo DS, Marlowe DB, Festinger DS. Secondary prevention services for clients who are low risk in drug court: a conceptual model. Crime Delinquency 2006;52:114–134.

35. Marlowe DB, Patapis NS, DeMatteo DS. Amenability to treatment of drug offenders. Fed Probation 2003;67:40–46.
36. Peters RH, Haas AL, Murrin MR. Predictors of retention and arrest in drug court. Natl Drug Court Inst Rev 1999;2:33–60.
37. Patterson CM, Newman JP. Reflectivity and learning from aversive events: toward a psychological mechanism for the syndromes of disinhibition. Psychol Rev 1993;100:716–736.
38. Petry NM. Discounting of delayed rewards in substance abusers: relationship to antisocial personality disorder. Psychopharmacology 2002;162:425–432.
39. Fishbein D. Neuropsychological function, drug abuse, and violence: a conceptual framework. Crim Justice Behav 2000;27:139–159.
40. Marlowe DB, Kirby KC, Festinger DS, Husband SD, Platt JJ. Impact of comorbid personality disorders and personality disorder symptoms on outcomes of behavioral treatment for cocaine dependence. J Nerv Ment Dis 1997;185:483–490.
41. Messina N, Farabee D, Rawson R. Treatment responsivity of cocaine-dependent patients with antisocial personality disorder to cognitive-behavioral and contingency management interventions. J Consult Clin Psychol 2003;71:320–329.
42. Silverman K, Wong C, Umbricht-Schneiter A, Montoya I, Schuster C, Preston K. Broad beneficial effects of cocaine abstinence reinforcement among methadone patients. J Consult Clin Psychol 1998;66:811–824.
43. Higgins ST. Some potential contributions of reinforcement and consumer-demand theory to reducing cocaine use. Addict Behav 1996;21:803–816.
44. Kleiman MAR, Tran TH, Fishbein P, Magula MT, Allen W, Lacy G. Opportunities and Barriers in Probation Reform: A Case Study of Drug Testing and Sanctions. Berkeley: University of California, California Policy Research Center; 2003.
45. Marlowe DB, Festinger DS, Lee PA, Schepise MM, Hazzard JER, Merrill JC, et al. Are judicial status hearings a key component of Drug Court? During-treatment data from a randomized trial. Crim Justice Behav 2003;30:141–162.
46. Marlowe DB, Festinger DS, Lee PA. The role of judicial status hearings in drug court. Offender Subst Abuse Rep 2003;3:33–34, 44–46.
47. McLellan AT, Cacciola J, Kushner H, Peters R, Smith I, Pettinati H. The fifth edition of the Addiction Severity Index: cautions, additions and normative data. J Subst Abuse Treat 1992;9:461–480.
48. DeMatteo DS, Festinger DS, Lee PA, Marlowe DB. Substance Use Patterns in Drug Court: No Problem? Paper presented at the 67th Annual Scientific Meeting of the College on Problems of Drug Dependence, June 2005, Orlando, Florida.
49. Harrell A, Cavanagh S, Roman J. Final Report: Findings From the Evaluation of the D.C. Superior Court Drug Intervention Program. Washington, DC: The Urban Institute; 1999.
50. Harrell A, Smith B. Evaluation of the District of Columbia Superior Court Drug Intervention Program: Focus Group Interviews. Washington, DC: The Urban Institute; 1997.
51. Goldkamp JS, White MD, Robinson JB. An honest chance: perspectives on drug courts. Fed Sentencing Rep 2002;6:369–372.

52. Satel SL. Observational study of courtroom dynamics in selected drug courts. Natl Drug Court Inst Rev 1998;1:43–72.
53. Cooper CS. 1997 Drug Court Survey Report: Executive Summary. Washington, DC: Drug Court Clearinghouse and Technical Assistance Project, Office of Justice Programs, U.S. Department of Justice; 1997.
54. Marlowe DB, Festinger DS, Lee PA, Fox G, Alexander R, Mastro NK, et al. Contingency Management in Drug Court. Presentation at the 67th Annual Scientific Meeting of the College on Problems of Drug Dependence, June 2005, Orlando, Florida.
55. Prendergast ML, Hall EA, Roll JM. Judicial Supervision and Contingency Management in Treating Drug-Abusing Offenders: Preliminary Outcomes. Poster session presented at the 67th Annual Scientific Meeting of the College on Problems of Drug Dependence, June 2005, Orlando, Florida.
56. Marlowe DB, DeMatteo DS, Festinger DS. A sober assessment of drug courts. Fed Sentencing Rep 2003;16:153–157.

23
Roadblocks to Success

Glade F. Roper

In many jurisdictions that consider the formation of a drug court, someone acts as a stumbling block. Frequently this has been the prosecutor, who is unaware of the true nature of a drug court and does not want to be considered soft on crime. Sometimes it is a law enforcement official who shares the same concerns. Law enforcement officers and prosecutors do not get their jobs by being perceived as lenient toward criminal offenders, including drug users and dealers. A sheriff may have an additional objection to the increased transport of prisoners that may be a consequence of operating a drug court.

Court clerks or judicial support staff may object to the additional paperwork involved in frequent court appearances. Judges may object for the same reasons. Holding a settlement conference and proceeding with a trial and sentencing will involve only three or four appearances; 18 months of drug court could involve 30 or more court appearances. In states where judges are elected, they also have political concerns about being viewed by the voting public as being indulgent of criminals. Many judges are former prosecutors who have a background of arguing for lengthy custody sentences and little regard for a "social worker" approach to criminal activity. Surprisingly, sometimes it is the public defender and defense bar that objects to implementing a drug court.

All of these objections can be effectively overcome to form a successful drug court. They have been raised before and are not unique to any jurisdiction. Most functioning drug courts have met and resolved many of them. This chapter discusses objections that might be raised by:

1. Judges.
2. Prosecutors.
3. The defense bar.
4. Law enforcement.

Judges

Some judges have resigned rather than impose mandatory minimum sentences they consider unjust and excessive in drug cases (1). Others have expressed serious concerns about the wisdom of sentencing drug offenders to lengthy sentences exceeding those imposed on violent criminals and murderers (2). Judges who have operated drug courts are generally advocates for the advantages of drug courts over the traditional criminal court approach. Having sentenced the same people to jail multiple times, it is rewarding to see them instead gain weight, get a job, clean up their appearance, get their children back from the child protective service, smile, and express gratitude for escaping the slavery of drug use. A judge in Fresno, California, expressed his satisfaction with participating in drug court: “Isn’t it great to be a part of helping people recover?”

The judge is a key element of a drug court, and without a judge willing to administer the process it cannot succeed. Although there is no unique personality that qualifies one to be a drug court judge, it does require a change of mind-set from the traditional criminal court process. The novelty and dissimilar approach can cause resistance in a judge who has experience in presiding over a criminal court. Judicial officers have voiced objections such as these:

1. Drug court is not real court.
2. Drug abuse cannot be treated.
3. Drug courts have unrealistic expectations.
4. Judges are not social workers.
5. Punishment and treatment should not be imposed on defendants who are not convicted.
6. Drug courts have not been shown to work.
7. Federal money causes loss of local autonomy.
8. Drug courts increase case loads.

Is Drug Court a Real Court?

Some judges have a philosophical objection to the blurring of traditional responsibilities of the various components of a court system. They may object to changing the traditional role of a judge as a referee into an active participant who deals directly with the defendants. Others have the distorted vision that unless a judge is handling trials, the judge is not doing real judicial work. Over 95% of all lawsuits filed in the United States settle before trial (3). Entire judicial departments are dedicated to pretrial settlement efforts in some court systems. It cannot be seriously argued that resolving cases short of trial is not legitimate work of a judge. One criminal trial for possession of a small amount of illegal drugs can consume up to 3 days and cost thousands of dollars. The cost of bringing in hundreds of citizens as potential jurors, the arresting officer sitting through the trial, the laboratory analyst testifying about the quantity and quality of the drugs, a prosecutor, a defense attorney, an interpreter if the defendant does not speak English, a court reporter creating a transcript, a court clerk to take the minutes of the proceedings and handle the evidence, a bailiff, and a judge to preside is a heavy burden on any jurisdiction. Although some of these are fixed costs, taking the officer off the street and paying for the laboratory analyst, the cost of the official transcript, and the jurors are all variable costs that are directly tied to the trial and can be avoided if there is no trial. With drug cases constituting a large portion of most criminal court dockets, reducing trials can mean reducing the number of courtrooms and attendant personnel. One 3-day trial can be the equivalent of hundreds of drug court appearances, so it does not take many avoided trials to offset the cost of a drug court.

Courts across the country are concerned about how they are perceived by the public. The Administrative Office of the Courts in California has commissioned elaborate and expensive studies solely to determine how the public views the courts (4,5). A public that is made aware of the benefits of drug court, including reduced expenses and recidivism, will be supportive and encouraged that the judges are doing something other than churning people through the jail and prison—something that really reduces crime and expense.

Can Drug Addiction Be Treated Effectively?

Some judges believe there is uncertainty about whether addiction is a disease and whether it can be successfully treated. Judges who have experience dealing with addicted repeat defendants may well be skeptical about their prospects for escaping the criminal whirlpool. Others doubt that addiction is anything other than an intense desire to use drugs and the lack of self-control to cease doing so.

The nature of addiction is enigmatic, and only in recent years have advanced brain imaging procedures yielded a glimpse into its etiology. Positron emission tomography scans and similar advances have allowed us to visualize how an addicted brain functions differently from a nonaddicted brain. There are marked differences between the neurons collected from the nucleus accumbens of addicted and unaddicted animals. The nucleus accumbens has been identified as the pleasure center of the brain (6). When a person becomes addicted, the actual structure of the neurons in the nucleus accumbens changes permanently. Contrary to the assertion that people are ever cured of addiction, all scientific and anecdotal evidence shows that an addicted person is never cured and that relapse is foreseeable, even probable, in addicted people years after they have ceased to use drugs unless they remain in a recovery program. For most people, the lifetime program consists of continued attendance at 12 Step meetings, maintaining contact with a sponsor, and practicing the 12 Step principles.

Certainly the great majority of people use mood- and consciousness-altering substances such as alcohol or other drugs and do not become addicted. That does not negate the fact that millions of people do become addicted; without treatment, they continue uncontrollable substance abuse despite horrendous consequences. Extensive research reported by the National Institute on Drug Abuse puts to rest any lingering questions about the reality of addiction (7). Addiction is similar to many other chronic, incurable, relapsing diseases such as diabetes, asthma, heart disease, and some cancers. They are treatable, but not curable. The rate of compliance with treatment among addicted people is about the same as the rate of compliance with treatment among diabetics (8,9). Yet no one would seriously suggest that diabetes should not be treated because some diabetics do not faithfully follow the treatment regimen. Recent studies have demonstrated that many people can be helped, and the experience of drug courts has shown that people coerced into treatment can greatly benefit from the treatment.

Realistic Expectations for Treatment

It can be argued that some drug courts allow only three or four treatment failures before terminating defendants and sentencing them to jail or prison, ignoring the reality of the disease concept of addiction. This is a valid criticism of drug courts that fail to distinguish between misbehavior and addiction symptoms. Some drug courts have adopted a hard-and-fast rule for sending people to jail for drug use. For example, one drug court in a western state adhered to the rule that a defendant would receive 30 days in jail for a first use, 60 days for a second use, and would be terminated for a third use. While it is clear and easy to implement, this approach is unrealistic and will result in skimming off the unaddicted recreational users while eliminating the addicted users from the program.

Most drug users have tried many times to stop using, and many have tried multiple treatment programs without success (10). In states like California, defendants who are convicted of drug use or possession offenses are given multiple attempts at treatment or educational diversion programs before any custody time can be imposed (11,12). The principal value of the drug court concept is the ability to constrain addicts to remain in treatment long enough to benefit from it. Terminating someone after two or three use episodes eviscerates the central purpose of a drug court.

The more rational and effective approach is to impose increasingly severe sanctions for failures to comply with the behavioral rules of the drug court and to prescribe increasingly potent treatments for failures to respond to treatment and to refrain from drug use. There are many levels of treatment available to addicts, including outpatient, intensive outpatient, residential, medically supervised inpatient, detoxification either in a treatment facility or in jail, and jail-based treatment. Not all drug courts will have every level, but they should use every level available before terminating a participant who is willing to comply with the treatment. Experience has shown that many participants who are not initially able to cease using drugs in an outpatient treatment program respond well to a stay in residential treatment.

Once they have a significant time away from drugs, their thinking clears, the cravings decline, and they are able to implement abstinence strategies. By definition, an addict cannot stop using drugs without help. Terminating someone from treatment because they cannot stop using drugs ignores the reality of addiction and defeats the purpose of a drug court.

Judges Are Not Social Workers

The traditional role of a criminal law judge is to sit as an impartial, unbiased referee, to watch truth and error grapple in the arena of a fair fight, and to impose appropriate punishment on a defendant who has been proven guilty beyond a reasonable doubt. The initial reaction of the author to the concept of drug courts was, "I'm not a social worker; I'm a judge."

A more educated view of judges shows that they are involved in social engineering with every decision. That is not to say that judges have unfettered discretion to steer society according to their notions of a better world. But no one can effectively argue that judges are mechanical automatons, mindlessly spewing out canned sentences and orders preprinted by "the law." Humans are complex, dynamic beings, and their interactions cause multifarious, labyrinthine disputes. Resolving those disputes requires skillful application of legal principles that cannot be accomplished by rote recitation of legal platitudes or imposition of standardized templates. Every case is different, every defendant unique. In a family law court, some parents have their children returned, others lose them forever. Some criminal defendants do community service work, others go to prison for life. Judges are charged with protecting the public and imposing terms that will facilitate the rehabilitation of criminal defendants under their jurisdiction.

Drug courts are an organized way to promote rehabilitation and reformation of criminal defendants. A properly organized drug court will rely on the participation of a prosecutor, a defense attorney, treatment specialists, and a probation officer to structure a plan designed to rehabilitate the offender. It is a far cry from a judge imposing his or her opinions based on unprofessional notions of social work or psychology.

Probation is designed to test a defendant and allow the defendant to prove that he or she will rehabilitate and abide by the law (13). A judge is allowed to impose any term of probation that is rationally connected to the offense and designed to promote the rehabilitation of the defendant. In a probationary drug court, the judge does not provide the treatment, does not supervise or analyze the participant, and does not do anything akin to social work. He or she administers and coordinates the input of all components and holds periodic reviews to ensure that the client is complying with the lawful probation orders of the court. Although the ambience and feel of a drug court may be different from a standard criminal courtroom, the function is essentially the same.

Imposing Requirements Before Conviction

There are three models for admitting a defendant into drug court, each having benefits and corresponding detriments:

1. Pre-plea.
2. Post-plea but prejudgment.
3. Postjudgment.

Pre-Plea

Some drug courts are based on a preconviction model. The accused agrees to participate in a treatment program and submit to sanctions without pleading guilty to the charges. If the treatment is fully complied with, the charges are dismissed. This model has a significant benefit of avoiding a criminal conviction record for the successful participant. Once a conviction appears on a record, it will follow the participant for life and can cause great difficulties in obtaining employment, professional licenses, grants, entry into education programs, and other benefits. Expunging a conviction is a laborious and taxing process that typically takes years and is sometimes impossible. Dragging a conviction throughout life will impair the ability of a reformed drug criminal to achieve a normal, productive life.

In this model, the defendant is frequently required to waive the right to a trial or stipulate that the matter can be tried on the police reports with no additional evidence. If the defendant either leaves the drug court voluntarily or is terminated for noncompliance, it is not necessary to then incur the expense of holding a trial on stale evidence.

Post-Plea, Prejudgment

The competing drug court models require the accused to be found guilty of the charges either by admission (through a plea of guilty or no contest) or by conviction in a trial. Most programs require a guilty plea, based on the philosophy that the first step in recovery is to admit that one has a problem and to take responsibility for it. This model rests on the theoretical advantage of tending to reduce denial because defendants who admit guilt are less likely to deny that they have a problem and resist treatment. Whether this theory is true in fact has not yet been determined, but the postconviction model has the additional benefit of being politically palatable. The defendant is placed on probation with the drug court agreement constituting the terms of probation.

Post-Plea, Postjudgment

A third model requires the accused to admit guilt through a plea of guilty or no contest and imposes the drug court terms as a condition of release from custody before judgment is pronounced. If the program is successfully completed, no judgment is entered, the plea is withdrawn, and the charges are dismissed. If the defendant fails to complete the drug court, judgment is entered and sentence pronounced. Depending on the jurisdiction, entry of a plea with pronouncement of judgment may constitute a conviction that will appear on subsequent inquiries into the person's criminal record.

In a pre-plea drug court, there may be resistance to imposing forced treatment on accused persons who have not been convicted of any crime. Certainly the U.S. Constitution protects against such abuses of government by requiring that guilt be proven to a jury, and all jurisdictions require that proof in a criminal case be proven beyond a reasonable doubt. Mere suspicion or accusation of guilt, no matter how strong the evidence may be, does not constitute a basis for punishment without a finding of guilt beyond a reasonable doubt.

Nevertheless, it seems apparent that when a defendant voluntarily agrees to terms of release from custody, which will ultimately remove the threat of criminal prosecution and result in a clean record, there is no violation of constitutional rights or due process. All defendants are faced with the choice of either admitting the charges and accepting a punishment or proceeding to trial and putting the government to its burden of proving the truth of the charges. Providing a third option, one that can ultimately improve the defendant's life immeasurably, lessens the threat to the defendant rather than increasing it. No one should be forced into a drug court, especially prior to conviction. Offering them treatment in lieu of prosecution is an advantage rather than coercion.

Imposing requirements on defendants prior to conviction is not a novel approach. Reasonable requirements of pretrial release have been an accepted practice in the courts for years. For example, when a defendant is charged with domestic violence, California requires that the defendant be ordered not to harm the alleged victim, not to possess any firearm, and to relinquish all firearms to a law enforcement agency or certified gun dealer pending trial. They may be ordered to move out of the house and have no contact with the victim or any potential witnesses. Similar requirements may be imposed in any criminal prosecution when it would promote a fair trial or protect someone involved. Gag orders may forbid discussion of the facts with any news media. A judge has wide latitude to impose orders to promote the ends of justice.

Such orders are not unbounded, and they must be rationally designed to promote acceptable ends of justice. Allowing a defendant to escape prosecution by completing a supervised addiction treatment program certainly falls within that stricture.

Evidence That Drug Courts Are Effective

Although 10 years ago it could be argued that no outcome studies existed that showed that drug courts are effective, this objection no longer holds water. Extensive studies by the states of New York and California, the U.S. Government Accountability Office, the Institute of Applied Research, the National Center on Addiction and Substance Abuse, the Center on Court Innovation, and other entities have concluded that drug courts not only reduce criminal recidivism but also save money over traditional criminal sanctions (14–16).

Federal Grants and Local Autonomy

Drug courts that are financed by federal grants are subject to federal control, with a resulting loss of local autonomy and ability to adapt to local needs. The choice of accepting outside money comes with strings attached. It is also a major mistake to create a drug court with grant money without building a sustaining element into the plan that will allow the program to continue after the grant is expired. It could be said that one who lives by the grant, dies by the grant.

If a grant is accepted for its intended purpose, to plan and implement the program, a grant need not hamstring the program permanently. Some grants come with built-in support systems and mandatory training that will allow creating the program without having to reinvent the process. Once it is fully functional, if sustainability has been planned in advance, grant funds are no longer needed and experience can teach what changes would improve the system and make it more responsive to local needs. The best approach is to use existing resources without the need to accept grants from outside sources.

Effect of Drug Courts on Caseloads

Properly supervising a drug court will require multiple court appearances, especially during the early stages when the participants struggle to maintain sobriety. The constant supervision of a judge, bolstered by rewards for compliance, is a strong motivator to those oppressed by the pain and discomfort of early withdrawal. Celerity (of response) is one of the key elements of effective rewards and sanctions. The best approach is to hold drug court review hearings no longer than 1 week apart during the early phases. These review hearings can become biweekly or monthly once the participants have stabilized.

Frequent reviews need not be an unbearable burden on the court. Although a judge can inspire, encourage, and discipline, judges are not treatment providers and should not substitute their judgment about the defendant's progress in recovery for the skill and training of the treatment provider. The review hearings should be to monitor compliance with the treatment plan, to lend encouragement and recognize achievement, and to provide correction for deviation from the treatment plan. If possible, the defendant should leave court feeling better about herself than she did when she arrived at court. Ordinarily, a short discussion of 2 to 5 minutes will suffice to achieve these goals. If the treatment provider has made an adequate report to the judge that is easily readable and in a standard format, the judge can review the report quickly, make appropriate comments to the defendant, and send her on her way to work or school. It will be necessary to spend more time on some cases, such as when a defendant has returned to drug use or violated a rule of the drug court, but for most status reviews when the defendant is in compliance, a short encouraging visit is sufficient.

This means that in one day, 80 defendants can easily be reviewed if each is given 5 minutes. The author routinely reviews 200 people in a drug court day, giving those who are doing well a minute or so and spending additional time with those who are doing poorly. This schedule is not an optimal arrangement but is sufficient to accomplish the goals of the drug court.

Initially, court clerks were wary of implementing the drug court, recognizing that seeing defendants every week would substantially increase the number of court appearances. They were right. It soon became apparent that the normal routine of clerical records would overwhelm them. Their first reaction was to throw up their hands and complain. After sitting down with the judge and analyzing what would happen at each appearance, they adapted their standard minute orders to a shortened form, allowing them to quickly check appropriate boxes and make short notes to track what happens at the hearings. As they observed changes in the participants' appearance, behavior, and attitudes over time, they became supporters of the drug court and came to value participating in the process of helping people escape their destructive drug use.

A single trial of a drug-related case can consume 3 or more days. If 15 cases per year are resolved by the availability of a drug court, the 45 days of trial time saved will offset an entire year of drug court weekly hearings.

Operating a busy drug court calendar can appear daunting, but experience has shown that if procedures are modified to standardize the reporting needed at each status review hearing, the paperwork soon becomes mechanical and routine. Clerks, probation officers, attorneys, and treatment providers can work together to shorten and simplify procedures.

Drug-abusing defendants frequently have multiple criminal cases that should be consolidated for review purposes so that the judge can handle fewer paper files. Additional case numbers can be annotated on the lead case file so that the judge is aware of the additional cases and can deal with them should the defendant violate out of the drug court. If the defendant commits new crimes, each court can decide whether to send the drug court cases to the regular criminal court judge hearing the new cases or whether the new cases should go to the drug court judge for resolution. Because the terms of a drug court agreement should specify that the defendant not commit new crimes, any new conviction can make resolution of the drug court cases simple, either in a violation of probation hearing or as the basis for a trial on a stipulated record. Although the goal is to rehabilitate the defendants and keep them out of custody, if they are not going to comply with the drug court requirements, they are easily sent to jail or prison. A study of the Tulare County, California Drug Court found that the fastest, least expensive way to send drug offenders to jail or prison was through the drug court if they demonstrated that they would not comply with the requirements (17).

Speaking at the 10th anniversary of the state of Virginia's drug courts, Virginia's Chief Justice, Hon. Leroy Rountree Hassell, Sr., said that he had observed firsthand the devastating consequences of drug addiction. He stated that he was proud of the Virginia Drug Court Association because it did not sit silently by and merely pontificate about the appropriate response from the judicial system because it organized and collaborated with each other (18).

Prosecutors

It is understandable why prosecutors might be skeptical of the drug court concept. Prosecutors are charged with protecting the community and enforcing laws. Their orientation is to seek convictions and punishment. For centuries their role has been one of arguing for increased incarceration to protect the community against criminals. Drug users wreak as much havoc on society as any other class of criminals, so it is natural for prosecutors to seek lengthy incarceration for drug offenders.

However, the advent of early release from jail and prison undermined the logic of this traditional paradigm. With overcrowded penal facilities in almost all jurisdictions, increasing custody sentences meant increasing the number of early releases. New scientific information about the nature of addiction and the efficacy of addiction treatment made it clear that it was not an effective use of prosecutors' time and resources to put addicted people behind bars who would respond to treatment.

The American Prosecutors Research Institute concluded that "Drug courts are one of the most effective means for ending the cycle of drug abuse and crime" (19). The National District Attorneys' Association adopted a resolution March 13, 1999, supporting drug courts as an effective means of reducing crime and enhancing public safety and advising that they must have prosecutorial leadership (20). Supporting and participating in a drug court is no longer a political risk or an unusual position for a prosecutor to take. Depending on the local legal culture, placing a defendant in a drug court may be the only way to retain control over the defendant.

In many areas probation has come to mean placing a file in a "banked caseload" (on a shelf in a back room) and a name in a computer tickler file. When probation is about to expire, the name is run to see if the defendant has been convicted of any new crimes, and, if so, a violation of probation is charged. Many probation departments have no funds to supervise criminal defendants with weekly or monthly visits and home checks. In those areas, placing someone on probation does essentially nothing to protect the community. Supervision in a drug court means frequent testing and judicial reviews. If a defendant is noncompliant, the judge will either deal with the violation at the next status hearing or, if the defendant fails to appear, issue a bench warrant for the defendant's arrest. Either way, the protection of the public is enhanced, and it is much more likely that the defendant will either be corrected or be behind bars quickly.

Some prosecutors have concerns that involvement in a drug court will consume considerable time sitting in court observing routine status hearings. This valid concern about use of a prosecutor's time can be alleviated by involving prosecutors only when their presence is necessary. For example, in some drug courts the prosecutor does not appear for regular status hearings. Arguably, there is no reason for the prosecutor to sit at the prosecution table and shuffle through the files only to hear that the defendants are doing well. Many drug courts find the involvement of the prosecutor to be a valuable part of the process, with the approbation of the prosecutor being an additional message to the defendant that society is invested in his rehabilitation and that the drug court is a place to get help instead of punishment. If a jurisdiction has sufficient prosecutorial resources to have an attorney sit in court for all status hearings, that involvement can be beneficial.

In jurisdictions where the prosecutors already strain to handle the existing caseload, there is no need that a deputy sit through the entire drug court every day. A much more limited involvement can be agreed to that will not be burdensome to the prosecutors yet will satisfy due process and properly represent the interests of society. For example, the prosecutor can attend a staffing session prior to the status hearings being called where she can give the prosecution's viewpoint on how problems should be handled and what action the judge should take. The drug court team can agree that the prosecutor need not be present if the judge will follow the agreed course or, if there is no agreement, whatever course the judge indicates she will follow. In the event new facts come to light that would justify a departure from the stated disposition, the matter can be postponed to the next drug court day or the prosecutor can be called to court if available. In the event that a significant violation of the drug court rules is charged, a designated time and place can be arranged to hold the formal contested hearings where the prosecutor is present to represent The People.

This process has worked well for years in the author's drug court where the prosecutor was initially opposed to the formation of the drug court. Once it became apparent that the drug court was not an easy, free get-out-of-jail option, the prosecutor saw no need to appear at all status hearings and now only appears for hearings involving significant violations that will jeopardize the continued involvement of the defendant in the drug court.

Defense Attorneys

Some defense attorneys oppose drug court because the programs constitute a heavier burden on their clients than a simple sentence of incarceration. This is especially true where the local legal culture imposes relatively light terms for drug offenses, and going to jail for a matter of weeks or months may be perceived as less onerous than a year or two years involved in a drug court. It is debatable whether a defense attorney should recommend a course of action to a client that is the easiest way out of the predicament if it is to the detriment of the client in the long run.

Considering the rates of recidivism among incarcerated drug users, one can make a strong case that obtaining a short jail term is not in the best interest of the client when compared to the long-term hope of effective addiction treatment. In any event, the decision is not the attorney's but the client's. The ethical issue is resolved by explaining the option of drug court to the client and allowing the client to make the decision. Adding another valuable alternative to the defendant's range of options should not be cause for any defense attorney to object to the implementation of a drug court.

In jurisdictions where the defendant would be facing long jail sentences or years of imprisonment for possessing drugs, it seems obvious that adding the potential for life-saving treatment instead of incarceration would be welcomed by the defense bar. Nevertheless, some defense attorneys, particularly public defenders, who seem to be always underfunded, are concerned about the additional burden on the attorneys of sitting through a drug court calendar. Just as this can be alleviated for prosecutors, a similar arrangement can be made for defense attorneys when resources will not allow them to appear at all status review hearings. If the client is doing well and in full compliance, there is no need to have a defense attorney present to protect the client's rights. In the vast majority of status review hearings, the defendant leaves happy and enthused, having been congratulated and praised by the judge and other court staff.

For those cases when the defendant needs to be corrected from an errant course, an appropriate response can be agreed to in the precourt staffing session with the prosecutor, defense attorney, probation officer, drug court coordinator, treatment representative, and judge present. The defense attorney can then either agree that if the selected response is implemented he will not appear with the defendant or, if this is seen as unacceptable, can come to the courtroom at a designated time when all matters requiring his presence will be called. There is no need to have a defense attorney sit through the entire drug court calendar.

In many post-plea jurisdictions, once a defendant enters a plea and is sentenced into the drug court, the defendant is no longer considered a client of the attorney of record. In such cases, the court should notify the defendants of the right to legal representation before any sanction is imposed. If the defendant chooses to invoke that right, imposition of any sanction can be postponed until defense counsel is obtained, either through private contract or by court appointment. In most cases, the sanction will be minor and the defendant will choose to waive the right to counsel and accept the sanction. For example, in the event of a significant violation such as attempted adulteration of a test, a sanction such as 15 or 30 days in jail might be appropriate. If the evidence is clear and the defendant knows that she is guilty of the offense, she may choose to accept the sanction rather than be incarcerated pending a formal violation of probation hearing that will require adequate time to prepare and may result in a longer jail stay than the sanction. If a minor custody sanction such as a night in jail is to be imposed, it will almost always be easier and more beneficial for the defendant to admit the violation and serve the short sanction rather than hold a formal contested hearing.

It is incumbent on the judge to ensure that defendants are not wrongfully sanctioned, and every reasonable precaution must be taken to avoid sanctioning defendants who have not violated the drug court rules. It is the author's experience that when the defense bar becomes satisfied that the judge will not impose sanctions heavy-handedly or without abundant, clear evidence of a violation, a trust is built and there is no need to hold formal violation hearings for minor sanctions. The defendants know the rules in advance, they know that they violated them, the reason and rationale for any sanction is fully explained to them, and they are ready to accept it. They know that they always have the right to contest any sanction and have legal assistance if they want it. It rarely happens.

California and other states have adopted different levels of treatment or education programs for drug offenses that are available prior to incarceration. The first is "diversion" or "deferred entry of judgment," consisting of a series of classes about drug use and abuse. If a first time offender is eligible for diversion, he may attend the classes, pay the mandatory fees, and, if he does not commit a new offense, have his case dismissed in as little as 18 months.

The second level was adopted by popular vote in 2000 as the Substance Abuse and Crime Prevention Act (adopted as Proposition 36). It provides addiction treatment lasting up to 18 months that, depending on the financial circumstances of the defendant, may be completely paid for by the state. Successful completion of the program also results in complete dismissal of the charges and expunging of the arrest.

In California and other jurisdictions with treatment programs available, people usually have extensive drug use and crime histories by the time they reach the drug court. Even the most staunch criminal defense attorney should recognize that the opportunity for her client to get effective treatment and halt the drug crime–incarceration cycle is usually far preferable to another term behind bars.

Law Enforcement Officers

Law enforcement officers share the prosecutors' responsibility to reduce crime and protect the community. They are naturally and justifiably skeptical of any program that releases recent arrestees from custody. Most officers have learned that when drug offenders go into custody, the number of burglaries drops.

In those jurisdictions where drug courts have been implemented, law enforcement officers have learned that drug and property crime goes down and they can see tangible benefits from their arrests. It is satisfying for an officer to see someone she arrested months before in an emaciated condition on the street, looking healthy, happy, and grateful for having been arrested and placed into a drug court. The arresting officer has the satisfaction of being part of a therapeutic intervention in the self-destructive life of a drug addict.

The author has heard dozens of drug court participants indicate that they had reached the limit of endurance, were ready to commit suicide, had decided how to do it, but in one final struggle to survive had prayed for deliverance from the horror of drugs, only to be arrested the next day. They attribute their arrest as an answer to their prayers and express sincere gratitude for the intervention of the police officer who made the arrest. Irrespective of one's belief in the efficacy of prayer, many drug court graduates are convinced that they are alive only because a law enforcement officer was sent by divine intervention to save them.

The Denver Colorado Drug Court was the twelfth in the nation, created in 1994. Judge William G. Myer presided over it for 2 years. Following his retirement, the other judges voted to disband the drug court, largely because they felt it increased their caseloads because law enforcement officers, having seen the positive benefits of the drug court, arrested more drug criminals. The *Denver Post* quoted Denver District Attorney Mitch Morrissey, who said that many people believe the drug court was effective and that without it "We've lost some ability to get inmates into the treatment track quickly" (21).

The newspaper explained that since the dismantling of the drug court, a greater percentage of serious drug cases resulted in prison time, increasing from 36.2% to 49.2%. In addition, the real impact was the time it took low-level offenders to get their charges resolved, meaning the defendants were stacking up in the city's jails, increasing the time to dispose of cases from 72 hours up to 90 days.

Although initially among the greatest skeptics, the police became some of the most vocal advocates of a return to the one-judge drug court. The *Denver Post* quoted Denver police Sgt. John Spezze as saying that drug court "made a huge difference in the neighborhoods and in the lives of the people who were arrested" (21).

Law enforcement agencies have endorsed and cooperated with drug courts all over the nation. Almost 60% of police chiefs polled, advocated judicially supervised treatment programs over other criminal justice options, and many police departments have assigned full-time police officers to assist with monitoring and supervising drug court participants (22). Many drug courts invite arresting officers to graduation ceremonies so that they can see the beneficial effects of their arrests. Too often police officers make arrests on the street and never know what happened to the arrestees until they see them committing a new offense. It is satisfying for them to see that they have been successful in their efforts to reduce crime and help people in a meaningful way.

An additional consideration is the impact on a sheriff or other law enforcement officers charged with transporting defendants in custody to court. It is inevitable that some defendants will flee the drug court and later be arrested on bench warrants. They will need to be returned to court for disposition, either reinstatement into the drug court or termination from the program and sentencing. Other defendants will commit various violations and have custody sanctions imposed on them. They will have to be returned to court for release or other hearings before the judge.

The experience of the author's county is that the drug court has reduced the inmate population of the county jail substantially, certainly enough to offset any additional transports of drug court participants. The sheriff is a major drug court supporter who attends all graduation ceremonies and publicly extols the value of the drug court.

Additional Roadblocks

Lack of available treatment can be perceived as a roadblock, and new research shows that various treatment modalities have differing efficacy in a drug court. Considering the abysmal results of incarceration, it is a fair assumption that almost any treatment will be better than incarceration at reducing crime, and at a fraction of the cost. Almost any community will have some form of substance abuse treatment, including treatment for drivers convicted of driving under the influence of alcohol. Although they may lack some expertise in treating drug addicts, many of the principles of recovery are common to both alcohol and other drug addicts. Every state has a Single State Agency Director in charge of all substance abuse programs in the state (23). They will provide direction and assistance in developing treatment skills.

Where treatment providers are available, they will likely welcome a drug court that will send them highly motivated clients and support their treatment with judicial authority. Treatment agencies that are not adequately trained will have the opportunity to develop new competencies for the facility and of the individual counselors who work for the agency.

Conclusions

Almost everyone knows someone whose life has been ravaged by drug addiction. The author is frequently contacted by people imploring him for any advice on how to help loved family members who are unable to escape the destructive shackles of addiction. Unfortunately, there is no magic answer. The options available to the average family are few: expend great sums of money in private treatment, sever all ties with the addicted family member, or allow their lives to be slowly and systematically destroyed while they suffer along with their loved one. The first option is not even available to most families, as private treatment can cost thousands of dollars every month, and treatment is a long process.

Experience has proven that in a jurisdiction with a functioning drug court, the seemingly undesirable option of seeing the affected family member arrested and thrown into the criminal justice system is a much better option. No matter how much they cry, beg, yell, argue, love, cajole, threaten, or plead, family members lack sufficient force to produce what Dr. Stalcup calls the "window of clarity" that can be the portal to freedom from drug use. Many times, it is only the arrest and subsequent court arraignment that shocks the drug user enough to produce this moment of clarity. If treatment is quickly offered, amazing results follow, what former Director of the U.S. Office of National Drug Control Policy General Barry R. McCaffrey called "one of the most monumental changes in social justice in this country since World War II" (24). For the first time in history, significant numbers of drug-addicted people are seeing major benefits from treatment, supervised by judges and law enforcement officers who care about the people they deal with and want to see significant reduction in crime.

Overcoming the barriers requires an open mind and a willingness to depart from staid, established legal culture and practices. The best way to become willing to undertake the process is to visit an established, functioning drug court. With almost 2,000 to choose from, everyone has access to a nearby drug court and can see firsthand what is being accomplished there. Any drug court would be delighted to invite observers to view their operation, and most, if not all, will offer technical support and freely share forms and ideas.

The National Association of Drug Court Professionals has numerous resources to assist in creating a drug court (24). Most states have a state drug court professionals organization that can offer assistance and guidance. Much of the hard work has already been done, and jurisdictions are not required to design a drug court from a blank sheet.

References

1. Federal justice resigns, calling judicial system unjust. New York Times, July 24, 2003.

2. See opinion of Judge Myron Bright in *U.S. v. Hiveley*, 61 F.3d 1358 at 1363; and of Judge Harold A. Baker in *U.S. v. Abbott*, 961 F2d 964 (Cent Dist Ill, June 22, 1993).
3. Hay B, Spier K. Litigation and settlement. In Newman P, ed. The New Palgrave Dictionary of Economics and the Law. New York: Macmillan; 1998: 442–451.
4. Judicial Council of California. Preserving Equal Access to Justice: Progress and Challenges of the California Judicial Branch. San Francisco: Judicial Council of California/Administrative Office of the Courts; 2004.
5. Judicial Council of California. Trust and Confidence in the California Courts: A Survey of the Public and Attorneys. San Francisco: Judicial Council of California/Administrative Office of the Courts; 2005.
6. Nestler EJ, Malenka RC. The addicted brain. Sci Am 2004;290:78–85.
7. U.S. Department of Health and Human Services, National Institute of Health. Prescription Drugs: Abuse and Addiction. Washington, DC: Government Printing Office; 2005.
8. Griffin SJ. Lost to follow-up: the problem of defaulters from diabetes clinics. Diabet Med 1998;5(3):S14–S24.
9. Littenberg B, MacLean CD, Hurowitz L. The use of adherence aids by adults with diabetes: a cross-sectional survey. BMC Fam Pract 2006;7:1–5.
10. National Institute on Drug Abuse. National Institutes of Health. Drug Addiction Treatment Methods. Washington, DC: National Institute on Drug Abuse; 2000.
11. Longshore D, Hawken A, Urada D, Anglin MD. Evaluation of the Substance Abuse and Crime Prevention Act: Cost Analysis Report. Los Angeles: UCLA, Integrated Substance Abuse Programs; 2006.
12. California Penal Code Sections 1000 et. seq. and 1210.1.
13. Dickey WJ, Smith ME. Dangerous Opportunity: Five Futures for Community Corrections. Washington, DC: Department of Justice, Office of Justice Programs; 1998.
14. United States Government Accountability Office. Adult Drug Courts: Evidence Indicates Recidivism Reductions and Mixed Results for Other Outcomes. Washington, DC: Government Printing Office; 2006.
15. Institute of Applied Research. A Cost-Benefit Analysis of the St. Louis Adult Felony Drug Court. St. Louis: Institute of Applied Research; 2004.
16. Rempel M, Fox-Kralstein D, Cissner A. Drug courts: an effective treatment alternative. Crim Justice 2004;19(2):5–11.
17. Lessenger JE, Lessenger LH, Lessenger EW. An Outcome Analysis of Drug Court in Tulare County, California. Visalia, CA: Tulare County Superior Court; 2000.
18. Virginia Drug Court Association. Chief Justice Hassel's Speech to the Virginia Drug Court Association. Richmond, VA: Virginia Drug Court Association; 2005.
19. Everitt T. Drug Courts. Alexandria, VA: American Prosecutors Resource Institute; 2005.
20. Resolution 99-01 SPR on Drug Courts, March 13, 1999. National District Attorneys' Association, Alexandria, VA.
21. Drug Court May Stage Comeback. The Denver Post. November 13, 2005.

22. Turner S, Longshore D, Wenzel S, Deschenes E, Greenwood P, Fain T, et al. A decade of drug treatment court research. Subst Use Misuse 2002;37:1489–1527.
23. The director for each state can be found at http://captus.samhsa.gov/home.cfm.
24. National Association of Drug Court Professionals. Press release: The National Drug Court Institute is created through a partnership between NADCP and ONDCP. Washington, DC: National Association of Drug Court Professionals; 1997.

24
Probation Strategies

Helen Harberts

Probation is a key partner in the drug court model. All drug court team members should understand the basic concepts of community supervision, the process of carrying out local community supervision agency work, and the need for community supervision to provide a support for recovery and accountability in a program.

An Overview

Following are the basic functions of community supervision:

1. Protect public safety.
2. Support recovery.
3. Confirm facts with objective information.
4. Inform the court on the current status of the client.

Community supervision generally refers to two primary agencies, probation and parole, that manage cases of criminal justice clients. Personnel in these agencies are knowledgeable about case management practices, strategies, and techniques. They are commonly trained in motivational interviewing, addiction principles, and treatment practices. They often have the power to arrest and conduct field services on clients.

The legal authority of probation and parole officers and policies on exercising that authority varies by jurisdiction. For instance, some officers serve a client base with limited jurisdiction, such as misdemeanors only, felony only, post-prison, pre-prison, or a combination of these areas. Some are sworn peace officers with the power of arrest. Occasionally, jurisdictions do not choose to exercise peace officer powers. Some jurisdictions arm their officers, some do not. Some are active in community-based field services; other agencies insist on performing their duties from an office setting (1). It is, therefore, very important to know what legal and policy limits are set on the local community supervision agencies. This will also assist the drug court in determining which supplemental community supervision partners can increase the supervision model to a 24-hour, daily operation. Drug courts thrive on good, rapid information that is shared across the entire team. The more information the drug court gets, the better the outcomes.

The Role of Probation

Probation departments play a prominent role in drug courts across the United States and internationally. Probation officers serve as court officers on the team to do the following:

1. Conduct field services.
2. Administer intermediate sanctions and incentives.
3. Arrest offenders threatening the public safety.
4. Conduct drug testing.
5. Work with families.
6. Advocate for additional services.
7. Perform assessments.
8. Meet with the clients frequently.

Some probation officers are trained in substance abuse treatment or are dual certified and conduct treatment services regarding addiction. Others perform treatment in life skills, correcting thinking errors, and running other cognitive behavioral programs that are required in addition to substance abuse treatment. In many jurisdictions, probation is the central case manager for the drug court, providing all of the information gathering and report writing for the judge.

In addition, probation plays a highly visible role in direct supervision within the community. Community supervision not only protects the public but also provides a supportive recovery environment through assertive field services.

In early recovery, refusal skills generally come from an external force. That force is often the thought of a probation officer showing up at your door to search and test you. Throughout this chapter are references to a central concept: probation supervision is a support to recovery.

Consider the tasks required of probation in the drug court structure being designed or improved. Caseload size is a crucial piece of the puzzle, and success of the program will depend on it. Consider what the court asks the officers to do and what else they are required to do for their jobs. Some questions to consider include the following:

1. How many people do they supervise?
2. What is the specific client base? Does this base justify low caseload levels because of unique characteristics of the caseload?
3. What will their supervision consist of?
4. Will there be a need for field services, and, if so, how often? What are the geographic impacts they may experience?

5. Will there be drug testing; if so, how often?
6. Will there be a need for office services; if so, how often?
7. What will be the form of coordination of services?
8. What will be the needs for case management and court reporting?
9. Will data management services be needed?
10. Are the probation officers going to work solely for the drug court, or will they have other duties?
11. What are their annual training requirements and other leave requirements?
12. Who will be the back-up officer when the one assigned to drug court is not available?

Although best practices recommend a dedicated, small caseload comprised solely of drug court clients, there is no magic number for the right number of clients per probation officer. Rather, the concept of workload must be considered. Examining the answers to these questions will help to determine how many clients one probation officer can realistically manage. In some programs, case management responsibilities may be shared with treatment or other drug court partners. Another consideration when deciding the capacity of a probation officer's drug court caseload is the type of client being served by the program. Some clients present greater needs; therefore, a smaller caseload is necessary. However, first time offenders or other groups may not need intensive case management. Family and juvenile drug courts often integrate more intensive contacts with collateral resources and additional family members (schools, athletic programs, boys and girls clubs, family counseling). Persons with concurrent disorders require additional time and case management. Persons who are assessed with high criminogenic needs should have at least 70% of their time structured. Therefore, if the drug court treats such clients, there is a need to have supervision that can monitor these clients constantly. As the program considers community supervision needs, it should consider program and budget issues, such as equipment costs, extra allocated overtime, and shift adjustments for field services outside of normal government hours.

Core Competencies

Probation officers assigned to drug courts should be experienced and not new staff. Working with this population can be taxing and requires a balanced approach to criminal justice and case management. Core competencies require knowledge of the following:

1. Principles of addiction and recovery.
2. The 12 Step programs and the traditions of the 12 Step community.
3. Basic cognitive behavioral programming.
4. Behavior modification principles.

5. Criminogenic factors and concerns.
6. Psychopharmacology.
7. Concurrent disorders.
8. Family dynamics.
9. Case management and supervision techniques.
10. Field service skills.
11. Peace officer training and skills.
12. Report writing training.
13. Assessments training and skills.
14. Cultural competency.
15. Drug testing interpretation.

In addition, probation officers (and all drug court team members) should be cross trained in each other's work within the drug court context. This promotes team building and understanding of the limits and strengths of the various professions on the team; it also reduces the possibility of exploitation of team differences by a client.

The Intake Interview

The abilities to interview people, assess them on the stages of change, utilize motivational interviewing, and collect essential information are required skills for intake and assessment. Various documents and criteria need to be taken into account by the officer in preparing intake reports. These items include the following:

1. Crime reports.
2. Defendant's statements.
3. Witnesses' statements.
4. Victim statements.
5. The criminal history (rap sheet) from local, state, and federal sources.
6. The drug use history from both self-reporting and from the criminal history.
7. Personal history forms from prior grants of probation. (How did he or she respond in the past when asked about drug use?).
8. Information on prior attempts at treatment.

Questions and issues to cover in the probation interview include the following:

1. Tell me about your current drug use.
2. Tell me about your current living situation.
3. What are the pros and cons of using drugs?
4. If treatment has been tried before, what about it has worked for you? What hasn't?
5. How long did you maintain sobriety after the last treatment episode?

6. Tell me which drugs you have used over time and which drugs you have had treatment for.
7. Tell me about your alcohol use.
8. Do you smoke or chew tobacco?
9. What are your past results of any urine testing to detect substance abuse?
10. Tell me if you have been treated for any physical injury (especially head injury).
11. Have you seen any doctors in the past year? Who? Where?
12. Tell me if you have seen any mental health professionals in the last few years. Who? Where? What happened? Were you given any medications? What are they? Are you taking those medications now?
13. Do you have any physical problems that are troubling you currently?

Note that it is also important to have intake and assessment results from other team members or other sources. Some clients are more truthful on a computer-driven self-assessment instrument. For some reason, the machine seems less threatening to some people. The best information comes from a blend of assessments taken over time.

An assessment gives you a starting point, but clients have no reason to trust the person doing the assessment and may not be entirely honest with the interviewer or with themselves about the depth of their problems. They may still be in early withdrawal or early recovery and may have memory deficits that impact their responses, particularly in methamphetamine users. Drug court clients may have prior experience, good or bad, with one of the team members or agencies that can impact the outcome of the assessment. It is important to consider the first assessments as preliminary. Continued assessment is important with clients. Drug courts are about change. Using continued assessment allows the program to monitor change and to determine areas where change is not occurring as expected.

Intake Forms and Information Sharing

Forms vary across systems and are subject to the requirements of local law and policy. As much as possible, best practices would suggest that we avoid duplicate information collection. The same basic data can and should be shared across the team. This is a cost saving, and it assists the client. Nobody wants to tell the same information to different folks over and over. In some cases, revisiting the same psychic injuries can inflame posttraumatic stress disorders or other injuries that are challenging for drug addicts to deal with until stabilized in recovery.

As a member of a drug court team, probation should always be part of the confidentiality waivers for treatment and medical information. Transmission of relevant information is critical to outcomes. This allows a better treatment plan and better responses to client behavior as they come up. Information should be shared when relevant to decision making. Note that many professions have ethical or legal obligations that may prohibit sharing certain information without an appropriate waiver. Some confidentiality restrictions can be waived, and some cannot. Some information is not necessary for the whole team to know, such as the timing of searches and arrests. Probation and criminal justice agencies cannot reveal rap sheets or criminal justice information that may be protected by statute. It is illegal in some states to reveal the existence of a search warrant, and it is dangerous to reveal when an arrest or field search is going to happen. On the other hand, it is critical for team members to know the results of drug testing as quickly as possible so that a therapeutic response can be developed quickly. It is critical for the team to know that a client is attending all treatment sessions as ordered and is "working treatment." It may not be necessary to share the details of what is being discussed in group. Thus, it becomes important for all team members to understand each other's professional responsibilities and limits.

Assessment

Probation is often responsible for some of the early and ongoing assessment of clients. This assessment may include risk assessment as well as needs and strengths assessment. Because probation officers are quite often the only members seeing the client in his or her home environment, they are able to offer invaluable information to the rest of the team. It is important for the entire team to understand the full picture of the client's life. This includes the client's home and work environment as well as his or her social activities and decision-making processes.

By going to a client's house, officers can assess the living environment. There are many reasons why clients may not report their situation objectively. Some may be embarrassed about how they live. Some clients may not know that how they live is not safe or acceptable. They may live as they always have, with no power, no sewers, and no water. Others may be afraid to reveal that they are being battered or that there are dangerous people in the home doing things that do not support recovery. By showing up at a home, probation officers can determine if it is a fraudulent address, if it is a safe recovery environment, or if the client needs to move to sober living or other safe facilities. Additional service referrals and assistance may be made from such a visit. All of the observed information, immediately delivered to the treatment staff, can make a significant difference in the treatment plan.

The American Society of Addiction Medicine has a patient placement criteria grid that is the standard used to determine minimum levels of treatment intervention for addicted persons (2). One of the criteria involves the recovery environment, which is a crucial element of treatment success.

Every drug court needs an objective, ongoing assessment of the recovery environment.

A probation officer dropping by and seeing unappealing new associates or a change in the living environment for the worse can detect a relapse pattern even if the use has not yet happened. It is critical that probation officers note and communicate the positive changes that are occurring in the client's home as well. Observing the positive or negative progress being made in the client's home environment and sharing this information with the team allows the team to respond in the most comprehensive and useful way.

There are many risk assessment instruments that can be used for a corrections population. It is important to get an instrument that allows use of objective information from outside reliable sources, such as rap sheets, and that is normalized for the criminal justice population. Some risk assessment instruments were normalized against college students who were not criminally involved. This does not give an accurate picture of the challenges facing a criminal offender. Commonly used risk and needs assessment instruments can be obtained from local criminal justice professionals in probation. Some instruments, such as the Level of Services Inventory, Revised, are proprietary, and some assessments have been developed for local regions, such as one for Maricopa County, Arizona. For a good discussion of criminal justice assessments with value for substance abusers, see Treatment Improvement Protocols 7 and 44 (3).

Probation officers may not be used to working in a team environment when developing a plan of action for a probationer. However, if drug court clients are on probation or are on a service contract as part of a civil case plan, their conditions of probation become part of the case plan that must be integrated with the treatment plan. After assessment, a case plan can be developed in conjunction with treatment and other partners in the program. Considerations of family, child custody or care, potential for violence or sexual exploitation, the presence of a concurrent disorder with the presenting addiction problems, criminal justice mandates, and public safety concerns all factor into the case plan. Indeed, a critical factor is the client's position on the stages of change (4). Drug court clients are part of the team and their input must be sought as well.

Community Supervision

Effective client monitoring must include more than simply checking to see if the client attended treatment sessions. Effective monitoring must include home and other field visits and, if possible, periodic searches. As mentioned earlier, the information gathered from a home visit can assist in developing an individualized treatment plan. Home visits offer an opportunity to learn information that can lead to rapid treatment intervention.

One of the most important functions of community supervision in a drug court is the concept of "catching the client doing something right." Praise and recognition of progress in addressing addiction are the great engines of change. This information is key to the team, and all positive news should be communicated to the team as quickly as possible. By performing community supervision, probation officers, while focused on accountability and public safety, are also uniquely positioned to see progress and to find improvements in the home, in the cognitive responses of clients, and in the overall progress of the client. Some of the positive changes that probation officers might expect to find are a more regular routine demonstrated, such as children attending school and not staying home without any apparent reason, meals being prepared and cleaned up, following a regular schedule (e.g., during a probation appearance at 11:00 am finding the client showered and dressed instead of in bed asleep).

As clients improve their choices or identify challenges themselves and as they begin to become the locus of control for their recovery, probation officers can see the changes and report them to the court team. This information, combined with the group and individual sessions with treatment, will form the picture of progress, or lack thereof, for the court team. Observing good changes and good decisions, followed by immediate reinforcement through praise, supports recovery.

Types of Contact

The types of contacts to be discussed in this section are home visits and searches, school and work visits, and enforcing the court's orders.

Home Visits or Searches

Home visits and home searches are two different functions. The home visit is a more casual and less intrusive appearance at the home of a client. Depending on the results of the home visit, a search may immediately follow. Home visits are done for the following reasons:

1. To confirm address accuracy.
2. To confirm that the address is not just a mailing address but a place where the client is living full time.
3. To learn who else may be living at the address.
4. To confirm the floor plan of the address for officer safety purposes and to determine if there are any dangerous dogs or surveillance equipment at the scene.
5. To provide an assessment of the needs and strengths of the client (because self-reporting by clients can be intentionally or unintentionally inaccurate, it is important to confirm information and inform the rest of the team about the findings).

6. To assess the recovery environment by evaluating the presence of supportive residents or the presence of inappropriate residents or substances.

Searches, on the other hand, include the activities of the home visit along with search activity. This may involve the following:

1. Field testing for alcohol or controlled substances through the observed taking of a sample.
2. Physical search of the premises, including all areas and items that are within the dominion and control of the client.

It is important to check all areas where controlled substances or other threats to officers or recovery might be hidden. Searches for alcohol should entail not only the cupboards and refrigerators but also receipts from liquor stores and empty containers around the premises, recycle bins, vehicles, and ice chests or other storage containers where liquor or evidence of liquor might be kept. Searches for controlled substances and paraphernalia take a similar methodic attention to detail. The areas where items can be stored are limited only by human imagination. In addition, officers would do well to look for evidence of attempts to defeat or alter urine testing, such as various products designed to alter tests, flush the system, or provide someone else's urine.

It is not uncommon for searches to reveal a sample of urine in a refrigerator or some bottles of urine ready in case of a random phone call to come test. Banned weapons, stolen property, and evidence of other criminal behavior such as forgery may also be found during searches. A search that turns up no contraband and demonstrates a good recovery environment is the best possible news, and this should be communicated to the team faster than bad news of finding contraband.

It is important to have a discussion with all team members about how home visits and searches are done. Many people have inaccurate, preconceived notions about how such visits are conducted. Because all of the team needs to be able to answer questions and comments by clients (and to avoid any misunderstandings among staff) all members of the team should understand the professional methodologies, why things are done in a certain way, and what the professional limitations of community supervision are. In addition, it is critical for all team members to understand that field services support recovery.

In early recovery, it is difficult for offenders to stay away from the people, places, and things that sustain their addiction. They have not developed sufficient refusal skills to support recovery. The knowledge that probation officers will come unannounced any time, day or night, with or without probable cause, is a good externally based refusal skill. The client can simply tell others, "I can't use drugs" or "I can't run around with the gang" because the probation officers in the drug court come by all the time. This is a socially acceptable excuse for not running with old associates. It works until the locus of control for recovery shifts to the client, who can then say "I'm not using drugs any more, and you have to leave."

School and Work Visits

No matter what target population your drug court serves, it is likely that your clients will have contact with schools. Adults may be working on basic literacy, GED, job skills, or career development courses. Children or juveniles should be in school. Family members may be pursuing education. If school staff are part of the case management plan or are part of a juvenile or family drug court, school will be a central component of the supervision strategy. Like treatment attendance, school attendance is a target behavior that must be monitored. Supportive services, encouragement, acknowledgment for improvements, and support if setbacks occur are critical for continued progress and ultimate success.

With juveniles, truancy, behavior, associates, and afterschool activities are important to monitor. Attendance can be monitored by having juveniles sign in with a probation officer before the beginning of school. Failure to appear for sign-in should immediately trigger a home visit. School visits should be done in close cooperation with school officials and in a supportive manner whenever possible. For juveniles, behavior and attendance are crucial; they must be monitored and addressed immediately if there is a problem. A school campus is the worksite of young people. It must be monitored as such, and the clear message must be sent that school is the highest priority.

In an effort to be comprehensive in service delivery, some teams pull students out of classes to deliver additional services, such as mental health appointments, group counseling, testing, or medical appointments necessary for medications. Clearly, one cannot succeed at school if one is not there. Every effort should be made by case managers to send the clear signal from the treatment team that school is high priority. This means that the team itself does not interrupt the school schedule. Appointments should be scheduled for after school. Pull-outs should be avoided at all costs.

Work sites of adults should also be monitored. It is important to verify that there is a job by examining legitimate pay stubs, for example. The approach of community supervision should be flexible and sensitive to the work environment. Decisions about having probation or other community supervision professionals wearing uniforms or high profile gear should be carefully considered. Clients rightfully may be concerned that they may lose their job if uniformed probation officers show up at their job site. Clients need to understand that probation visits to work are a possibility. The team also needs to understand that it is not always necessary to visit work sites but that it may become necessary. If the law requires reporting to an employer that someone is on probation for a specified offense, the client will need to work on how that news is delivered. This is common with truck drivers and controlled substance violations. In the experience of many, employers will work well with drug court clients if they are informed about the program and how it works.

It is important for a careful discussion to occur regarding the nature of the client's work. If the work site is not conducive to recovery, it may well be a part of the case plan to change employment. Because steady employment is a goal of many programs and clients, it is important to consider which jobs might not be a good idea for persons in recovery. Bartending, for instance, is a poor idea. Many drug courts ban clients from entering casinos for any purpose, thus ruling out employment at such locations. People who work in an addiction-heavy environment such as construction, may need to change employers. The challenge of dealing with people, places, and things is an overwhelming task for early recovery. Supervision needs to assess these things for the team.

Enforcing the Court's Orders

Curfews, geographic limitations ("don't go to the downtown park because it is a known location for drug sales"), and prohibitions against entering alcohol establishments must be enforced if they are ordered. Phone calls with identifying questions may help address curfew concerns. Similarly, surveillance, both personal and electronic, can enforce curfew and geographic limits. Community-based field services are essential. A common tactic to enforce these terms is for the supervision team to visit those places during banned hours or to enter into bars and other places looking for clients. It is simple to have an entry team walk in the front door with a couple of officers waiting at the back door in case the clients suddenly exit the rear. During these activities, high-profile gear such as shirts saying "PROBATION" is effective. One advantage to such activities is that only a few people need to be caught violating parole for effectiveness. Word will quickly spread among everyone else in the program, and they will realize they are vulnerable too.

Addiction is a cruel and deceptive disease that impairs decision making. Clients make poor choices at first. The thought of being caught helps them resist the temptation to slip. Failure to enforce the orders of the court does not support recovery. If failure to enforce the orders is a pattern and practice, due process concerns may make the attempt to enforce court orders on selected troublesome clients invalid.

There are other considerations regarding searches that must be discussed by the entire team. Search activity must fall within the limitations of the law. Every jurisdiction has slightly different policies or interpretations of the law, and probation officers must strictly follow the rule in their jurisdiction. In some instances, searches are not allowed because of the civil nature of the case, such as some dependency cases. If officers conduct searches, their searches are limited by the law and by the exact terms of the search authority ordered by the court. To provide uniformity, many programs condition admission on a full waiver of the fourth amendment rights of the clients. As long as the executions of the searches are not arbitrary, capricious, or harassing, they will be considered lawful in most jurisdictions.

Probation Office Visits

The office visit is the ideal time for the following activities:

1. Planned confrontations.
2. Continued written assessments.
3. Confirmation of treatment attendance.
4. Confirmation of self-help work.
5. Confirmation of 12 Step work.
6. Confirmation of other court-ordered tasks, such as education, employment, health visits, collateral treatment requirements for co-occurring disorders, or other needs as defined by the assessments.
7. Catching up on paperwork requirements with clients.
8. Catching up with client feelings, progress, and needs and encouraging continued progress.
9. Advising clients on what is coming next in their program, and working with them to determine where they are in the stages of change.
10. Encouraging clients to keep motivated through this difficult and arduous process.

How to Search

This section reviews the search of the residence of a drug court client or another location where the client may be present.

First Rule: Search with Respect

Drug court clients may have had bad experiences with law enforcement in the past. Whether or not this is true, the prospect of officers searching one's home, person, vehicle, or any property under one's dominion and control is intimidating. It is important to be sensitive to these feelings and to practice courteous, professional behavior when conducting searches. Remember that officers will be back many times to monitor progress. Relationships of trust and mutual respect will need to develop. The court team models the behavior that clients are expected to learn as members of society. While most agencies are highly professional about their practices, there are others who may not be. Rules need to be clearly spelled out at the highest levels.

Officer Safety Is Paramount

Although the probation officer may know the clients and may have searched their homes many times, these situations are unpredictable. A client who has begun using drugs or alcohol again has reason to keep the information from those searching. Even the client who is in recovery may have an uninvited guest who has a warrant or who otherwise may want to deter probation from their visit.

The following are key points to remember:

1. Weapon sweeps are important.
2. Do not let people sit or stand where you have not searched first.
3. Wear gloves, take a flashlight, and do not put your hands where you cannot see first.
4. Practice universal precautions at all times. Often these homes are full of needles, broken glass, and used personal supplies and are profoundly unclean. Good search technique requires caution.

After an area has been searched, another officer should follow behind. It is easy for the eye to overlook things, and a second set of eyes may pick up something that was missed. Officers need to look everywhere and learn from others where hiding places might be.

Develop Guidelines for Officer Action

The supervision agency will need to develop guidelines for officer actions when problems are detected in the home environment. For example, some agencies have bright line policies about when offenders go into custody during field visits. Examples of situations in which rapid custody is warranted include finding an offender who is participating in a driving-under-the-influence court with measurable alcohol in his body during a field visit. That person, who has a demonstrated propensity to drive when he has been drinking, goes into custody immediately. Clients who are pregnant and using drugs may be taken into custody on a bright line rule. Other agencies leave the decision up to the officers in the field. It is critical for drug court team members to understand what mandates probation has and then to develop policy around those mandates. As is true with each team member, there should be parameters within which a team member may make autonomous decisions.

Practice Good Field Precautions

No matter what, it is important for community supervision and for the team to clearly understand the importance of good field safety practices. Field work is dangerous. It is not for those who have insufficient training or equipment. Depending on the drug of choice or on the nature of unknown associates, a simple home visit can quickly turn into a very dangerous situation. The nature of the community and the availability of back-up assistance all factor into safety decisions. It is necessary to train frequently and to have good officer safety techniques, including management of assaultive behavior, continuum of force, self-defense, arrest techniques, radio training, weapons training, understanding how to unload a seized weapon, and arms training if armed. Simple entry tactics and search technique training are a must. Evidence seizure training is also critical.

If an environment looks unsafe, officers should not enter it. They should come back with more people and better preparation. The real danger for community supervision is a place that looks safe, has been safe in the past, and suddenly presents something on the other side of the door that is unexpected. As noted earlier, an officer may have a splendid relationship with a client but has no relationship with parolees or others who may just show up and move in. A client, particularly a gang member, may not have a good enough foundation in recovery to withstand the pressure of collective behavior. Caution is always the underlying rule. Officer safety always comes first.

Have Appropriate Equipment

Some agencies develop field gear that combines a local drug court logo with a badge or other professional logo. The search kit should include latex gloves, some hand cleaner, evidence tags, evidence bags, chain of evidence forms, seizure receipts, a digital camera, pen or pencil, a small ruler to place near objects to be photographed, and some protective eyewear. A first-aid kit should always be on hand. Before leaving, the team should develop a list of addresses to be visited and the route to the nearest emergency room. Report forms should be developed so officers can note critical facts for discovery and recordkeeping purposes.

What to Look for During the Search

Entry into a home and the initiation of a home visit or search entails a great deal of detail. Depending on the jurisdiction, many concerns immediately come to mind. Many jurisdictions are battling methamphetamine, and the danger of accidentally finding a clandestine laboratory is great. Knowing what is, or what may be, a laboratory is important. Strange chemicals can cause fires, explosions, poisoning, and death.

Elder or child abuse or neglect may be present. Field service officers are generally mandatory reporters. It is important to be trained to look for the signs of such abuse. Especially in methamphetamine areas, it is critical to examine for drug-endangered children and to immediately take action if they are detected.

Substance abuse and domestic violence often go hand in hand. Officers should assume that domestic violence, with all of the officer safety risks that it carries, may be present at any field visit.

Searches should look for the presence of alcohol. Alcohol use is a commonly misunderstood area of drug courts. Many clients do not make the connection between drug abuse and alcohol abuse. They will argue that they have a drug conviction or addiction but not an alcohol problem. Studies have demonstrated that people who drink alcohol while in recovery are 20 times more likely to relapse on their primary drug of choice (5). It is important for officers to make that connection clear to friends, family, and the client. When a court says no alcohol in the home, the judge means everyone in the home must not have alcohol. Until clients understand the full concept of addiction through treatment, this is a difficult concept for them to grasp.

It is important to distinguish between homes that are unclean or disorganized and homes that are unsafe. One is a problem to be addressed through case management, and the other may constitute an emergency that requires rapid intervention. A home with no heat in winter may be unsafe. A home with no working plumbing may be unsafe. Exposed electrical wires, fire hazards, explosive materials, and spoiled food are unsafe. These things need to be acted on with all due speed. Cleaning issues are not solved with shame. Shame-based responses do not create lasting change. As supervision is done, it is important to keep focused on safety versus cleanliness.

When Probation Searches Are Not Possible

Some dependency or family drug courts may not have the capabilities of probation officer searches, and some drug courts may not use fourth amendment waivers. In either case, it is important that a drug court perform as many field services as possible to allow an assessment of the recovery environment. However, unless people are trained and legally authorized to act as officers, the best practice would be to notify residents before the visit and only conduct simple home visits. Generally, the officers may not learn as much or be as effective overall, but they have a better chance of getting home at night. This is the most important thing. If the program does not include supervision when it is begun, the directors should work toward partnerships that can expand the activities or authority. Police can be asked to join a social worker on a visit, and fourth amendment waivers can be pursued as a condition of participation in drug court.

Probation as Case Managers

Treatment providers may perform some case management functions. On a team, it is not uncommon for every member to be conducting some function of case management. However, the performance of major case management functions for both adult and juvenile drug courts is generally left to treatment, probation, or a case management agency (6,7). With so many team members performing some portion of the case management responsibilities, coordinating the case management activities becomes a challenge. Preferred practice in many jurisdictions is to have probation perform the central case management function, that is, to be the repository of all available information and data for the court and to deliver the collected case information from the other partner agencies to the judge in an easy-to-manage report format (8). Drug court programming for recovery is based on assessing and addressing strengths and deficits of criminally involved drug addicts.

Whenever possible, it is important to understand the concept not only of treatment and service matching but also of probation officer matching. Issues of communication, culture, and gender can impede progress. The goal of drug court programs is positive change, and anything that impedes positive change is not the preferred practice. Sometimes probation officer matching is not an option, for example, in small jurisdictions, but, when possible, it is the best practice. Traditionally, probation supervisors have not considered the importance of the right fit for caseload assignment, but for the drug court program to be most effective, they should consider this issue.

Cultural proficiency and competence are strong components of community supervision. There is a youth culture, a culture of poverty, a culture of addiction, a culture of sobriety, and a number of other cultures that come into play in a drug court and through the progression of a client's stay in drug court. Effective community supervision incorporates cultural competence into all functions in order to improve outcomes.

Supplemental Law Enforcement Assistance

The drug court team should enlist the assistance of as many local law enforcement agencies as it can to support its drug court supervision activities. For example, some drug courts use the local highway patrol or sheriff to stop by and conduct random unannounced breath testing. Other programs have their clients' names entered into central law enforcement dispatch so that anytime a client is identified by the police, the officer knows he or she is in drug court and can act accordingly. Officers are trained to ask about step work that is part of the 12 Step self-help movement and drug court phases and to report both good and bad news to the court.

Reporting

Whenever possible, co-locating offices is an excellent way to provide drug court client services. Transportation is a difficult challenge for clients. One-stop shopping helps to cut down travel, saves time, and improves communications. Day reporting centers work well when they are the center of intensive outpatient treatment, life skills education, supervision, and testing. Co-location sends a highly visible message that treatment and supervision work closely together at all times. This provides more opportunities for contact and eases the burdens on offenders and their families.

Reporting to probation officers must be frequent and timely. Aside from criminogenic concerns, clients in drug courts often have acute life skill challenges that delay entry or success in the workforce. Teaching clients how to keep a calendar, show up on time, dress appropriately, and engage with the team are program elements that equate to job skills. It is necessary for clients to learn and practice these skills in order to achieve success in life after sobriety.

Case Studies

The following case studies, based on actual events, demonstrate how probation's involvement at various points in a client's program can support recovery.

Case Study 24.1

Keisha (not her real name) is 24 years old, has been in drug court for 9 months, and is in phase three. She has tested clean for just over 7 months and is in weekly group treatment for another 3 weeks before beginning aftercare. Keisha has found part-time work, is studying to take the GED, and is currently one of the model clients in the program.

She had difficulty early in the program, specifically stating that she had "stayed clean before" and therefore believed that she could "figure out my own program." She was initially resistant to working with treatment or probation in developing a plan and was concerned that the requirements of the program would make it impossible for her to take care of her two children, aged 2 and 6 years. The children's father has been in prison for the past 2 years and has recently been paroled.

Although Keisha tested positive for methamphetamine and marijuana off and on during her first month in drug court, she attended treatment and probation visits and gradually came to understand how the program could help her get off drugs and alcohol. Probation officers randomly visited her home weekly when she first came into the program and on two occasions took her into custody because she was under the influence of methamphetamines; her case was placed on the next drug court calendar so that her noncompliant behavior could be addressed. On both occasions, her children were staying with her mother. Once she began testing negative for drugs and alcohol, the home visits and searches became less frequent and, at this point, she has not been visited for over 2 months.

Recently, Keisha asked her probation officer if it would be possible to have a home visit and search. This seemed like an unusual request, but upon further discussion Keisha revealed that for the past week her ex-boyfriend and father of her children had been staying at her house despite her repeated demands for him to leave. He was officially paroled to his mother's home and was finding that environment too confining. He was sleeping on Keisha's couch most nights. Keisha was sure he was using drugs again. Keisha reported that she had told him more than once that drug court officers could show up anytime, but he did not believe her. She was now asking for some help. Two probation officers showed up at Keisha's residence and began the search. Within minutes the ex-boyfriend packed some things in his duffel bag and left.

What did the probation officer do in this case study?

1. Monitored the home environment.
2. Immediately responded to violations.
3. Provided support and refusal skills.

Case Study 24.2

Phillip (not his real name) is a 17 year old who has been in juvenile drug court for 6 months. Although most of the other kids in the program primarily use marijuana and alcohol, Phillip's drug of choice is methamphetamine, which he has been using for almost a year. He is also the only youth in the program with a diagnosis of chemical dependency. Phillip has a 1-year-old son and continues to date the mother of his child despite continual arguments. He reports mixed feelings about being a father, saying that it is one of the best things that has happened to him. At the same time he feels totally overwhelmed at times. Phillip works part-time at a drive-through lube shop and is taking classes to earn his GED. He reports finding it difficult to manage all his responsibilities.

Because of severe overcrowding at the juvenile hall, few custody sanctions are used in this juvenile drug court. Phillip's situation has warranted juvenile hall time on one occasion since he was admitted. Probation officers in this program do not have the authority to search clients' homes. However, during a routine home visit after just 3 weeks into the program, probation officers found marijuana and a smoking pipe on Phillip's dresser. Phillip was at school at the time of the visit, and his mother reported to the probation officers that she was not aware of the marijuana or pipe and that she does not go into Phillip's room because she wants to "respect his privacy." The probation officer in charge of Phillip's case was able to have a discussion with Phillip's mother about the importance of monitoring her son's behavior and gave her some practical tips for talking to Phillip about what privacy he could expect.

Phillip was contacted at school to discuss the contraband found at his house, and during the meeting he admitted to possessing a small amount of methamphetamine that was currently in his locker. The probation officer called local sheriff's deputies who arrested Phillip and booked him into juvenile hall until his case could be heard the next day in juvenile drug court. Phillip was also drug tested by the probation officer at the time of his booking, and the sample was sent to the laboratory. The result, which was positive for methamphetamine and marijuana, was available 24 hours later, in time for his case to be heard by the drug court judge.

When Phillip was released 48 hours after being booked, he met with his probation officer and treatment provider. Together, they discussed the events leading up to his arrest. Prior to the arrest, he had tested clean for over 2 weeks. Phillip admitted to using methamphetamine on the weekends because, based on what other clients had told him, he was fairly sure no one would test him until after group on Tuesday night.

Phillip was honest with his probation officer and treatment provider, saying that sometimes he thinks he is ready to stop using drugs and alcohol and he knows he should do it for his son, but there are other times when he just feels like it is too hard. He says that there are many opportunities to buy methamphetamines from coworkers, although he does not feel pressured in any way to do so. Phillip is asked what needs to change for him to stop using and what help he needs. At first he says he is not sure, but then he says that maybe he should look for a different part-time job to avoid the drug-using situations. In the meantime, the probation officer suggests working on refusal skills, ways of saying no or avoiding situations. The treatment provider agrees to work on this in his individual sessions and to revise his treatment plan to address the recent drug use. The probation officer agrees to help Phillip practice the refusal skills during their office visits. Some other strategies are discussed, including some time management techniques, and then the probation officer brings Phillip's parents into the meeting to determine what they can do to help Phillip.

What did the probation officer do in this case study?

1. Monitored the home environment.
2. Provided support to the parent.
3. Detected drug use early and imposed an immediate sanction.
4. Collaborated with local law enforcement and with treatment providers.
5. Worked with the youth to develop a revised plan.
6. Employed motivational techniques.

Case Study 24.3

Gina (not her real name) is in an adult drug court and was admitted 7 weeks ago. She is 34 years old and has been using heroin and oxycodone for almost 10 years. She reports drinking and using marijuana at age 11 and most other drugs throughout her adolescence and adulthood. Gina has been in residential treatment three times and in intensive outpatient treatment five times but has failed to complete the program in each case. She has a 16-year-old daughter who lives with Gina's parents in another state. She has been on probation for misdemeanor drug offenses for most of her adult life, and her current offense is a felony charge of drug possession.

When Gina first met with her drug court probation officer she was reluctant to try the program, saying "I'm not ready to quit using, and besides, I've tried before and it never worked." The probation officer agreed with Gina, telling her that he was aware she had not been successful at her previous treatment attempts but also that he was impressed by her continued attempts. He suggested that she might make the best choice possible if she talked to her attorney again. The probation officer briefly went over the program requirements and told her to call or come by the office for more information if she needed it to help her make her decision. According to the probation officer it seemed to shock Gina that there was no argument or attempt to talk her into entering the program. Ultimately, Gina did talk to her attorney and agreed to enter drug court.

During the first week in the program, Gina failed to attend half of her commitments, including two treatment sessions and a drug test. In one case, the probation officer went to her home and found her asleep at 11:30 am. Gina was belligerent and refused to go with the probation officer. At one point Gina was screaming and throwing things and tripped over a box causing her to hit her head, which started bleeding. The two probation officers on the scene called 911 and Gina was taken to the emergency room where she was given stitches and released. Gina was taken home to rest and she agreed to report to the probation department the next morning at 9:00 am.

The probation officers made an unannounced home visit and search of the home the following weekend and found two recently filled prescriptions, one for oxycodone and the other for hydrocodone. The prescriptions were from different doctors and were filled by different pharmacies. Both bottles were half full. Gina admitted to seeking out these prescriptions because of the pain her head injury was causing her. She denied that there was anything inappropriate about her actions. Her probation officer reminded her that her signed drug court contract required her to report any new medication to the probation officer and that the emergency room had already prescribed a non-narcotic pain reliever for her. Gina said that she would have reported these new prescriptions the following week. The probation officer also pointed out that she had taken well over the prescribed dosage of both medications. Gina stated that it was possible that some of the pills had fallen down the drain.

The probation officer then did a set of field assessment tests to determine if Gina was under the influence of controlled substances and found that she was. Gina was then taken into custody for a violation of her probation. Her case was put on the next drug court calendar for review and response. When the probation officer returned to the office, he left a message for the treatment provider and asked to meet before the review hearing. A report was also prepared and distributed to the entire team.

The probation officer and treatment provider met the morning before the drug court hearing and discussed the specifics of Gina's case and what had happened over the weekend. The treatment provider and the probation officer agreed that there was some hope that Gina could make it in the program if she could become stabilized, but this did not seem likely if she remained an outpatient. The entire team then met and agreed that Gina should be placed in a residential treatment program until she could be stabilized. Some team members, however, were initially opposed to the idea of residential treatment, stating that she had tried it before unsuccessfully.

Gina's attorney asked if the probation officer and the treatment provider would join him in discussing this with her. Gina did decide to enter residential treatment and is expected to be discharged after 1 week into intensive outpatient treatment. She has been visited three times by her probation officer to provide urine samples and to discuss her expectations and concerns for discharge.

What did the probation officer do in this case study?

1. Employed motivational techniques.
2. Monitored the home environment and provided timely information to the entire drug court team.
3. Responded to missed treatment sessions immediately.
4. Provided monitoring during nongovernmental hours.
5. Detected drug use early and imposed an immediate sanction.
6. Collaborated with treatment providers and her attorney.
7. Provided support through her residential treatment stay.

References

1. Center for Civic Innovation. "Broken Windows" Probation: The Next Step in Fighting Crime. Civic Report No. 7. New York: Manhattan Institute, Center for Civic Innovation; 1999.
2. American Society of Addiction Medicine. The American Society of Addiction Medicine Patient Placement Criteria, 2nd ed, rev (ASAM PPC-2R). Chevy Chase, MD: The American Society of Addiction Medicine; 2001.
3. Substance Abuse and Mental Health Administration. Treatment Improvement Protocol, No. 7. Rockville, MD: U.S. Dept of Health and Human Services, 1994.
4. DiClemente C. Addiction and Change: How Addictions Develop and Addicted People Recover. New York: Guilford Publications; 2004.
5. Marr JN. Interrelationship Between the Use of Alcohol and Other Drugs: Summary Overview for Drug Court Practitioners. Washington, DC: Bureau of

Justice Assistance, Drug Court Clearinghouse and Technical Assistance Project; 1999.
6. Substance Abuse and Mental Health Administration. Treatment Improvement Protocol, N. 27. Rockville, MD: U.S. Department of Health and Human Services; 1999.
7. Taxman FS, Shepardson ES, Delano J, Mitchell S, Byrne JM. Tools of the trade: A Guide to Incorporating Science Into Practice. Washington, DC: U.S. National Institute of Corrections, Department of Justice; 2003.
8. U.S. Department of Justice. Implementing Evidence-Based Practice in Community Corrections: The Principles of Effective Intervention. Washington, D.C.: National Institute of Corrections, U.S. Department of Justice; 2004.

25
Relapse

Timothy J. Kelly, James M. Gaither, and Lucy J. King

Substance dependence, like diabetes, asthma, hypertension, and many other diseases, is a remittent illness (1). When a patient with diabetes, for example, is found to have very low or very high blood sugar, adjustments in medication, diet, and daily activities are made in the treatment plan in order to minimize long-term complications. Unfortunately, because of the stigma involved, an individual who has been abstinent but has relapsed to abusing drugs and alcohol is more likely to receive a lecture rather than a treatment plan. This chapter addresses factors leading to relapse and appropriate ways of preventing and dealing with relapse.

Natural History of Relapse

The diagnoses of major disorders in the *Diagnostic and Statistical Manual of Mental Disorders*, fourth edition (DSM-IV) (2), have been based, in part, on long-term, prospective studies of large numbers of individuals during the 20th century. Such studies have shown that when an individual is carefully diagnosed with substance dependence by DSM criteria, he or she will very likely have periods of partial or full remission but will also be at risk throughout life for relapse to drinking and using drugs (2).

In a series of studies over several decades, Vaillant and colleagues have delineated several patterns of the fluctuating course of alcohol and other substance dependence (3), for example, a progressive course of worsening relapses to earlier than expected death from substance-related causes; a continuing fluctuating course of less severe or less frequent relapses; or stable abstinence.

In confirmation of the 12 Step principles, research indicates that the ability to maintain long-term moderate substance use without return to dependence in someone whose symptoms at one time met criteria for substance dependence occurs only in a very small percentage of individuals, usually those with later age of onset, fewer problems from use, and lack of physiological dependence. In contrast, individuals with substance dependence who maintain abstinence for at least 5 years are highly likely to remain abstinent for the rest of their lives (4).

Correlates of Relapse

Why is relapse possible throughout life in those who become abstinent? Kalivas and Volkow (5) reviewed the literature, including their own research, and outlined three components:

1. Genetic (inherited) condition.
2. Additional changes in neurons and neurotransmitter function if heavy use is initiated and continued.
3. Maintenance of some of these changes in the brain during abstinence so that environmental triggers can lead to craving and relapse even after years of abstinence.

Genetic Influences

Substance dependence is highly heritable. A number of genes in complex relationships are involved; some predispose to dependence on any addicting substance and others to dependence on specific classes of addicting drugs. Different genetic influences appear to affect different stages of the progression from initiation of use to maintenance, to heavy use, to dependence, and finally to the various complications of dependence. Although much progress has been made in the past decade, not all of the genes have been discovered as yet nor are their functions fully understood (6–8).

Additional Changes in Neurons and Neurotransmitter Function

Motivated behavior involves attaching salience (importance) to a particular stimulus. The salient stimulus leads to a behavioral response that results in a reward (5). In substance dependence, the stimulus might be seeing favorite alcoholic drinks or addicting drugs, or pictures of them, or being in an environment in which they are consumed. The behavioral response might be going to a liquor store or finding a cocaine or heroin dealer and then using the substance obtained. The reward is a high from use.

Three areas of the brain are especially important in any motivated behavior, including addiction: the nucleus accumbens, amygdala, and prefrontal cortex (5). When a salient stimulus is perceived, dopamine from the ventral tegmental area is released into the nucleus accumbens. On repeated reward of stimulus-induced behavior, this pathway is involved in establishing a pattern of learned behavioral response to the stimulus. Once an individual predisposed to substance dependence repeatedly experiences environmental triggers that suggest alcohol or drug use, carries out behaviors to obtain and use addicting substances, and is rewarded by highs, he or she will respond to those triggers with behavior that leads to use.

The amygdala monitors the salience of multiple sensory perceptions from inside and outside the body and controls resulting behaviors. It sends glutamate pathways to the nucleus accumbens and to the prefrontal cortex. Certain parts of the prefrontal cortex participate in directing whether a behavioral response occurs and how intense it will be. Activation of these areas is related to how likely the reward is to occur. Glutamate pathways from the prefrontal cortex connect to the nucleus accumbens and complete circuits among the amygdala, nucleus accumbens, and prefrontal cortex.

When addicting substances are repeatedly and heavily used, neuron structures and neurotransmitter functions in these areas are reorganized to establish the compulsive behavioral patterns of addiction. Glutamate pathways become more important than dopamine pathways (5). There is an overwhelming craving to use drugs and alcohol.

Dopamine release in the nucleus accumbens is required for the high and for the transition from use to addiction. Continued use leads to gradual involvement of glutamate pathways from prefrontal cortex to nucleus accumbens. These changes gradually become more long-lived. Vulnerability to relapse in end-stage addiction endures for years and results from equally enduring cellular changes (5).

A patient with end-stage alcoholism once said, "Doc, the cure for alcoholism would be if you could give me a shot in my arm, and after that I would always be able to go into a bar, have one drink, and leave." He was right. The difference between an alcoholic or addict and someone who never has difficulties with addicting substances is that the first has the chemical changes outlined above and cannot easily turn off the behavioral cycle whereas the second can stop after one or a very few drinks or hits.

Maintenance of Some of the Changes in the Brain

Some of these changes in the brain are maintained during abstinence so that environmental triggers can lead to craving and relapse even after years of abstinence. A recent study of methamphetamine-dependent men was able to predict relapse on the basis of functional magnetic resonance neuroimaging in early recovery (7). Brain activity as subjects performed a decision-making task showed deficits in cerebral cortical areas related to decision making in those who would soon relapse. One possibility is that, in the absence of higher decision-making functions in those who relapse, previous behavioral habits come into play such as compulsive alcohol- and drug-using behavior.

Some of the connections among brain, body, and the external environment occur via the hypothalamus, a brain area that maintains constant balance in functions such as body temperature, blood pressure, and blood sugar and oxygen supplies. For example, there are hormonal feedback loops that operate somewhat like thermostat controls among the hypothalamus, the pituitary gland at the base of the brain, and glands like the adrenals.

Cortisol, a stress hormone, is secreted by the adrenals in response to stress. It travels through the blood to the pituitary and receives back a controlling hormone from the pituitary. In turn, there are hormonal connections between pituitary and hypothalamus that complete the hypothalamic-pituitary-adrenal axis.

The hypothalamus sends stimuli to various areas of the brain, including the amygdala. Thus, the motivation–reward circuits are connected to hormonal responses to stress. When there are environmental stressors, the hypothalamic-pituitary-adrenal axis becomes imbalanced. Readjustment then occurs. In individuals with substance dependence, this readjustment leads to craving. These individuals are likely to relapse under stressful conditions (9).

We have now defined two important environmental factors in relapse: triggers for craving that a substance-dependent individual perceives will be rewarded by obtaining and using alcohol and drugs and stress that can activate motivation and reward circuits in the brain via the hypothalamus. No lecture from a physician, family member, or religious advisor will change the biologic and environmental correlates of compulsive use of addicting substances. More sophisticated and longer term methods of behavioral change are required.

Treatment and Prevention of Relapse

Any method to prevent or minimize relapses must address triggers and stresses. Achieving and maintaining abstinence provides an opportunity for improvement in both physical and psychological health as well as better social function in the family, at work, and in the community. As a result, psychosocial modalities focus not only on abstinence but also on developing social skills and coping mechanisms that lead to a productive life and rewarding relationships.

Some commonly used methods for addressing potential or actual relapse are discussed below. They are not mutually exclusive and often employ similar concepts. Combinations are used to good effect. Until we fully understand all the intricacies of how relapses develop and how they can be treated, it is best to provide a number of approaches and ultimately select in each case those most useful to particular individuals.

Twelve Step Fellowships

For over seven decades, 12 Step programs have provided hope and help for the addicted. The only requirement for membership is a desire to become clean and sober. They suggest avoidance of "slippery" people, places, and things by eliminating triggers to use until stable abstinence is achieved. An acronym for identifying potential relapse during stress is HALT for hungry, angry, lonely, and tired.

There is emphasis on the need for working the steps with a sponsor who has established stable abstinence. This work plus regular attendance at meetings with others who are striving to achieve and maintain abstinence gradually brings about behavioral change in many areas of life. One who has achieved sobriety without losing other destructive behaviors is considered a dry drunk in need of working the steps further.

Constructive ways of managing stress and relationships are found through a higher power as each individual defines that. Helping others struggling with addiction helps members when they become sponsors. Families are helped through groups like Al-Anon and Nar-Anon. Most alcohol and addiction programs in the United States today encourage involvement in 12 Step programs.

Double Trouble groups use 12 Step principles for individuals with co-occurring substance use and psychiatric disorders. There are other, more recently established self-help groups such as Self-Management and Recovery Training (SMART).

Psychosocial Therapies

Relapses are not sudden events that fall out of the blue. Patients need to learn the chains of events and behaviors that lead to their relapses. Triggers and stresses are often highly individual. They must be identified in each person in order to help him or her learn to prevent or minimize relapses.

Cognitive-Behavioral Therapy

Cognitive-behavioral therapy methods were originally designed by Beck and his colleagues. Their research and that of others has demonstrated the efficacy of this approach (10). A patient learns to understand his false beliefs (cognitive) that lead to use and by changing these becomes able to change how he deals with craving (behavioral). Adaptations of the basic principles have been devised by these and many other authors and applied to group therapy, marital and family counseling, and other modalities.

Like any other successful therapy, cognitive-behavioral therapy depends on empathy of therapist for patient. The therapist in this situation must also be knowledgeable about addiction. Through a series of Socratic questions, a therapist gradually helps a patient understand what false beliefs about self, others, and addicting substances are leading to behaviors that result in use and its consequences.

Relevant questions to be asked about cravings or relapse might include such comments as, How were you feeling that day? That week? What was happening at home? At work? What were you thinking and feeling about all that? Common patient answers to questions might be "The boss chewed me out, so I thought I might as well drink." "My wife is always on my case, so I decided to show her." "I had one joint at my boyfriend's house and decided that, if I had already done that, I might as well go on a binge." "I was feeling great and thought I no longer needed to worry about relapse." Advantages and disadvantages of such beliefs in the patient's life are examined.

Once false beliefs are understood, changes in behavior are devised by the therapist and patient working together so that the patient can avoid the behavioral response of using addicting substances when there is craving. The following pattern changes:

Trigger/Stress → Craving → Obtaining Alcohol/Drugs → High

becomes

Trigger/Stress → Craving → Productive Behaviors →
Long-Term Rewards of Being Clean and Sober

Homework assignments are used so that the patient can examine everyday problems and try different behaviors to deal with them. Results of behavior changes are examined and modified until the patient has developed the most productive behaviors to avoid use and to deal with stresses. Patient responsibility is emphasized (10).

Motivational Interviewing; Trans-Theoretical Model of Intentional Behavioral Change

Miller and Rollnick have developed methods of leading patients through stages of change from being unaware of the need to address substance dependence (or other problems) to realizing of the need for change, to taking appropriate action, to maintaining behavioral change.(11–13). An individual's own motivations for change are delineated and emphasized by a therapist to implement behavioral change.

As always, relapse is a possibility, especially in an environment filled with triggers. A slip or lapse (brief return to use) is not considered a failure but rather a need to move back into earlier phases of the cycle. Thus, the individual's self-efficacy does not erode, and hope is not lost. A therapist can help to make sense of the relapse and encourage the patient to revise previous actions in terms of the cycle of change (13).

Relapse Prevention

A variety of treatments have focused specifically on helping patients prevent relapses or at least terminate them rapidly and effectively. These include various combinations of educational, cognitive-behavioral, motivational, and self-efficacy and coping skills training. Research has indicated that these approaches are effective in reducing the number and severity of relapses (11). Explanations at a patient's level of understanding of neurobiological data and the definition of alcoholism and addiction as a disease can help to educate patients. Pharmacologic adjuncts directly dealing with substance dependence or with associated medical or psychiatric disorders might be used as well. Psychotherapy and counseling have been found to be most effective when combined with random urine testing or other laboratory methods to document relapse (12).

If a patient has been able to prevent relapse despite triggers and problems, he should be complimented. If she has had a few drinks or used drugs briefly, methods that helped terminate the lapse can be examined and emphasized as can ways to anticipate and prevent relapses. All of this assumes that a patient feels free to contact his or her therapist (counselor, probation officer, supportive friend, 12 Step sponsor) as soon as possible when cravings arise or at least contact the therapist when a brief lapse has occurred.

A patient must believe that his or her therapist will not be judgmental or impose immediate sanctions, and the therapist must confirm this belief by how the patient is treated. If a serious relapse occurs, elements of the original treatment plan need to be reevaluated, perhaps after appropriate inpatient or outpatient treatment. The days of harsh confrontation and immediate dismissal from substance dependence treatment are, fortunately, gradually disappearing. Therapists must provide encouragement that there is hope for recovery (3).

Recovery Management

A great deal of outcome research has shown not only that a variety of combinations of treatments are effective but also that the longer patients stay in treatment and the more sessions they attend, the better the results in terms of long-term maintenance of abstinence (14). There is increasing research evidence that a public health model is useful for individuals with substance dependence. Long-term outcomes can be improved by ongoing monitoring of patients after discharge and reducing the time from relapse to reentry into treatment (15).

A continuum of care is provided. If a patient has a serious relapse, inpatient or intensive outpatient treatment might be needed. If there are less serious lapses or increased cravings, increased frequency and intensity of sessions is provided. If stresses like death of a loved one or job loss occur, a patient can be seen more frequently and encouraged to attend more self-help meetings.

In other words, the intensity of treatment is tailored to the individual patient's current status, as in any other area of medicine. Specific modalities such as individual, group, marital, or family counseling and educational or vocational training are used when indicated. Community resources can be called into play. Twelve Step or other self-help groups are encouraged. Case managers or recovery coaches are valuable in ensuring that each patient has the treatment resources necessary to prevent relapse or to treat relapse as soon as possible when it occurs.

Pharmacologic Treatments

Medications such as methadone (Methadose), buprenorphine (Suboxone), acamprosate (Campral), naltrexone (Revia), and disulfiram (Antabuse) help patients to keep clean and sober until longer term psychosocial treatments begin to have effect. Random urine screens for drugs and breath analysis for alcohol not only help to monitor a patient's progress but also serve as an incentive to remain clean and sober.

Identification and Treatment of Medical Illnesses

Chances of relapse are greater if patients are in pain or are suffering from symptoms of disease. Substance dependence contributes to disorders in all the organs of the body. As individuals with substance dependence age, they develop diseases typical of older age groups. Aging baby boomers are coming into treatment with a history of having used a multiplicity of drugs that contributes to their medical problems.

Avoiding use of addicting medications unless absolutely necessary is crucial. Also helpful are nonpharmacologic modalities such as physical therapy, occupational therapy, relaxation training, and psychosocial therapies. Managing physicians must be knowledgeable about substance dependence.

Co-Occurring Psychiatric Disorders

Bipolar disorder, schizophrenia, major depression, panic disorder, and social phobia are more likely to occur in individuals with substance dependence than in the general population (16). Antisocial personality disorder and attention deficit hyperactivity disorder (associated with conduct disorder) predispose to substance dependence (2).

All too often these disorders are overlooked in the chaos of substance dependence, especially mood and anxiety disorders and attention deficit disorders. Difficulties in differential diagnosis are compounded by the fact that intoxication and withdrawal from various addicting substances can mimic almost all psychiatric syndromes. Diagnosis during intoxication, withdrawal, and early recovery is very difficult.

It is crucial that co-occurring psychiatric disorders are differentiated from substance-induced disorders as soon as possible because failure to treat co-occurring disorders contributes to relapse. Past history can be helpful when a patient is stable enough to give a good history or when old records or other informants are available: Which came first in the patient's life, substance use or psychiatric symptoms? Were there psychiatric symptoms or was psychiatric treatment necessary during periods of several months or more of abstinence? Do psychiatric syndromes continue or get worse as recovery and abstinence continue?

First, it is important to rule out the most serious general medical conditions and psychoses. These are characterized by changes in memory and intellectual function persisting into recovery and include delirium, dementia, amnesic (memory) disorders, and cognitive disorders. These require medical and neurologic evaluation.

Evidence of psychoses, including hallucinations, delusions, and bizarre behavior, must be appropriately treated. Schizophrenia, by definition, is a psychosis and has additional characteristic negative symptoms. Psychotic symptoms might be seen in delirium and dementia, are sometimes seen in mania, and occasionally are present in major depression. These require immediate psychiatric attention, perhaps hospitalization.

Other common disorders to be ruled out are mood disorders, including major depression and bipolar disorders, and anxiety disorders, including panic attacks and social phobias. Consider psychiatric hospitalization when there is a possibility of suicide (most likely in major depression, bipolar disorder, and substance dependence but possible in schizophrenia).

Fortunately, antipsychotics, antidepressants, and mood stabilizers are not addictive. Antianxiety medications, primarily benzodiazepines, are addicting, but anxiety disorders can be treated with antidepressants. There are nonaddicting medications for attention deficit hyperactivity disorder. There are few instances in the treatment of psychiatric disorders in which addicting drugs would be necessary. In sum, pharmacologic treatment of co-occurring disorders in substance-dependent patients is possible.

Research at the New York State Psychiatric Institute, Columbia University School of Medicine, has developed and tested a brief screening instrument for assessing the possibility of psychiatric illness. This questionnaire has been tested in a number of substance abuse and mental health treatment settings and found to have good reliability and validity. It does not provide diagnoses but rather indicates which individuals might need further diagnostic evaluation.

Social Factors

Family issues, housing, education or vocational training, employment, and a variety of legal concerns are obvious sources of stresses that can be involved in relapse. Social workers are invaluable members of the treatment team, providing individual, group, marital, or family therapies and interventions. Case managers, or recovery coaches, are able to provide contacts with community resources and follow up to be sure patients are using them and that the resources are providing the needed assistance.

When Relapse Prevention Does Not Prevent Relapse

Experienced addiction treatment specialists in all disciplines are familiar with patients who seem unable to avoid heavy use of addicting substances more than briefly for periods of years. Assuming that all of the above factors have been considered and a number of treatment modalities have been employed through multiple relapses, what should be done?

This is the time for the entire treatment team, hopefully in communication with one another throughout, to meet to discuss options and then to present them to the patient, obtaining his or her input as to what changes in the treatment plan might work. Dismissal from treatment is a last resort. It can be carried out with the option to return to treatment under specific conditions that are made clear to the individual. Like every other aspect of treatment, such meetings and plans should be carefully documented in the records.

Drug Courts and Relapse

It has become increasingly clear that treatment of substance dependence and prevention or minimization of relapses also decreases recidivism in the criminal justice system (17). The methods described in this chapter have been utilized in various ways by drug courts. The participant becomes abstinent, attends treatment, and is involved in relapse prevention (17–19).

The judge in a drug court, in addition to the usual judicial role, assumes to one degree or another the roles of individual counselor, treatment team leader, and case manager. In comparison with addiction treatment settings, there are both advantages and disadvantages in dealing with potential or actual relapses. For example, a drug court judge can impose penalties like incarceration that are unavailable to addiction counselors. On the other hand, an addiction counselor can be more lenient in individual cases of positive urine screens than a judge when laws require harsher punishment. However, a drug court judge should consider carefully the consequences of incarceration and not allow traditional notions of "tough on crime" court reactions to interfere with the effective use of treatment. For example, it is not necessary or desirable that a participant be incarcerated for every drug use episode.

Relapse prevention, as in any other setting, involves identification of triggers and stresses for each individual. Because frequent and prolonged follow-up, as in recovery management, is part of the drug court system, treatment team members can help participants to identify potential relapses and to utilize appropriate behaviors to avoid relapse.

If a relapse occurs, it is not unusual for a participant to arrive in court having already discussed the problem with the treatment provider and a probation officer or court coordinator, who will present a recommendation to the judge. This recommendation might involve jail time, increased meetings, and/or increased urine tests. When participants themselves propose the sanctions, they are more likely to comply with them and not to feel coerced by the system or the judge (18).

Participants, ultimately, must assume responsibility for their own actions. The structured system of drug courts with straightforward education about substance use and coping with life problems assists participants who have previously been involved in criminal behaviors to learn lawful responses to life situations. Relapse prevention is a unifying concept whether the problem is substance dependence, psychiatric disorder, or criminality (17).

Sexual offenders present a special problem. Although brief relapses in substance dependence can be tolerated, crimes such as rape or molestation of children demand absolute prevention of relapse. Available data suggest that one half to two thirds of sex offenders are substance abusers, and many were intoxicated at the time of the crime. The lack of impulse control of habitual sexual offenders is worsened by use of addicting substances (17). This lack of control might well relate to some of the neurobiologic factors discussed earlier.

Although treatment for habitual criminal sexual behaviors and treatment for substance dependence is best performed by experts in each field, such treatments can be coordinated. Unfortunately, treatment teams in each of these areas do not always recognize the necessity of assessing the possibility of problems in the other area (17). Nonetheless, criminal justice settings are increasingly using sophisticated behavioral methods, including preventing relapse to substance abuse, to try to prevent these tragic behavioral patterns.

Conclusions

Drug courts, utilizing a team approach to treatment of substance dependence, have developed ways to use psychosocial therapies and medical treatments to diminish recidivism for many individuals in the criminal justice system.

References

1. McLellan AT, O'Brien CP, Lewis D, et al. Drug addiction as a chronic medical illness: implications for treatment, insurance, and evaluation. JAMA 2000; 284:1689–1695.
2. American Psychiatric Association. Diagnostic and Statistical Manual of Mental Disorders, 4th ed, text rev. Washington, DC: American Psychiatric Press; 2000.
3. Vaillant GE. Natural History of Alcoholism, Revisited. Cambridge, MA: Harvard University Press; 1995.
4. Vaillant GE. Natural history of addiction and pathways to recovery. In Graham AW, Schultz TK, Mayo-Smith MF, et al, eds. Principles of Addiction Medicine, 3rd ed. Chevy Chase, MD: American Society of Addiction Medicine; 2003:3–16.

5. Kalivas PW, Volkow ND. The neural basis of addiction: a pathology of motivation and choice. Am J Psychiatry 2005;162:1403–1413.
6. Schuckit MA, Smith TL. An evaluation of the level of response to alcohol, externalizing symptoms, and depressive symptoms as predictors of alcoholism. J Stud Alcohol 2006;67:215–227.
7. Paulus MP, Tapert SF, Schuckit MA. Neural activation patterns of methamphetamine-dependent subjects during decision making predict relapse. Arch Gen Psychiatry 2006;62:761–768.
8. Uhl GR. Addiction genetics and genomics. In Madras BK, Rutter JL, Colvis CM, et al, eds. Cell Biology of Addiction. Cold Spring Harbor, NY: Cold Spring Harbor Laboratory Press; 2006:15–28.
9. Kreek MJ. Endorphins, gene polymorphisms, stress responsivity, and specific addictions: selected topics. In Madras BK, Rutter JL, Colvis CM, et al, eds. Cell Biology of Addiction. Cold Spring Harbor, NY: Cold Spring Harbor Laboratory Press; 2006:63–92.
10. Beck AT, Wright FD, Newman CF, Liese BS. Cognitive Therapy of Substance Abuse. New York: Guilford Press; 1993.
11. Daley DC, Marlatt GA, Spotts CE. Relapse prevention: clinical models and intervention strategies. In Graham AW, Schultz TK, Mayo-Smith MF, et al, eds. Principles of Addiction Medicine, 3rd ed. Chevy Chase, MD: American Society of Addiction Medicine; 2003:772–785.
12. Mercer D, Woody GE, Luborsky L. Individual psychotherapy. In Galanter M, Kleber HD. Textbook of Substance Abuse Treatment, 3rd ed. Washington, DC: American Psychiatric Publishing; 2004:343–352.
13. Miller WR, Rollnick S. Motivational Interviewing: Preparing People for Change. New York: Guilford Press; 2002.
14. McLellan AT, McKay JR. Components of successful addiction treatment. In Graham AW, Schultz TK, Mayo-Smith MF, et al, eds. Principles of Addiction Medicine, 3rd ed. Chevy Chase, MD: American Society of Addiction Medicine; 2003:429–442.
15. Scott CK, Dennis ML, Foss MA. Utilizing recovery management checkups to shorten the cycle of relapse, treatment reentry, and recovery. Drug Alcohol Depend 2005;78:325–338.
16. Regier DA, Farmer M, Rae D, et al. Comorbidity of mental disorders with alcohol and other drug abuse: results from the epidemiologic catchment area (ECA) study. JAMA 1990;264:2511–2518.
17. Center for Substance Abuse Treatment. Substance Abuse Treatment for Adults in the Criminal Justice System. Treatment Improvement Protocol (TIP) Series 44. DHHS Publication No. (SMA)05-4056. Rockville, MD: Substance Abuse and Mental Health Services Administration; 2005.
18. Carlson HB, Hora PF, Schma WG. Special issues in treatment: drug courts. In Graham AW, Schultz TK, Mayo-Smith MF, et al, eds. Principles of Addiction Medicine, 3rd ed. Chevy Chase, MD: American Society of Addiction Medicine; 2003:445–449.
19. Winick BJ, Wexler DB. Therapeutic jurisprudence. In Graham AW, Schultz TK, Mayo-Smith MF, et al, eds. Principles of Addiction Medicine, 3rd ed. Chevy Chase, MD: American Society of Addiction Medicine; 2003:550–552.

26
Law Enforcement and Drug Courts

Ronald R. Thrasher

Placing or replacing a law enforcement officer on a drug court team offers unique challenges and opportunities. Police administrators struggling with personnel shortages must justify deploying an officer to yet another outside project. Drug court directors worry about the acceptance of a "gun-toting" enforcer to a group of legal, social service, and treatment-oriented professionals. Police officers struggle with conflicting roles, ethics, and image, and everyone worries about the clients' reactions to a law enforcement officer whom many of them blame as the source of their problems.

The drug court officer represents municipal, county, state police, probation, parole, or any variation of law enforcement. For purposes of this chapter, law enforcement includes any sworn individual with the power and responsibility of arrest. The specific duties and roles vary between jurisdictions, but the goals, general philosophy, and ideology remain the same.

Every drug court is unique. Many well-established program teams developed without a law enforcement member while others began with one. Over time, and with experience, it has been learned that law enforcement offers a valuable contribution to the drug court philosophy.

This chapter explores the often uneasy relationship between the various members of the drug court team and the law enforcement member. The chapter concludes with a discussion of the future of the partnership between law enforcement and drug courts.

The Police Administrator's Concerns

Some experienced chiefs, sheriffs, or marshals, having seen hundreds of new ideas or programs come and go, need convincing of the usefulness of drug court. Other administrators embrace such an obvious and applied approach to community policing. Regardless, administrators face many common concerns when deciding to deploy a drug court officer from an otherwise overworked patrol or investigative force.

Justification of the Expenses

Money is the first issue and often the issue heard loudest by city managers, commissioners, mayors, and community leaders. Few courts possess available discretionary funding for salary, mandated continuing training, equipment, and benefits for a police member. Even with the lower salaries paid in the South and Midwest, communities estimate total costs of personnel, equipment, and training to be $200 to $500 per hour for each police officer (1). Partnership and grants are the most obvious sources of funding. Although grants vary in purpose and availability, the drug court model provides ample justification for funding. The same arguments provide justification for assignment of an existing officer from a law enforcement agency.

Drug courts report half the recidivism of felony drug use of traditional prisons. Drug court programs range in costs from $2,000 to $4,000 per client-year compared with incarceration costs ranging from $16,000 to $50,000 per offender-year (2,3). These figures fail to consider the latent cost savings not re-arresting the same offenders or continually providing other social services to the offender families and victims.

The argument that, "when these drugged criminals are locked up, they aren't out committing crimes," fails to consider costs associated with this type of crime prevention. Incarcerated offenders do not commit robberies, burglaries, check frauds, and other drug-related crimes while institutionalized. However, because of prison overcrowding, these offenders are far more likely to be found in diversionary programs, including work-release, probation, parole, community supervision, or some other type of nonconfining personal-recognizance program. Depending on the drug of choice and the type or area of the community or county, these nontreated, diversionary program offenders can easily commit over $50,000 worth of crimes per offender-year. Drug court clients save money through fewer new offenses, reduced recidivism, avoided additional criminal justice and incarceration costs, all while clients pay for fees and services (4).

The justification of saving money by deploying a law enforcement officer to the drug court program is used to convince either a funding source for grants or a public body to support diverting an officer to the drug court effort. After all, even if there is not a prison in town, the criminals eventually come home as soon as they are released, to offend again. If nearly half the clients graduate, drug courts save money (5).

Overcoming Obstacles

Police administrators face other issues. Creating a new specialty position may require union approval or specialty pay. The position itself may require policy revisions. How do you evaluate an officer whose success may be measured by client compliance rather than by the number of arrests, tickets, or cases made? Is it fair to evaluate a single officer by the drop in drug-related crimes when so many other factors also play a role?

Drug courts often encompass multiple jurisdictions that may require interjurisdictional agreements. What about liability concerns when a lawsuit arises from an officer working in another jurisdiction while conducting a consent home visit under the supervision and direction of a treatment plan and a civilian drug court director?

What selection criteria are used for this unique position? Must a particular specialty assignment be offered based on departmental seniority? Does the police labor contract require officer bidding? Is specialty pay required, available, or an option or enticement for the position? Is the opportunity for advanced training an incentive? Can the chief just pick someone? Can the drug court team participate in the selection process, and do they want to?

Finally, what about the position itself? Many law enforcement agencies utilize some type of peer review or peer panel as promotion boards. Will assignment to a drug court team spell promotion poison or will it put a newly selected officer seeking advancement within their agency on the fast track?

These issues just scratch the surface of the many concerns facing the law enforcement administrator. Individual issues vary between jurisdictions. It remains important for each drug court member to consider and be sensitive to the problems of the chief or sheriff. After all, it is the chief or sheriff who makes that (sometimes long) trip to the city manager, county commission, or state legislature seeking money and manpower. Although the concerns seem overwhelming, solutions are often found in the course of everyday business.

Multijurisdictional Agreements

Increasingly, small and rural departments survive by multijurisdictional agreements. Many states provide legislation allowing law enforcement officers and agencies to assist in routine and emergency situations when requested by other agencies. Administrators look to interagency agreements traditionally used for covert narcotics investigations, drug task forces, and, more recently, antiterrorism task forces for interagency cooperation models. Other government interagency agreements are found with firefighters, utility providers, and state licensing bodies that allow counselors, psychologists, and other medical personnel to practice in another state following a terrorist attack or natural disaster. Any of these documents may provide a starting point for a law enforcement–drug court agreement. Facilitators for these agreements may be law enforcement heads, governing bodies, district attorneys, or state or federal agencies.

Many agencies address issues of officer selection and evaluation through job descriptions, departmental policies, and interagency agreements. Take advantage of existing policies. Those new to the drug court concept can send off a half dozen requests to other agencies within the state or jurisdiction asking for copies of their drug court policy. Law enforcement Internet bulletin boards and mailing lists can be useful, as are state chief's or sheriff's associations, the appropriate state or federal accrediting organization, or an agency such as the International Association of Chiefs of Police (IACP). Most law enforcement policies are public record, and agencies typically like to share. For an administrator, if a policy is challenged and several other agencies are using the same or similar policies, the umbrella against liability suddenly gets a whole lot bigger.

Administrators might form a committee within the department that includes interested officers, union leaders, and the director or a member of the existing drug court team. Provide sample policies to the committee and wait for the results. Share committee draft policies with area agency heads, government leaders, and legal representatives for questions and feedback. Feedback goes to the policy committee for consideration and possible revision.

Administrators may also look to nontraditional sources for comments and suggestions. Provide a copy of the policy and multijurisdiction agreements to the local defense bar or county bar association. Diverting their clients to therapeutic drug court programs often presents not only a service but possibly a new revenue opportunity for local trial attorneys. The more people who are involved in the process, the more people who become invested in the outcome. Those who have a part in its creation want to have a part in its success.

The Drug Court Director's Concerns

Just as the law enforcement administrator faces many concerns, so does the drug court director. How will valued, long-time members of the drug court team react to a law enforcement officer? How is the officer used on the team; what will this person do? How does one control a "John/Jane Wayne" "book-em or bury-em, lock-em up and throw away the key" stereotypical cop? How do team members work with someone who carries a gun, has the authority to use deadly force, and has the power of arrest? Who supervises this person and how? On some level, these issues present themselves to the drug court director whose only goal is to make it all work better.

For the director, the drug court model works by close supervision and immediate intervention following repeated relapse. What can the law enforcement officer contribute to this model? The son of a police officer recently said in a college speech class that he always possessed an immediate response for not using drugs, "My dad's a cop; every cop in the world calls him when they see me, and he always knows every time I try to lie."

Immediate accurate information and intervention (sometimes called sanctions and incentives) is the essence of the drug court model. The best use of a law enforcement officer on the drug court team requires understanding of the law enforcement culture, particularly the concept of sharing and trust within the law enforcement family.

Traditional law enforcement neither trusted nor communicated within or among agencies. Police officers did not trust or talk to each other. Investigators refused to disclose information to patrol officers, and narcotics officers did not talk to anyone. "I'll trust you with my life; just don't ask the name of my informant." This began to change with the advent of information technology, training, and success in identifying and apprehending the violent traveling serial offender. It began with the Federal Bureau of Investigation (FBI).

In the mid-1930s, the FBI developed the National Academy, an in-residence academy just outside Washington, DC. For the very few, mid-career law enforcement supervisors selected to attend, this meant 3 months away from home and family. Mostly men, they passed the time between classes by telling war stories. Occasionally, academy instructors heard the same war story from students from different parts of the country. These stories particularly concerned *modus operandi* or the way in which a particular violent rapist or murderer committed their crime. Agent instructors began telling students, "You might give Lt. Jones a call at the Somewhere Police Department. He was in the 160th Session and told pretty much the same story you just told." As officers graduated and returned to their home jurisdictions, they made the calls.

Major criminal cases were solved when one jurisdiction had fingerprints with no suspect and another jurisdiction had a suspect but no physical evidence. Who would have thought that a truck driver or traveling salesperson might be committing crimes throughout their route of travel? This information sharing has facilitated programs in which officers and agencies contribute information to national shared databases. These efforts and successes fostered a new age of openness and cooperation on local, regional, and national levels to drug court programs.

The drug court model relies on close supervision and immediate intervention. Law enforcement agencies, particularly police departments, work 24/7. How important is it to the drug court team to know if a client was just seen "doing nothing wrong" in the alley behind a bar at 3:00 am while visiting with a known drug dealer? This represents the type of information known by the beat cop working that area. To be effective, the beat cop must possess the drug court client list just as the drug court must possess the law enforcement agencies' field interview information. It is all about trust and sharing—something that the law enforcement team member facilitates.

Even small law enforcement agencies utilize computer-aided dispatch (CAD). As dispatchers send officers to a call, the call information is entered into CAD. In general, the CAD accepts the address or name of the reporting person and the suspect or citizen contacted. The system then searches for additional names and checks these names and addresses against prior arrests, contacts, outstanding warrants, past incidents of violence or weapons, criminal associates, or any other information important to responding officers. The CAD references vehicle information on traffic stops just as it does on suspicious persons and field interview and may also reference persons at a residence to associate lists and even utility records of a particular person or place. What is my client doing at a place where a known drug dealer pays the electric bills?

With the cooperation of law enforcement, client lists and identification can be entered into CAD using an information sheet, and data files can be attached to these flagged clients. For example, an officer sees someone he or she had previously arrested standing on a street corner in the middle of the night and checks the individual either by radio or from the computer in the patrol car. The individual comes back flagged as a drug court participant with an attached file. The officer clicks on the file link and sees that the client is under a court restriction not to be out after dark and, if seen, is authorized by Judge Jones to be arrested. The officer makes the arrest with little paperwork other than a computer-generated arrest report that automatically routes to the judge and the drug court team. Supervision becomes 24/7 with immediate sanctions and notifications.

Home Visits

Most successful drug court programs include home visits, which should *never* be conducted alone. Having previously consented to a search of their residence and person as a condition of their drug court participation in a performance contract, clients feel particularly vulnerable and threatened during a home visit. Many drug courts utilize law enforcement as one member of the home visit team.

Law enforcement possesses vast experience and training in a variety of useful skills. Cops immediately survey environments and individuals for weapons, behaviors, and other indicators of violence. Cops excel in techniques of search and seizure and the legal requirements to get the evidence to court if necessary. Law enforcement carries back-up just a radio call away. Equally important, law enforcement is often most aware of the latest recipe for "cutting horse" or "cooking crank" and any safety concerns associated with a particular drug or manufacturing process.

Finding an Officer

How does one find the right law enforcement officer and then groom that officer for a drug court assignment? One answer is training and involvement. Police supervisors and administrators, along with judges and prosecutors, can narrow the field with their knowledge of innovative officers who seek hard work and new challenges. Once identified, these officers should participate in the chief's committee to help develop policy for drug court participation. Once a policy is in place, formal selection begins. Regardless of the process of selecting the law enforcement drug court team member, serious concerns remain for the new officer assigned to the drug court team.

The Drug Court Officer

For many people, the rite of passage to becoming a sworn officer is the oath of office, often including the law enforcement officer code of ethics. This document illustrates many of the conflicts the drug court model offers the newly assigned officer.

Even as law enforcement continues to professionalize, many states require only a high school education, graduation from the state's basic police academy within the first year of employment, and little, if any, continuing education or training. Given the power and responsibility provided to peace officers and often low levels of formal education, issues of ego and insecurity often emerge when officers become equal team members with highly specialized and highly educated professionals on the drug court team.

Cops trust their lives to anyone wearing a gun and a badge. How does a cop trust someone who makes four times his or her salary, drives a fancy car, lives in a gated community, and travels in very different circles of perceived privilege? These issues are real. The drug court officer must be welcomed as a full team member with unique and valuable assets. Equally important, officers must realize their value to the team.

Transitioning to a drug court team also offers many challenges to a law enforcement officer whose training consists of recognizing a violation of the law, arresting an offender, and preserving the chain of evidence necessary for prosecution in a criminal court. These challenges require new understandings of due process, confidentiality, sanctions and incentives, client relations, and a clear perception of the officer's role and responsibility on the drug court team. For the officer, these concerns become serious issues while performing specific, sometimes very different, duties on the team.

Several issues may emerge during the home visit. The officer may be teamed with drug court personnel, a social worker, or a treatment provider during a home visit. Safety remains the officer's primary responsibility. Once the residence or the immediate area is secure, the team may or may not conduct a warrantless search of the premise. In situations in which the team has previously decided that a search would not be conducted on this particular visit, the officer's observation of behavior or of artifacts such as drug paraphernalia or residue may warrant an unexpected search of the premise or client. This could even lead to an unexpected urine test. An officer may recognize a possible weapon not seen or recognized by the social worker. The treatment partner may be in the best position to decide if arrest or recommending additional sanctions to the court is in the best interest of the client and the community.

Officers in some jurisdictions find it strange to conduct a search, find dope, seize dope, place dope in property custody (preserving the chain of custody if later needed in court), release the client, then write a report recommending sanctions for the otherwise criminal offender. In the end, the home visit team must become a team effort. The members must develop equal trust and respect for the abilities brought by each member. Comfort levels will develop with experience and client staffing meetings.

Staffing meetings usually occur just prior to court and often include the entire team. In these meetings many officers feel insecure, as if they have little to offer in a meeting seemingly dominated by therapists, lawyers, the director, and judge. However, given the situation, the officer often holds client alternatives not recognized or available to other members of the team.

Drug courts represent one of the basic ideal types of community policing. From this perspective, the officer represents one of the most connected and informed of community resources with the ways or means to mobilize those resources.

The officer knows that for juveniles, the big deal is the local high school or college sporting team. Sometimes it takes a cop to get a sideline pass, a signed ball, or tickets to the big game. Sometimes it takes a cop to match the right kid to the right merchant to sweep the business floor, leading to a part-time job. Sometimes it takes a cop to get the court order to divert unclaimed bicycles from the police evidence locker to clients with lost driving privileges. Sometimes it takes a cop to tell the staffing team that something just does not smell right and the seemingly perfect client may need an unannounced home visit or urine test the day after court rather than the customary precourt test.

In the end, trust and respect within and between the officer and the drug court team is a two-way street. Roles, duties and responsibilities develop with time and familiarity. Confidential information can then be trusted and shared for the benefit of the client and the community. Officers recognize that when an arrest must be made from the warrantless search or the late night encounter, this also provides the officer with the opportunity to sell the drug court process and program to the uninformed officer assisting with the arrest and booking.

So how does the officer sell the drug court concept to the otherwise cynical cop who sees the program as nothing more than another "soft-on-crime, hug-a-thug" program? Whether they know it or not, most cops are closet classic criminologists.

The theory states that punishment changes behavior and has three components (6). The two most important components are the swiftness and the sureness of the punishment. If potential offenders know that they will be punished and the punishment will occur immediately, they are less likely to commit the crime. Every cop knows, believes, and supports this. It is waiting over a year for a case to come to trial and waiting through countless hearings and postponements that frustrate police. The third component of punishment is the severity. Even the most hardened officer knows that shaming or rewarding an individual (particularly a kid) often holds a greater impact than the severest punishment.

A typical street cop conversation might be: "So you arrest this guy on a felony possession of crank, what happens?"

1. He spends the night in jail.
2. He is arraigned the next morning and released.
3. He is sentenced a year later.
4. He gets a deferred or suspended sentence for less than 5 years, and,
5. If there is any supervision it is infrequent, Monday through Friday and 9 to 5, and he is never tested for drugs.

You arrest the same person and he goes to drug court:

1. He spends the night in jail.
2. He is arraigned the next morning and released.
3. Within a week he is back before the judge where he pleads guilty and is deferred to drug court.
4. Now he is accountable 24/7.
5. He can be randomly drug tested, his home randomly searched, and he has a curfew and other restrictions that, if violated, can warrant an arrest on the spot.
6. He has to get a job and pay for his supervision and treatment.
7. If he messes up, he is back before the judge the next day where the judge sends him to jail for 1 to 30 days, no questions asked.
8. And, when he does something good, it is really something to see him break down and cry just because the judge gave him a gift certificate to take his wife out to eat or a couple of passes to take his kid to a ball game.

Invite officers not involved with the program to a drug court session. Even the most skeptical officer tears up when watching a long-time addict cry when given a coffee cup for a month of sobriety or an addicted kid receive a movie pass for a week of clean urine tests. The same skeptical officer becomes sold when a client comes to court with alcohol on his or her breath and is immediately taken away for a night in jail, no questions asked.

The Treatment Provider's Concerns

Some drug courts provide treatment in-house while others contract or outsource treatment services. Many of the same concerns arise regardless of who provides client treatment. Confidentiality of medical records represents one of the most serious concerns for the treatment provider (7). Regardless of the particular specialty or field, the Health Insurance Portability and Accountability Act of 1996 (HIPPA) or client's rights to confidentiality of medical records represents a topic for every mandated continued education training for treatment providers.

Law enforcement represents additional concerns. For many treatment providers, providing medical information to a presiding judge or program director is one thing, but providing medical information, much of which could be legally incriminating, to a law enforcement officer is quite another. This issue, although serious, is easily overcome with a disclaimer on the medical intake form that states that all records are made available to the entire drug court team.

Although petty on the surface, there is one issue that undermines many drug court team efforts. For many teams, the treatment provider is the most educated member of the team. After completing a 4-year degree, a psychologist may spend another 7 years completing coursework and internships leading to a PhD. In the same state, the law enforcement officer who may have completed thousands of hours of specialized training may academically hold a GED. Although never spoken, it is often difficult for the officer and the doctor to overcome this discrepancy in education, applied training, income, and street experience. In successful drug court teams, members recognize the values and contributions of each team member and know that every contribution betters the recovery chances of the client.

Field Training for the Drug Court Officer

What does a law enforcement representative to the drug court need to know? What are the expectations for this role? The law enforcement representative is expected to do the following:

1. Review the mission of the program.
2. Review the organization chart of the agency.
3. Review client steps to get into the program.
4. Review the entire program step by step from intake to graduation.
5. Conduct background investigations (local, state, and federal) and maintain criminal history files on clients.
6. Track and follow up on defendant/client re-arrest, police contact, and program compliance.
7. Assist with home visits and address verification.
8. Assist the court with the development of programs for eligible offenders and assist with referrals.
9. Participate in staffing.

10. Provide the drug court team with the newest findings and methodologies in drug testing, altering tests, drugs of choice, forms of usage, susceptible communities or populations, and prevention models.
11. Educate peer professionals and community leaders about drug court.

Where does the newly appointed officer get the training to contribute to the team? If you are that officer, do a ride-along with officers assigned to established drug courts in your area. Contact the National Association of Drug Court Professionals (NADCP) and ask about publications and upcoming training. Seek, lobby, or beg for funds for your entire drug court team to attend the NADCP annual training conference, where they can network and talk.

Discuss your role and possible contributions with each member of your drug court team. Talk to other officers, trial attorneys, and community leaders about what they know and think about drug courts and what they think would make them better. Finally, talk to clients. You know who made it; you know who failed the drug court program; talk to both. Surprisingly, they will tell you what works and what does not. They will tell you that recovery is easier with closer supervision and more frequent drug testing.

Finally the day comes when you have made it as a drug court officer. It is usually when you least expect it. For me it happened at Wal-Mart. The dutiful husband that I am, I was pushing the cart for my wife. With my shoulders rolled, back slumped, and feet dragging, I trod through the endless aisles of groceries and women's apparel, until I was stopped by a suspicious person.

I immediately thought, "I really should carry an off-duty gun," as I was hugged by the rough, soiled individual. With tears in his eyes and concern in my wife's, he began to thank me for arresting him and saving his life. He talked of a life of crime and addiction, about my arrest, and his experience with the drug court. He talked about 1 year of sobriety, a new job, and the opportunity to see his children for the first time in years. He remembers me as the one who saved his life.

He walked away for the first time feeling comfortable talking to a cop and finding the cop he wanted to thank. I walked away still not remembering the man or the arrest. But now I carried a new-found pride as I continued to push the cart. My wife cried.

References

1. About Policy Services; Police Departments. Available at: http://www.aboutpolicy.com/direct/reports/police_dept.htm. Accessed April 12, 2006.
2. McMahan T. Officials working to expand drug court. The Daily Oklahoman. February 20, 2006.
3. National Association of Drug Court Professionals. The Facts: Facts on Drug Courts. Alexandria, VA: National Association of Drug Court Professionals; 2006.

4. West HC, Freeman-Wilson K, Boone DL. Painting the Current Picture: A National Report Card on Drug Courts and Other Problem Solving Court Programs in the United States. Washington, DC: Bureau of Justice Assistance, National Drug Court Institute; 2004.
5. Belenko S. Research on Drug Courts: A Critical Review. New York: The National Center on Addiction and Substance Abuse at Columbia University; 2001.
6. Beccaria C. On Crime and Punishment, 1764. Young D, ed. Indianapolis, IN: Hackett Publishing; 1986.
7. National Drug Court Institute. Federal Confidentiality Laws and How They Affect Drug Court Practitioners. Washington, DC: Drug Court Program Office, Office of Justice Programs, U.S. Department of Justice; 2004.

27
Record Keeping and Statistics

Cary N. Heck and Aaron Roussell

Drug court research and evaluation has improved greatly since the advent of the first program in 1989. The initial successes were fueled by anecdotal evidence and testimonials, but the expansion and sustainability of the model depend on solid research and evaluation techniques. It is in this arena where drug courts have the most growing to do. This chapter uses the drug court logic model to describe process and outcome measurement. It also focuses on a standardized method for keeping the records important for evaluation and research purposes.

Process evaluation is primarily a tool used by program managers to evaluate and improve their own program. As the name suggests, process evaluations focus on the process and its related indicators, not on the theoretical final product of drug courts, the sober, crime-free citizen. These evaluations measure several things, the first being the program' s goals. As a drug court is established, each program is created to address specific community goals. The extent to which the program is meeting those goals is the target of the process evaluation.

Policy implementation is another important objective of the process evaluation. Drug courts are established according to best practices that represent research-tested means of achieving goals. A process evaluation finding that a drug court is following literature-based recommendations and implementing them in an efficient and effective manner should give an indication that the program is reaching its potential.

Drug courts are goal-driven criminal justice programs oriented toward the expected outcomes of reduced criminality, cessation of substance abuse, and improved citizenship. Outcome research moves beyond a simple counting of outputs, that is, those hours of treatment completed, drug screens administered, or sanctions imposed. Outcomes generally refer to the effects that the program has on its participants. The assumption is that these will be largely positive, and research on sobriety and recidivism bears this out (1).

The Logic Model

The drug court logic model is a key concept for designing research and data collection strategies (2). A logic model is a tool used to break a process into its component parts to allow analysis of the whole based on these parts. Logic models are based on the actual operation of programs as well as the theoretical underpinnings related to the intervention. Generally, logic models for social interventions include the following:

1. *Inputs*: client characteristics and program staff.
2. *Process elements*: the actual workings of the intervention.
3. *Outputs*: number of hours in treatment or supervision.
4. *Outcomes*: the changes in the clients who participate in the program.

Inputs

Inputs into the drug court system typically are clients and program staff. When considering clients as outputs, they can best be described by their demographic and personal characteristics as they relate to the intervention. It is important for evaluators and researchers to identify the social and psychological conditions that clients bring to the process. For example, addiction severity is important to consider as a client-level variable related to subsequent programming.

One means for categorizing these important client variables is through analysis of risk factors. Important social risk factors include client criminal records and personal drug use history. People who begin their criminal offending or drug use at an early age tend to persist in that behavior well into adulthood (3). Clients with more serious criminal histories and more extensive addiction problems tend to do poorly in programs designed to curb this behavior. Drug court literature specifically addresses the issues of prior treatment failures and the current age of the client (younger clients tend not to do as well) as social risk factors.

Psychological risk factors related to client success are also important. People with antisocial personality disorders tend to have better outcomes when they meet regularly with the judge (4). Likewise, the diagnosis of co-occurring disorders will likely play a role in client performance and should guide the program activity.

The second type of input is the availability of program staff for the implementation of the drug court model. Often clients need psychiatric or psychological services that are difficult to obtain. Furthermore, drug courts rely on services that can only be provided by contractors, program staff, and those on loan from other agencies. For the evaluator or researcher it is valuable to know how much time is available for client service.

Process Elements

The structure of the drug court process has three main components:

1. Treatment.
2. Supervision.
3. Coordination.

Treatment

Substance abuse treatment data are generally captured using measures of dosage, including counseling attendance and length of stay. To document these variables in a meaningful manner, the program must report service referrals and actual attendance. Clients who remain in treatment for a longer period of time tend to have improved sobriety outcomes (5). In this logic model, treatment is not limited to substance abuse therapy but also includes adjunctive services such as medical and mental health services. Both referrals and attendance are critical variables to capture. It is not enough for a program to simply refer clients to treatment. They must also ensure that clients take full advantage of the services offered based on need.

Supervision

Supervision variables are composed of client visits, including those at drug court, the probation office, the clients' homes, schools, or places of employment. Theoretically, such visits promote an environment of watchfulness that helps clients to maintain prosocial activities.

Additionally, supervision variables include those related to the behavioral model espoused by drug courts. This model relies on a system of incentives and sanctions based on client behaviors that is designed to elicit improved conduct over time. The effectiveness of incentives and sanctions is based on three major behavioral constructs: celerity, certainty, and severity (6). Celerity refers to the time period between the precipitating behavior and the court response. This time period should be minimized in order to create a clear link between the action and the response. It is important to fully document the date on which the action occurred as well as the date the court response happened. Certainty refers to the likelihood that a behavior will result in a court response. The greater the likelihood a response will occur, the more of an impact this response will have on future behavior. Severity refers to the proportionality of the response. The response of the court must reflect the action taken. It is important to document not only that a response occurred but also the nature of that response.

Drug and alcohol screening is another form of supervision. The tests given to clients should be recorded in a consistent and uniform manner that includes the test dates, types, and results. These test results serve as a foundational measurement of client sobriety and also relate to the behavioral model mentioned above.

Coordination

Coordination variables are more difficult to document but are highly important. Drug court coordination includes the bringing together of various program components (i.e., prosecution, defense counsel, supervision) in a manner designed to elicit support and input. Although the roles of these agencies outside of drug courts are adversarial, the drug court model requires all participants to work in a cooperative manner. The best way to measure such cooperation is by looking at progress reports, court liaisons, and case reviews. It is important to consider the timeliness of responses to requests for information, as well as the actual participation in case review and court sessions. It is valuable to assess the program staff' s sense of how well the team works together in the best interest of the client. Imbalances can lead to a shift in the program' s focus from the drug court model to strongly punitive or treatment-oriented models.

Outputs

The outputs of the system consist of the descriptive numbers that can apply to several parts of the drug court:

1. *Clients*: number in the system, number graduating.
2. *Supportive services*: number of services, number of clients in each service.
3. *Drug testing*: number of tests done, number per client, number positive.
4. *Staff*: numbers in each court or position.
5. *Judges*: numbers in each court.
6. *Drug treatment providers*: numbers of provider organizations and numbers of providers in each organization.

Outcome Measurement

Outcome measurements in drug courts are typically expressed as fractions or a number compared to another number, such as the number of clients graduating per the number of clients entering the program. To truly draw conclusions about outcomes, the researcher must find appropriate measurement tools and be able to compare the drug court client outcomes to some other group.

Outcome analysis has traditionally focused mainly on recidivism. The required information is already in a database for criminal justice professionals to access and policymakers tend to seize upon it as the sole measure of the effectiveness of a criminal justice intervention. The logic model for drug court implies the importance of substance abuse and related psychosocial indicators in affecting the criminality of an offender, so it is incumbent on courts to examine other indicators as well (7).

Performance measurement is an easy way to do this to the satisfaction of state and federal partners and the drug courts team. Performance measurement, more than any other aspect of evaluation, should be seen as an ongoing process rather than as an event that, once completed, can be dealt with, archived, and forgotten. Constant reports on these measures can assist administrators in understanding their own programs and comparing data with other programs. This is ultimately in the interest of the local program, in terms of funding, increased credibility, and legislative advantages.

Outcomes can be disaggregated by looking at short-term and long-term measures. Short-term outcomes tend to refer to those effects that the program has on the participant during the time that they are in the program. In-program recidivism is a classic example in the literature; evaluators record the return to criminal activity while under the supervisory care of the drug court (8). A lower recidivism rate than those traditionally reported is usually viewed as a measure of success. Sobriety, as determined by clean urine screens and measured by consecutive clean days, is another. Even a reduction in problem days when the participant is uncooperative (but not to the point of invoking an official sanction) can be considered by treatment and supervisory staff as a positive outcome. Short-term outcomes are perhaps the best documented because the client is under the watchful eye of the program. Drug screens are required; parole and probation officer contacts are constant; treatment is mandatory; and the judge can personally watch the actions of the individual. Because the client remains under the threat of legal sanction, compliance is an outcome in and of itself.

It is also valuable to consider other measures that may be less obvious, such as consumer satisfaction. If the program has the goal of improving the outlook for clients through treatment and other types of interventions, it is important to capture the extent to which the clients feel that these interventions are actually meeting their needs. Although this research method is attitudinal, it is often an excellent means for judging the cultural competency of a program.

Long-term outcomes are more difficult to obtain because they require the tracking of individuals after termination (positively or negatively) from the program. Drug courts have always presented themselves as long-term solutions to drug abuse and related criminality, and long-term outcomes must therefore be considered. The only reliable indicator is recidivism, which can be tracked through state databases and the National Crime Information Center.

Process Evaluation

Process evaluations can be highly effective methods for program management. Although often associated with unpleasant changes, an independent evaluator consulting with program staff can both affirm existing practices and recommend more effective ones.

In evaluating processes, everything that the court does from its screening intake to case management is available for appraisal. When drawing up an evaluation plan, the spectrum of possibilities is so large that an evaluator must narrow it in two ways:

1. By deciding on the most critical elements to be considered.
2. By consulting with the program staff to determine their concerns about the program and what issues might deserve more attention than the evaluator might otherwise give.

Critical elements to consider for process evaluation include the following:

1. Target population.
2. Substance abuse treatment.
3. Judicial/court supervision.
4. Provision of services.
5. Cooperation between disparate agencies.
6. Community support.
7. Outcomes.

The structure of the drug court is not always entirely determined internally or even by local authorities. State and federal funding can complicate the structure and processes of the program through statutory requirements and funding conditions that may have no relationship to best practices or literature-based recommendations for effective management. This is partially checked, however, by the fact that enabling legislation often utilizes the 10 key components established by the National Association of Drug Court Professionals (9). Although these components are expressly part of the drug court structure, their fidelity to the model should be enumerated and examined. The best way to address these issues is through a well-designed and executed process evaluation.

Target Population

Determination of the target population is the most crucial element for overall success. An examination of the target population is also a crucial ingredient to a thorough process evaluation. The intended interventions of substance abuse treatment and other services are planned around a specific type of offender; if a program is ill-suited to serve a client, it would be counterproductive to admit him or her to the program (10).

Most programs do have some hand in setting their own goals, and drug court evaluators should scrutinize client intake in terms of those stated goals, framing the discussion in terms of resource limitations as well as the universe of those who could be eligible for the program. Ideally, target population goals defined at program genesis would become the backbone of screening and eligibility requirements for clients around which treatment and ancillary services will be built.

Substance Abuse Treatment

Substance abuse treatment encompasses philosophies such as zero tolerance and harm reduction and modalities such as 12 Step programs and cognitive-behavioral therapy. Research dating to the federal Special Action Office for Drug Abuse Prevention in the 1970s suggests that different treatment is effective for different personalities, different ethnic and racial groups, or different drugs of choice. Although the full panoply of choices in treatment is available to very few drug courts, an acknowledgment of these options and the populations for which they are best suited is important (11).

It is crucial that baseline measures of client addiction at program entry be considered. Because documenting sobriety is a significant feature to any evaluation, documenting client use prior to the program enables accurate comparison throughout the program and thus should lead to exciting evaluation findings. Although assessment instruments differ widely, any instrument should contain measures of past and present prevalence and incidence of drug use, addiction severity, and drugs of choice. An instrument must demonstrate such basic qualities as reliability and validity, essentially the ability to actually measure addiction and dependence and the ability to do so reliably across clientele.

Judicial and Court Supervision

Like all programs, drug court is a process, functioning with the court as its focal point. Activities from first contact to follow-up programs contribute to the success of the drug court and are worthy of analysis. Such basic processes as intake, phase advancement, graduation, and drug testing are prime candidates for evaluation. Hold-ups in phase advancement, bottlenecks in graduation, and drug-testing problems are examples of concerns that might go unnoticed in the day-to-day operations of the court.

Perhaps the most important aspects of the court process are the status hearings and supervision contacts, as they are the regularized contact between the client and court system. Certainty of response is the most important factor in shaping client behavior in drug court. Thus, measuring the relationship of client behaviors to programmatic responses is critical. Both the perceived magnitude of incentives or sanctions and the application schedule should be reviewed in accordance with the principle that response plans should be individualized based on client history, demographics, and personality (11). Furthermore, the coordination of service application falls under the court processes. Questions should be asked about information sharing and team involvement in the decision-making process.

Provision of Services

Drug courts offer a variety of ancillary services to clients in their programs. An evaluation should establish not only which services are offered but also how they are utilized and whether the clients are satisfied with them. It is important to document service referrals as well as actual participation. An examination of the intake process may reveal indications of need for services not yet provided. It is important to document those services that were included in the treatment plan and those that actually were delivered to the intended clients.

A unit of service is an easy way to document supplementary benefits provided by the court. Included in this documentation should be medical and psychological services, job training, placement services, education, and any service to which the client was linked by program staff. Measurement is largely linked to billing; inpatient treatment is easiest to measure in days, outpatient treatment in hours, and doctor' s appointments by visit.

Cooperation

Drug courts, by their very nature, are collaborative enterprises that harness the power of cooperative, rather than adversarial, relationships in their attempt to treat addiction and co-occurring crime. Although measurement of cooperation can be complex, one simple method involves questioning team members individually as to their perceptions regarding the extent to which their input is considered when decisions are made by the drug court team.

Community Support

Many team members are responsible to the voting public for their positions, local businesses may be supportive in providing incentives and job placement, and local action groups may assist in funding. There is clear value in exploring the community reaction to the drug court and assessing the support of stakeholders, community leaders, and the general public. This can be done with a survey or questionnaire that asks specific questions about their understanding of the model and its implementation. As with all evaluation findings, the results can be used to continue the program in a successful vein or to fix problems that are discovered.

Outcomes: Performance Measures

Outcomes are the best performance measures in drug court because outcomes of individual programs are measured for funding, and, in a broader sense, the entire drug court movement is assessed by them. The following outcomes are typically measured:

1. Retention.
2. Sobriety.
3. Criminal recidivism.

Retention

Retention refers to the ability of a drug court program to maintain and eventually graduate its clients. Treatment has proven to be effective in combating drug addiction but only when received in sufficient dosages. Research supports the use of criminal justice coercion to gain this level of dosage. Retention is thus a crucial indicator of the success of a program. In the short term, retention refers to maintenance and advancement in the program; in the longer term, it refers to graduation.

Retention should be calculated as a ratio or percentage: the retention rate is the number of people who complete or remain in the program divided by the number that enter the program during a particular time period. The time period is crucial because all those who enter the program during that time period (usually 6 months to a year), including those who abscond, voluntarily withdraw, and are expelled, should be included in the denominator and are thus part of the cohort. Overall program retention should be the ratio of those who complete the program or are still enrolled in the program divided by those who enter the program during the time frame under consideration, generally 6 months to 1 year.

Because some participants who are still enrolled when a court decides to assess retention may ultimately drop out, the retention rate may need to be recalculated once the entire cohort has departed the drug court, either successfully or unsuccessfully, to obtain the graduation rate. For example, a program requires clients to complete 12 months of continuous participation in treatment and court activities. Fifty clients entered the program during the first 6 months under consideration; this is defined as the retention cohort. At the end of that first 6 months, a retention rate could be calculated using 50 as the denominator. In this case, 5 clients opted out of the program and 5 more were dismissed from the program, leaving 40 clients from that 6-month period who eventually graduated (even if it took longer than 12 months to graduate) or were still in the program. The retention rate would then be 40/50, or 80%.

Sobriety

Another measure of program success, sobriety, is also time frame specific. Over the course of a program, a general trend should be apparent: the number of dirty drug screens should decrease more as clients progress. Overall program performance can be documented using the average length of sobriety during a specific time frame. Self-reported drug use during the program without a formal drug screen result is not considered a reliable measure. All drug screens and the results thereof, both positive and negative, should be documented, as well as those that are missed, excused, tampered, stalled, and inconclusive. Drug courts should be able to document both the average length of continuous sobriety and the average number of failed tests that a client has during the program or during a particular time period. Both the trend and the averages will prove useful measures of program performance.

Criminal Recidivism

Recidivism has traditionally been a contentious subject in drug court research. The term simply means a return to criminal activity by someone who has already been adjudicated guilty or delinquent. The methods available to measure recidivism are diverse. Arrest is not a flawless indicator because all people in a jurisdiction are not at the same risk for re-arrest. Risk factors depend largely on such things as race, neighborhood, and policing strategies. Nevertheless, arrests are preferred by drug court scholars over other measures because of the ease of documentation and the accelerated turnaround time for processing documentation not found with other common methods, such as conviction (12). Maintaining records of both arrest and conviction is useful for research purposes, but the associated complications of conviction render it less useful than arrest for program evaluation purposes. In considering in-program recidivism, researchers should remember that more clients will be arrested and charged with a crime during the program than will actually be convicted. Therefore, arrest is a better measure for evaluation purposes.

Recidivism is the one performance measure that could plausibly be considered after program completion. Graduates can potentially be tracked for years, depending on available evaluation resources. It is recommended that, to the extent possible, programs develop methods to track clients after program participation to examine this, using information from the local justice process as well as state and National Crime Information Center databases. Doing so allows drug courts to build on sample data collected by the National Institute of Justice and the Urban Institute to continue to refine our understanding of drug court recidivism at the national level (13). The use of a comparison group enhances this type of research, but the data are certainly useful on their own and should be collected even in the absence of such a group.

Some programs track graduates through alumni groups and thus have the ability to pursue further research. While this sort of follow-up is admirable, any alumni group is likely composed of the most recent and most committed graduates, thus marginalizing it for research purposes.

Programs are well served simply by tracking the recidivism of their clients. No comparison group is necessary for performance measurement. Should the court decide that comparison group study is best, however, there are some important considerations to bear in mind.

It is widely recognized that the real-world criminal justice system is a poor arena for experimental laboratory research. If a treatment is thought to be successful, it is unfair to withhold it from one group and provide it to another. Random assignment to different kinds of treatment is the foundation of experimental research. By randomly assigning qualified individuals to a treatment group (drug court) or a control group, the effects of the program intervention can be shown to cause the observed differences in behavior. Because of the ethical problems, however, this is rarely possible (14).

The next best option for real-world evaluation is a quasiexperimental design using a comparison group. Sometimes called matched groups, comparison groups are structured to be highly similar to the drug court population on key factors identified by the literature, such as age and criminal history. It is incumbent on the evaluator to ensure that the two groups are statistically similar in these important ways (15).

The ideal comparison group would be a set of offenders from the same jurisdiction arrested at the same time as the drug court group and equally eligible who never entered the program for bureaucratic or logistical reasons. Although it is possible to use a group that turned down the drug court option, such a group might have motivational differences that would make it unsuitable for comparison. It is ideal to gain as much information as possible (such as substance abuse history and substance dependence) to ensure an adequate comparison, but obviously this is not always possible.

If there is no group similar to the drug court population in a jurisdiction, there are still other possible comparison groups to be considered. Historical comparison group evaluation, known as a "pre–post design,"involves using groups of offenders arrested in the time frame immediately before drug court was established. The assumption is that they would have been eligible for drug court had it been available. For pre–post designs to produce valid data, the policing and adjudication policies of the jurisdiction must have remained constant over the course of both time frames.

Even more care must be taken with the other available options. Demographically similar jurisdictions without drug courts can produce comparison groups. Again, however, policing and adjudication policies must be closely scrutinized to ensure that there are no significant differences in chance for participant re-arrest, which would severely compromise the value of the comparison. That group of offenders found ineligible for drug court is highly flawed as a basis for comparison unless the reasons can be conclusively proven not to affect comparability. Most important, drug court failures are not an appropriate comparison group. Just as schools do not prove their teaching effectiveness by comparing "A" students to "F" students, drug courts cannot learn anything about their effects on recidivism from this comparison, and to do so is fundamentally bad science.

Conclusions

Regardless of the modality selected for drug court evaluation and research, two overriding principles should guide these activities. First, the evaluation and research must be useful to the consumers. Process evaluations should help program managers and stakeholders to improve their programs for their clients. Furthermore, drug court research should serve to inform the field. Marlowe and his colleagues (10) recently published an article outlining important research questions that are the most pressing in the drug court environment. This research agenda can be used as a tool for selecting pertinent research questions to analyze.

Second, it is of the utmost importance that drug courts continue to develop and disseminate scientifically valid research that can be relied on to inform policy and programmatic decision making. To accomplish this, researchers must continue to adopt and utilize empirical methods when studying drug court activities and outcomes. As the drug court movement continues to gain momentum, it will be these research products that help to shape the field for future generations of practitioners to improve outcomes for clients.

References

1. Roman J, Townsend W, Bhati A. National Estimates of Drug Court Recidivism. Washington, DC: National Institute of Justice, U.S. Department of Justice; 2003.
2. Marlow DB. Drug Court Logic Model. Philadelphia: Treatment Research Institute; 1998.
3. Cullen FT, Gilbert KE. Reaffirming Rehabilitation. Cincinnati, OH: Anderson Publishing; 1995.
4. Marlowe DB, Festinger DS, Lee PA. The judge is the key component of drug court. Drug Court Rev 2004;2:1–34.
5. Satel SL. Drug treatment: the case for coercion. Drug Court Rev 2000;1:1–43.
6. Skinner BF. Science and human behavior. New York: Macmillan Publishing; 1950.
7. Marlowe DB, Heck C, Thanner MH, Casebolt R. A national research agenda for drug courts: plotting the course for second-generation scientific inquiry. Drug Court Rev 2006;2:1–32.

8. Belenko S. Research on Drug Courts: A Critical Review: 2001 Update. New York: National Center on Addiction and Substance Abuse at Columbia University; 2001.
9. National Association of Drug Court Professionals. Defining Drug Courts: The Key Components. Washington, DC: Office of Justice Programs, U.S. Department of Justice; 1997.
10. Marlowe DB, Festinger DS, Lee PA, Dugosh KL, Benasutti KM. Matching judicial supervision to clients' risk status in drug court. Crime Delinquency 2006;52:52–76.
11. Marlowe DB, Kirby KC. Effective use of sanctions in drug courts: lessons from behavior research. Drug Court Rev 1999;1:1–31.
12. Dinkins DN. Does quality-of-life policing diminish quality of life for people of color? Crisis, July 1997.
13. Roman J, Townsend W, Bhati A. National Estimates of Drug Court Recidivism. Washington, DC: National Institute of Justice, U.S. Department of Justice; 2003.
14. One of the few exceptions is Gottfredson DC, Najaka SS, Kearley B. Effectiveness of drug treatment courts: evidence from a randomized trial. Criminol Public Policy 2003;2:171–196.
15. Rempe M. Recidivism 101: evaluating the impact of your drug court. Drug Court Rev 2006;2:83–112.

28
Policy Options for the Future

James P. Gray

Drug Policy Options

This chapter explores 10 policy options for future drug laws in the United States, from my perspective as a judge with 22 years on the California State bench and my previous service as a federal prosecutor and Naval Judge Advocate General officer. These options are 1. increased zero tolerance, 2. ending drug prohibition, 3. drug treatment, 4. drug rehabilitation programs, 5. drug maintenance programs, 6. needle exchange programs, 7. overdose prevention programs, 8. de-profitization of drugs, 9. education, and 10. federalization.

Before discussing the policy options, it is necessary to establish what our drug policy goals should be. The overall goals for the United States should be to reduce crime, improve public safety and health, prevent the loss of civil liberties, and decrease the recreational usage of mind-altering drugs.

Increased Zero Tolerance

"Zero tolerance" for any contact with drugs of abuse is the policy in place today in the United States and in many other countries, such as Singapore. One policy option would be to continue to utilize even more strict zero tolerance programs by increasing the use of mandatory minimum sentences; making further attempts to search people, trucks, and ocean shipping containers as they enter our borders; and utilizing even more wiretaps and police sting operations in attempts to intercept illicit drugs. However, increasing efforts for an even more strict zero tolerance approach would simply amount to doing more of what has already been shown not to work. In no way is this intended as a criticism of law enforcement agencies. They have a difficult and dangerous job, and they are doing it more successfully than we have a right to expect.

Today the United States is convicting increasing numbers of highly placed drug dealers in court, seizing larger quantities of drugs, and giving longer prison sentences for the offenders than ever before. However, no corresponding decrease in drug use or sales has resulted.

Any intelligent approach should analyze what has been done in the past that has worked and not worked and change policy to programs that are shown to be effective. It is also productive to look at what has worked and not worked in other countries and attempt to emulate the successes. Considering the results of the present U.S. drug policy, where increasingly victory is defined as simply slowing down the pace of defeat, it is my opinion that we could not do it worse if we tried.

Ending Drug Prohibition

The biggest contributor to the problems caused by the presence of illegal drugs is the policy of drug prohibition. The arguments positing in favor of drug prohibition are summarized in five points: 1. crime reduction, 2. availability of drugs, 3. financial costs, 4. collateral damage, and 5. corruption and upheaval abroad.

Crime Reduction

Homicides decreased by 60% in the United States within a year after alcohol prohibition was repealed (1). The same phenomenon would be seen when the United States repeals drug prohibition. Every dollar the United States invests in the investigation and prosecution of drug crimes is a dollar not spent to investigate and prosecute crimes such as burglaries, homicides, rapes, and frauds. As a result, the "tougher" the United States gets on drugs, the "softer" it becomes on other crimes.

Availability of Drugs

Drugs are already fully available to anyone who wants them, including children. In fact, most prison wardens will acknowledge that prisoners can get all the drugs they want; it just costs them more in prison than on the street.

Financial Costs

The cost of drug abuse to the United States has hovered between $30 and $40 billion per year between 1992 and 2000. During the same period of time, the cost of the War on Drugs increased from about $80 billion in 1992, to about $140 billion in 2000 (2). The exponential increase in the cost of drug abuse has been maintained despite the fact that the U.S. Drug Enforcement Agency's budget had doubled in only 7 years to $1.6 billion in 2002, while the agency "is unable to demonstrate progress in reducing the availability of illegal drugs in the United States" (3).

Collateral Damage

Many other things have gone wrong as a result of a failed drug policy. The United States leads the world in incarceration, in both numbers and per capita. In fact, more than *six times* as many people are incarcerated in the United States as in all 12 of the countries of the European Union, even though there are 100 million more people in those European countries (4). In addition, about half of the convicted drug offenders in the United States are incarcerated for nonviolent and nonserious offenses, and a disproportionate number of them come from poor, minority communities (5).

The problems with violent street gangs are also increased because gangs are largely financed by the sale of illicit drugs. Gangs use the sale of drugs as a recruiting tool, encouraging young people to join the gangs so that they can be a "part of the action." The result has been the spread of the gangs from large cities to smaller towns across the country because these new areas present new business opportunities for the gangs.

There are tens of thousands of people with serious injuries and illnesses that are in unnecessary pain because their physicians are so intimidated by the U.S. Drug Enforcement Agency that they hesitate to prescribe sufficient pain-reducing medication containing opiates. Statistics do not begin to take into account the tragic loss of civil liberties caused by attempts in the United States to enforce our nation's War on Drugs and the almost universal loss of respect for the nation's laws.

Corruption and Upheaval Abroad

Today most of the fighting among warlords in Afghanistan comes from efforts to establish and control the sales of the opium poppy for the heroin trade (5). This was also true during the civil war in Lebanon. The same result has been seen in Mexico, where the same amount of foreign currency flows into Mexico from the exportation of illegal drugs as comes from the exportation of oil. This activity is so lucrative that there are serious allegations that the Mexican army is actively assisting the smuggling of drugs into the United States (6–9). In Colombia, drug money corruption has deeply infected the police and army, endangering public safety and everyday life (6,7).

Historically, virtually every rogue government in the world has raked in huge amounts of money from dealing in the illicit drug trade. This includes Muammar Kaddafi in Libya, Erich Honnicker in East Germany, Manuel Noriega in Panama, and Fidel Castro in Cuba. Entire governments have been destabilized by guerrilla organizations that are almost completely financed by the sale of illicit drugs, including the Shining Path guerrillas in Peru and the Serbs and the Kosovo Liberation Army in the former Yugoslavia. The U.S. military believes that the present government of North Korea is subsidizing its nuclear weapons program by illicit drug sales between \$100 and \$500 million every year (10).

Drug Treatment

According to a Rand Corporation report, taxpayers get seven times more value for their tax dollars with drug treatment than they do from incarceration, even for heavy-using, drug-addicted people (11). Because incarceration is the most expensive option, and in most jails and prisons nothing is done to help drug-addicted people address their problems, drug offenders released from custody are almost predestined to fail.

All drug treatment programs are successful for some people and unsuccessful for others. Because each person is unique, the impact that different drugs have on specific people in unique situations can be quite varied. So, the best approach with treatment is for society to have as many different approaches as possible.

The approach of the criminal justice system to those offenders should be, in combination with an appropriate period of incarceration for their antisocial conduct, to address their drug addictions with programs like drug courts. These programs are positive revolutions in the criminal justice system not only because they are effective but also because they force judges, prosecutors, and probation officers to treat drug-addicted people as individuals. Prior to drug courts, drug offenders almost always were only treated as statistics or "prison fodder." Now the people in authority realize that drug-addicted people also have needs, desires, and hopes, as well as failures, just like all the rest of us.

It makes sense to devote scarce prosecutorial resources to address the problem of drug users, because their drug usage is a threat to public safety. There are only so many resources to spend in the criminal justice system, and they are best utilized addressing those who are a threat to public safety. The drug use by nonproblem users may very well be a threat to their own medical safety, but those potential harms can best be addressed by education, drug treatment, and programs such as drug testing.

Drug Rehabilitation Programs

Many people, if they are removed from the environment in which they associate with drug use, are able to depart from their lifestyle of drug abuse.

Delancey Street Program

One of the most successful programs of redirection of this kind is the Delancey Street Program, started in San Francisco by psychologist and criminologist Mimi Silbert (12). The focus of this live-in program is to teach job skills and a work ethic to people at the very bottom of the social ladder. This training is also combined with instruction in social discipline, personal responsibility, and social skills. Clients are placed in one of the businesses owned by the Delancey Street Foundation, including a moving company, a catering business, and an advertising specialties company.

Ms. Silbert is the only professional involved in the program. The rest of the people in charge are ex-felon graduates of Delancey Street, many of whom have an extensive history of violence. The strictly implemented program requires that all of the participants be well groomed, dress for dinner, learn at least three marketable job skills, and earn the equivalency of a high school diploma. Violence or the use or possession of any nonprescription, mind-altering drugs, including alcohol, is cause for immediate removal.

Eighty percent of the participants successfully complete the requirements of the program for the prescribed 2 years, plus an added 3 months during which they live at the facility while holding a job in the community. Thereafter, they come back to the center as volunteers to help mentor and assist the new "recruits." Of the program, it has been written (12),

> Ms. Silbert explains that the goal of the program is to show that the "losers" in our society can be helped and empowered to help others. She describes the client population as part of an underclass. Fully one third of the clients were homeless, and the average resident of the program comes from a family that has been in poverty for four or five generations and has had members in prison for two or three generations. The clients have been hard-core dope addicts and are unskilled and functionally illiterate. They have experienced horrible violence and have been violent themselves.

Donovan State Prison

Positive results similar to the Delancey Street Program have been seen at Donovan State Prison in San Diego County, which has conducted a small drug treatment program for its problem drug users since 1990 (13). The Donovan program addresses job skills, anger management, individual responsibility, parenting skills, health, and an honest appraisal of the risks and benefits of using drugs. This training is combined with the availability of a support group upon their release from prison. The results of this program are also remarkable; within 1 year of their release from prison, only 16% of these problem felon drug users who successfully completed the program, as well as the after-release support group, were re-arrested for a new offense or parole violation, as opposed to 65% of those similar problem felon drug users who had not been involved in the program (14,15).

Drug Maintenance Programs

Drug maintenance is the maintaining in a controlled manner of a client on the drug that he or she is addicted to. The prototype is heroin maintenance.

One of the drug treatment options being used in several countries in Western Europe is a medicalized approach to heroin usage. For example, in 1994, Switzerland began a 3-year pilot program with a medical clinic in each of seven cities (16). The clinics were staffed by a medical doctor, a registered nurse, and a social worker. These professionals went into the community to find heroin users and encouraged them to obtain drug treatment. The users would be placed in a program if they could satisfy each of three criteria:

1. The person was at least 22 years of age and had failed drug treatment at least twice.
2. The person was addicted to heroin.
3. The person would be crime-free.

Patients at the clinics were given prescriptions for heroin that are filled at pharmaceutical prices, and the heroin is injected by the users under medical supervision at the clinics.

Given that none of the presently illegal drugs is expensive to produce, the only reason they are expensive is that they are illegal. Even the heaviest using drug-addicted person can support a habit for a maximum of $10 a day. The Swiss program does not become an orgy of heroin usage because the clients are screened by a physician to determine what their daily normal tolerance level is and are kept at that level. Accordingly, the dosage is not strong enough to provide a high or euphoria; however, it is strong enough to keep the person from going through withdrawal.

Within 1 year of its beginning of the program, the Minister of Health of Switzerland held a press conference and said that, because of the positive results, they were not going to wait for the full 3 years to expand the program nationwide. For example, the programs resulted in a major reduction in crime in the neighborhoods surrounding the clinics.

Burglaries, thefts, prostitution, check offenses, and other street crime of almost every kind decreased. If clients are arrested, they are off the program, and they know that this would put them back into the hustle of trying to get the money for their drugs, locating their supplier, and dodging the police. As a result, the clients stay away from crime so that they can continue with the program. The merchants in the surrounding neighborhoods experienced a sevenfold decrease in shoplifting (17).

Another result of the program was that drug usage in the neighborhoods surrounding the clinics was also substantially reduced. Fewer people were selling the drugs in the communities, and therefore fewer people were using the drugs. Employment of the clients in the programs increased by about 50%. They began to support themselves and their children; they were no longer a drain on society, and they began paying their taxes. The drug addicts' other medical problems began to be under control because not only was their drug usage not harming them as much because of the medical supervision, but the health care professionals were able to address their other medical problems as well. Large numbers of the drug-addicted people began to take that extra step by requesting treatment in order to get off heroin completely because they had developed a relationship of trust with the health care professionals and had developed confidence in themselves (17).

Today the heroin maintenance program has the full support of the Swiss Government, and in March 2003 the National Council voted 110 to 42 to extend it until the year 2009 (18). A nationwide plebiscite to abolish the heroin maintenance program failed by more than 80% of the voters. The Swiss people saw a program that was working, and they voted in overwhelming numbers to keep it.

Opponents in the United States argue that drug maintenance would "send the wrong message to our children." What is the right message? The message being sent now is, "Go ahead and die. It's okay if you contract AIDS from dirty needles, or die from the unknown strengths and impurities of the drugs, or get killed from the violence associated from illegal drug sales."

Drug addiction is a medical issue that must be addressed by medical professionals and the drug-addicted people themselves. Doctors can address these medical issues far better than the criminal justice system can, leaving the criminal justice system to do what it does best: holding people accountable for their conduct. That is the message the Swiss have given to their children, and I think they are clearly on the right track.

Needle Exchange Programs

Another medicalization program that works is a needle exchange program that allows a person to exchange a dirty needle and syringe for a clean one. No money changes hands, and no questions are asked. Studies demonstrate that these programs do not increase drug usage, but they do not decrease it either. However, needle exchange programs reduce the incidence of AIDS and hepatitis C in drug abusers by 50% (19).

Dirty needles also represent a health threat to the public. When they can no longer be used, they are often discarded in parking lots, public parks, along railroad tracks, in children's sandboxes, or in trash cans that other people sometimes tamp down with their hands. They can infect people with terrible diseases if they accidentally get pricked by them. If a dirty needle can be exchanged for a clean one, then it has value, so it very likely will be recycled, thus greatly reducing health threats to everyone concerned (20).

In Holland, where the government has formally adopted a drug policy of harm reduction, most of the drug-using communities are served by needle exchange programs. Such countries have found that the more "user friendly" the program is, the more successful it is. As such, the needle exchange sites are clean, safe, warm, lighted, and open 24 hours per day.

Many locations are found in police stations, because that satisfies all of the appropriate criteria (21,22).

Drug Substitution Programs

A program that works enormously well for some people, fairly well for others, and not at all for the rest is called *drug substitution*. In these types of programs, one drug, usually methadone, is substituted for another drug, usually heroin (23).

The first methadone maintenance program began in Shreveport, Louisiana, in the early 1900s but was forced to close down with the passage of the first national laws of drug prohibition in 1914. They were reinstituted in the United States during the early 1960s (23).

Methadone is an addictive, synthetic opiate that has almost no mind-altering effects, but methadone has the benefit of satisfying the body's cravings for heroin without intoxication. People who are taking methadone are mostly able to live normal lives. Usually methadone is taken in liquid form, which means that the problems related with injections are overcome. In addition, the effects of methadone are much longer lasting than those of heroin, so it can be taken only once per day.

A major criticism of methadone programs in the United States is that the federal government has taken a "hands-on" approach to the management of these programs. This approach has resulted in all methadone patients, regardless of the responsibility they have shown in their everyday lives and the amount of time they have been on the program, being required physically to come to the clinic and swallow their dose every day at the site while being observed. The process becomes cumbersome and difficult, especially for those clients who are working or going to school. Furthermore, many methadone clinics are in back alleys and the more rundown parts of town. The clients are required to line up for hours, in many clinics. The process becomes demeaning for the clients and is not at all conducive to recovery.

While only about 20% of the heroin-addicted people in the United States participate in methadone programs, over 60% participate in the more user-friendly programs in Amsterdam, where they employ buses as roving methadone clinics (23). Where the U.S. government greatly limits the number of medical doctors authorized to prescribe methadone, Holland and Spain have thousands, and Germany and Belgium authorize general medical practitioners as a principal source of methadone distribution.

The U.S. government is so concerned about the possible misuse of the methadone that it requires strictly applied procedures to be followed. However, the countries in Western Europe maturely understand that there are always going to be some abuses in any program. Therefore, they take steps to maximize the beneficial use of methadone and understand that it is less dangerous for people to misuse methadone than it is to misuse heroin.

Overdose Prevention Programs

In 2003, almost 3,600 drug users died in California alone because of overdose, an increase from 2,050 in 1990 (24). This means that more people died in California by drug overdose than from firearms or AIDS and makes overdose second only to automobile collisions for fatalities.

In attempts to reduce the numbers of these overdose deaths, the cities of New York, Chicago, and San Francisco have set up programs to distribute syringes containing naloxone to drug-addicted people. Naloxone counteracts the respiratory failure caused by drug overdoses, which enables the person to begin breathing regularly within minutes. The intent is that drug-addicted people will use the naloxone on others if they overdose. Since San Francisco began its naloxone program in 2003, the number of deaths from overdose per year has dropped below 100, which is the lowest it has been for 10 years. Each naloxone kit costs about $3. The risks are minimal, because naloxone itself has no mood-altering capabilities and is unlikely to be abused.

De-Profitization of Drugs

There is a definite difference between "drug crime" and "drug money crime." Without a doubt, illicit drugs have harmful results, but making the drugs illegal clearly has some harmful results as well, both in the United States and abroad.

For example, today, if Budweiser has a distribution problem with Coors, it does not send its thugs to shoot it out on the streets with its commercial rivals. Instead, Budweiser files a complaint against Coors and resolves the matter peaceably in court. Certainly we still have problem alcohol users in our country, but at least they are not prostituting themselves or burglarizing homes to get the money to buy their drug of choice. In addition, the "bathtub gin" problems where the impurities in the illegal booze seriously injured or killed large numbers of people during alcohol prohibition no longer exist.

People at all levels of our society have been corrupted by the allure of the large amounts of cash to be made by the sale of illicit drugs. This includes the poor and the rich, males and females, people at the lower ends of society and the upper, people in positions of responsibility such as the police, attorneys, and health care professionals, as well as children. This is not to mention entire governments of other countries in the world, such as Colombia, Mexico, and Afghanistan, where money from the trade in illicit drugs has corrupted safety and security. Governments will never be able to keep people from selling small amounts of drugs for large amounts of money.

Winners in the War on Drugs

There are five groups who have been winners in the War on Drugs: large-scale drug dealers, government officials designated to fight the drug dealers, politicians, private industry that makes large amounts of money from the fight on crime, and terrorists.

Large-Scale Drug Dealers

Large-scale drug dealers are making hundreds of millions of dollars per year and consider seizures of their goods as a small cost of doing business.

Government Officials

People in government are paid large amounts of tax dollars to fight against the large-scale drug dealers. Seldom in history has there been such a linkage of benefits for the "good guys" and the "bad guys" to perpetuate the status quo. Government bureaucracies continue to grow through every failure, and government has been able to convince the taxpayers to continue to pay more and more money for what has been demonstrated over the past decades simply not to work.

Politicians

Politicians continue to get elected and re-elected by talking tough about drugs. As two congressmen told this author privately, "Most politicians in Washington realize that the War on Drugs is not winnable, but it is eminently fundable. And politicians are addicted to the drug war funding."

The Private Sector

The private sector makes large amounts of money as a result of increased crime, including the people who build prisons and those who staff them. Some of the strongest lobbying groups in most states are the prison guard unions. It also includes people who make and sell burglar alarm equipment and security services. It also includes newspapers, because the more crime there is, the more newspapers are sold.

Terrorists

Terrorists all around the world obtain a large part of their funding from the sale of illicit drugs. Realistically, there will always be radical and psychotic people in the world who want to inflict injury and pain, but they will be far less dangerous if they do not have money.

Proposals for De-Profitization

Marijuana can be treated like alcohol and become a test case of what might be expected if other drugs are de-profitized. If adults want to buy, use, or possess marijuana, they could. As with alcohol, these people will be held accountable for their actions.

There would be five positive results:

1. The taxpayers would save about $1 billion every year that is spent to eradicate marijuana and to incarcerate nonviolent marijuana offenders.
2. The marijuana could generate billions of dollars a year in tax revenues.
3. Marijuana would be *less* available for children than it is today. Under the present system it is easier for young people to get marijuana than it is to obtain a six-pack of beer because the alcohol is regulated and controlled by the government and the illegal marijuana is controlled by illegal dealers who do not enforce age restrictions.
4. The historically important product of industrial hemp would reemerge, providing an opportunity for farmers to compete more equally around the world (25,26).
5. The entire medical marijuana dispute would disappear.

The question remains, should the United States use a program of strictly regulated distribution for other presently illegal drugs like that now used for alcohol? All drugs were legal in the United States prior to 1914, with no particular ill effects. However, no one truly knows what would happen if the United States were to return to that system.

Education

No matter what problem area of society one wants to discuss, education is an important part of the remedy. This is true with regard to health problems, teenage pregnancy, and drunk driving, and it is also true with regard to drug policy. It is critically important to understand that education will be utilized regardless of which policies are implemented. Every suggested option I have ever heard of contains an important provision for education.

The value of education has been shown graphically with regard to the biggest killer drug in the world: tobacco. The estimates are that about 400,000 people die in our country alone every year because they use tobacco. Significant progress has been made in the reduction of smoking by presenting the public, particularly children, with full and honest information about the benefits, dangers, and risks of tobacco use.

If tobacco were to be made illegal, we would simply pave the way once more for people like Al Capone to enter the tobacco smuggling and distribution business, with all of the crime, violence, corruption, and other lawless behavior that would accompany it. Education, along with the ability to regulate and control the use of tobacco, has resulted in a longstanding downward trend of tobacco usage (1).

There has never been a society in the history of humankind that has not had some form of mind-altering, sometimes addicting drug to use, misuse, abuse, and become addicted to. So no matter what we do, we will always have these potentially harmful drugs in communities.

Education programs need to be truthful and honest to make potential users face reality. As with anything else, there are risks and benefits from taking drugs. It is silly to think otherwise; if there were no benefits to taking drugs, people would not take them. There are people who take presently illicit drugs just as I take alcohol, and do so responsibly and in moderation, and they do not need drug treatment either.

Our education efforts must recognize that even though we have made some drugs illegal, they are still present in our society and always will be for anyone who wants to obtain them. Therefore, we must draw distinctions between harms caused by the drugs themselves and harms caused by drug money. We must understand that there are differences between drug use, misuse, abuse, and addiction. We must also understand that some drug usage can be harmful even though the drug is not illegal, and some drug usage is not particularly harmful even though the drug is illegal.

We need to understand the difference between those people who are harming others, as opposed to harming only themselves. If people drive a motor vehicle under the influence of drugs of abuse, we should use the resources of the criminal justice system to hold them accountable for their actions. The same is true for people whose drug usage results in burglaries, assaults, thefts, or other offenses. We should rightfully put them in jail for an appropriate length of time and also use the criminal justice system to coerce them into drug treatment so that they will not return to such harmful behavior. If they persist in being a threat to the health and safety of others, then they should be removed from society until that threat substantially diminishes.

The pivotal plan of action should be to use the criminal justice system to hold people accountable for their actions, not to try to control what they put into their bodies, just like we do with alcohol. The current system is enormously expensive, and we will never run out of problem drug users.

"Just Say No" is not a policy. This is true particularly for children. Children are inquisitive, and after they pass the age of 12 years, they are at an age of taking risks. As a result, "Just Say No" will sometimes become "Just Say Maybe," or even "Just Say Sometimes." Unfortunately, with some children it will also become "Just Say Yes."

Generic approaches like "Just Say No" and indoctrination approaches only work when people do not have access to contradictory information. Obviously most people today, including youth, have access to abundant and almost uncontrolled amounts of information through the Internet, so these approaches fail. Children have discovered that adults are often so frightened by illegal drugs that they will resort to virtually any tactic to get them not to use them, including telling them things that are not true. When we preach to them, for example, that marijuana is addictive and will cause them to lose their abilities to succeed, and then they see, either from their own experiences of from their observations of their peers, that we are untruthful, we lose our ability to guide them. This in turn causes them to disbelieve us when we actually tell them the truth about more harmful drugs such as methamphetamines and cocaine, often with disastrous consequences. Everything we teach to our children, even to our young children, must be truthful, thoughtful, verifiable, practical, and reasonable, or it will be counterproductive.

My strong suggestion to parents about how to talk to their children on the issues of drugs is to follow the approach of my friend Marsha Rosenbaum of the Lindsmith Center in San Francisco, who wrote a letter about the usage of drugs to her high school-aged son Johnny and then published it in the newspaper (27). She began by reiterating truthful information about various drugs and the dangers of using them and again discussing with him why she encouraged him to abstain from them completely. However, she then closed her letter by advising her son that if he ignores her warnings and does decide to use drugs, that he research them, learn as much as he can about them, and use them in a safe manner. She urges her son to observe his friends using them and note that each person responds differently to drugs and to always remember that there are consequences to all his actions, including sex.

This is truthful education. It is forceful, but not hypocritical, and it identifies the issues squarely and shows our legitimate concerns. Parents must be a source of good examples and accurate information for their children, not a source of scare tactics and indoctrination. Marsha Rosenbaum's approach does this and also keeps our foremost goal in sight, namely, that the overall safety of children is the most important thing. It also shows that the use of many of these drugs is risky, harmful, and unattractive. Instead of "Just Say No," the real thrust of our efforts in education to our youth should be "Just Say Know."

The Concept of Federalism

Many people agree that the policy of drug prohibition is not working, but what is the answer? No one knows, but the best way to find out what works is to go back to the concept of federalism. In fact, the United States was founded upon this concept. We should get the federal government out of the equation—it certainly has shown beyond question that it does not have the answers—and allow each state to address this difficult area in the manner that it believes will work best for its people.

Actually, this is what happened when we finally came to our senses and repealed alcohol prohibition. We did not say that everyone could then buy, possess, and drink alcohol. All we did when alcohol prohibition was repealed was to say that each state could determine what was best for its people, and the federal government was restricted to assisting each state in enforcing its chosen laws. Some states allowed alcohol to be sold in various private stores under programs of strict regulation and distribution; others formed government package stores for its sale; and other states or counties therein remained "dry."

In effect, there would be 50 "crucibles of democracy" experimenting with various feasible programs, all the while learning from each other. Maybe one type of program or combination of programs would work for cities but would not work as well for agrarian areas. Over time each area could formulate a program that would best meet its needs.

This type of trial and error, or even reasonable risk taking, is what made America great, and it is what we should employ in the difficult area of drug policy. Will there be some mistakes by some of the states? Probably. However, nothing the states could do would be worse than what we are doing now. Our present drug prohibition/zero tolerance policy directly results in increased crime, violence, prison populations, disease, loss of civil liberties, and the corruption of adults and children. It also results in enormous corruption and de-stabilization of entire governments worldwide.

References

1. Thornton M. Policy Analysis: Alcohol Prohibition was a Failure. Washington, DC: The Cato Institute; 2006.
2. Office of National Drug Control Policy Study. Economic Costs of Drug Abuse in the United States 1992–2000. Washington: Government Printing Office; 2001.
3. Schrag P. For feds, a pyrrhic victory in pot war. Orange County Register. 2002 February 14, 2003.
4. Butterfield F. Number of inmates reaches record 1.8 million. New York Times. March 15, 1999:A12.
5. Schiraldi V, Ziedenberg J. Incarceration of all offenders is not the right answer. Los Angeles Daily Journal. January 21, 2000:5.
6. Ramirez E. Unintended effect of war on drugs found in study. Los Angeles Times. September 20, 2002:A24.
7. Moreau R, Yousafzai S. Flowers of destruction. Newsweek. July 14, 2003:33–34.
8. Pot smugglers in uniform escape back to Mexico, officials say. Los Angeles Times. January 25, 2006:A20.

9. Marosi R, Lopez R, Connell R. Reports cite incursions on U.S. border. Los Angeles Times. January 26, 2006:A1.
10. Paddock R, Demick B. N. Korea's growing drug trade seen in botched heroin delivery. Los Angeles Times. May 21, 2003:A1.
11. Rydall CP, Everingham SS. Controlling Cocaine: Supply Versus Demand Programs. Santa Monica, CA: Rand Corporation; 1994.
12. Whittemore H. Hitting bottom can be the beginning. Parade Magazine. March 15, 1992:4–6.
13. Colby A. Working to kick criminal habits. Los Angeles Times. June 3, 1995: B15.
14. Editorial. Attacking the drug/crime link. Los Angeles Times. January 7, 1999: B8.
15. Yablonsky L. Link between drugs and crime. Los Angeles Times. January 16, 1999:B9.
16. Buechi M, Minder U. Swiss Drug Policy: Harm Reduction and Heroin-Supported Therapy. Vancouver: The Fraser Institute; 2001.
17. Farrell M, Hall W. The Swiss heroin trials: testing alternative approaches. BMJ 1998;316:639.
18. MacPherson D. Comprehensive Systems of Care for Drug Users in Switzerland and Frankfurt, Germany. Vancouver: Social Planning Department of Vancouver, Canada; 1999.
19. Leary W. Report endorses needle exchanges as AIDS strategy. New York Times. September 20, 1995:A1.
20. Lurie P. When science and politics collide: the federal response to needle-exchange programs. Bull NY Acad Med 1995;72:380–396.
21. Recer P. Study finds needle exchanges don't promote illegal drugs. Orange County Register. September 20, 1995:7.
22. The Committee on Drugs and the Law. A wiser course: ending drug prohibition. Rec Assoc Bar City New York 1994;49(5):521, 562–563.
23. Nadelmann E, McNeely J. Doing methadone right. Public Interest 1996;123: 83–90.
24. Editorial. Just the right dose. Los Angeles Times. January 30, 2006:B10.
25. Ackerman E. The latest buzz on hemp: U.S. farmers want the ban on cultivating the plant lifted. U.S. News & World Report. March 15, 1999:50.
26. Turner C. New hemp isn't meant for smoking. Los Angeles Times. May 16, 1994:A1.
27. Rosenbaum M. A mother's advice about drugs. San Francisco Chronicle. September 7, 1998:A23.

29
Case Study of Drug Court Intervention

Glade F. Roper

Sara had been addicted to heroin for over 30 years and had been committed to numerous terms in jail and state prison, spending over 22 years behind bars. Her numerous convictions included possession of drugs, being under the influence of drugs, prostitution, disorderly conduct, petty theft, and grand theft. Every one of her crimes and incarcerations resulted directly from her drug use. Every time she was released from incarceration, she immediately returned to heroin use. Her preferred method of use was intravenous injection. She also frequently injected a combination of heroin and cocaine, commonly referred to as a "speedball." She developed numerous disfiguring scars and deep pits from "skin popping" and "mainlining" (intravenous injections) on her arms, hands, and neck from repeated injections.

A transient, Sara lived wherever she could obtain shelter. Whenever possible, she sought residence with someone, frequently an older male, who would support her. Because of her frequent incarcerations, she was usually unable to establish a stable home and spent much of the time homeless and living on the streets.

In 1998 she was sent to state prison for the second time for grand theft of jewelry stolen in order to purchase drugs. In 2000 Sara was released from state prison, absconded from parole, and resumed injecting heroin. On February 20, 2000, she purchased a 3-day supply of heroin and, after the first injection, felt a burning sensation in her left arm. The burning persisted and she began to experience pain in her arm but continued to inject heroin. After 3 days she realized that the infection in her arm was serious and that it would not go away without medical help. She went to the emergency room of the local hospital to seek treatment. Upon observing the extent of the damage to her arm and shoulder, the treating physician took a photograph (Figure 29.1) and told Sara that she had necrotizing fasciitis, commonly referred to as "flesh-eating disease," that was progressing so rapidly that there was no way to stop it and that she would die within a few days. He asked if there was anyone who should be notified or if she wanted a priest to administer last rites. He told her that had she come 1 hour later she would not have lived to make it to the hospital.

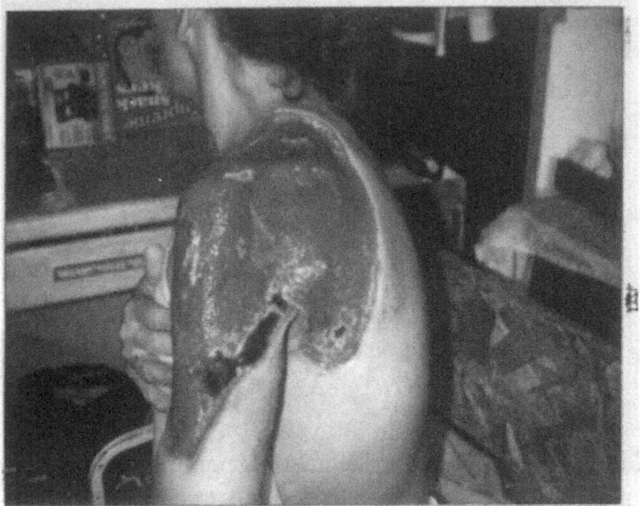

FIGURE 29.1. Necrotizing fasciitis of the shoulder caused by an embolism from an injection and the subsequent infection.

Upon hearing the news from the doctor, Sara looked upward and said, "Thank you God, it's finally over." She felt gratitude that she would be freed from the lifestyle of devoting every effort to seeking and using heroin and going in and out of jail and prison. She felt no fear of death and saw it as a means of escape from a previously inescapable situation.

Sara was rushed to emergency surgery, where the necrotic tissue was excised. The incision was irrigated with antiseptic and antibiotic solutions, and she was aggressively treated with intravenous antibiotics. Because of the extent of the damage, several square inches of skin had to be removed from both of her thighs and grafted onto the gaping wound in her shoulder.

Sara recovered from the surgery, to her surprise and to the surprise of the physicians who thought for sure she would die. The physician explained that had the progress of the infection been toward the front rather than the rear of the shoulder, it would have invaded the pericardial sack surrounding the heart, and she would have died quickly. Because the progress was toward the rear, they were able to remove all infected tissue through debridement and arrest the infection.

Sara spent several days in the hospital and several months under a physician's care. During that time she did not return to heroin. She was determined not to return to drug use. After about a year, she failed in her determination to remain abstinent and resumed using heroin, mixing it with cocaine whenever possible and injecting it into her veins. She was arrested for two additional charges of possession of drugs and paraphernalia, was cited to appear in court, and released.

As is so often the case with people caught in the cycle of drugs, she failed to go to court for her arraignments. When she was arrested for her third charge on April 26, 2001, 12 days after her second charge, she was retained in custody and appeared in shackles for arraignment on all her charges. While she was in custody, she was also detained by the parole agent for violating her parole from prison. She admitted to violating parole and was sentenced to an additional 7 months in prison.

When she appeared in court for arraignment on the new charges on April 30, 2001, she pled guilty to all charges and asked to be placed in the drug court. She was referred to the drug court probation officer for an interview. At the interview, she readily admitted her addiction and asked for help. The probation officer contacted her parole agent, who said, "If you put her into the drug court she will run."

Nevertheless, the probation officer recommended that she be placed in the drug court, noting on the form, "Defendant is in need of treatment. However, her extensive drug use history may be beyond the capability of traditional outpatient drug treatment. Nevertheless, I feel she is suitable for drug court."

She was referred to the drug court judge for sentencing on May 4, 2001. After reviewing her five voluminous files, the judge expressed skepticism about her ability to participate. Sara pleaded with him saying, "I need help. I almost killed myself, and I can't stop using. Please let me in the drug court."

When asked if she was being held in custody for anything but the new charges, she stated that she was serving a 7-month sentence for the parole violation. The judge had her criminal record in front of him and could see that she was going back to prison. Since her four pending cases were misdemeanors, he told her that she would be given concurrent custody time on the new charges rather than being placed in the drug court.

She responded, "Please let me into the drug court. I can't stop using and I want help. Please let me into the drug court."

The judge explained that concurrent time meant that she would not do any additional custody time by pleading to the new drug charges and her sentence would be served at the same time as the prison sentence. Sara responded, "Judge, I have spent 22 years behind bars. I know what concurrent time is! I don't want to do concurrent time. I need help! I almost killed myself. I want to do the drug court when I get out of prison."

Sara had no apparent means of support, a lengthy criminal record, and over 30 years of active addiction. She did not appear to be a good candidate for the drug court, but she was adamant in her insistence and apparently sincere in her desire.

In front of a courtroom full of people the judge said to her, "Sara, I am going to place you in the drug court, and you need to come back here as soon as you are released from prison. You have a lengthy criminal record.

There are only two people in this room who believe that you are going to be successful in the drug court. Do you know who they are?"

She responded, "Yes, me and God."

The judge replied, "No, I said two people. I can't speak for God."

Sara responded, "No, I can't imagine who the other person is."

The judge replied, "It is you and me, and I am the judge, so nobody else matters. I believe that you can do this. I expect to see you back in 7 months and you can stop using drugs. You can change, and you will never have to go back to prison if you will do everything we tell you to."

A review date was scheduled for November 5, 2001, shortly after Sara's expected release date. The jail failed to release her to the Department of Corrections on time, and, because of the delay, Sara's review date was changed to November 28. The Department of Corrections sent a letter to Sara giving her the new release date.

Sara was supported by the judge's expression of faith in her. She thought about it every day during her prison stay and it was a major impetus in refraining from drug use while in custody. The stated expectation of the judge was a motivator and a source of hope for the future. She learned that her release date would be postponed and wrote a letter to the judge giving her new release date of November 29. In her letter she wrote, "I am truly sorry for this inconvenience and I will be out and at the court on 11-29-01 if I don't hear from you. Thank you very much. Truly yours, Sara."

Released from state prison November 29th, Sara missed the court date the judge had scheduled. She later stated that when she was released from prison it took her 3 days to make it back to town and she was afraid to go back to court. She thought the judge would reject her from the drug court because she had missed the scheduled date. Despite her fears, she summoned courage and came to the court clerk's office on December 5, 2001 and asked to be placed on the court calendar.

Sara was scheduled the same day and with trepidation went into court. The judge was surprised to see her but expressed appreciation for her appearance and readily accepted her explanation for not appearing earlier. She enrolled in treatment December 7 and appeared at her first regular drug court review hearing December 12.

Sara found a job cleaning and repainting apartments from 4:00 am to 8:00 am to pay for her treatment. She immediately began to comply with treatment requirements. She sought friends in recovery and attended enrichment activities such as bowling nights sponsored by the treatment facility. At the April 3, 2002, drug court hearing, she proudly displayed her newly acquired driver's license and asked permission to go out of town to purchase a secondhand car. She moved through the phases without delay and the reports from her treatment provider contained numerous notations of her commitment to recovery and bettering her life.

Sara got another job working at the local swap-meet. She obtained her high school diploma equivalency and went on to study human services in the local community college. At the July 31, 2002, court hearing, she proudly reported that she had made the Dean's List at the college. She began to visit her mother whom she had not seen for years.

Because she was required to pay for treatment, Sara experienced financial struggles but was determined to finish the program. She married an old friend and became pregnant. She was happy about the pregnancy but suffered a miscarriage in May 2003. Although saddened by the news, she accepted the development and continued with her addiction treatment. A July 2003 treatment report noted that she "appears to be setting boundaries with people in her life. Client shares openly with her group and her counselor. Client appears to be doing well." The next report noted, "Client is a joy to work with. Sara has excelled in everything she has done in recovery and treatment."

During her tenure in drug court, Sara consistently tested negative on a multidrug panel. Each test was done once or twice a week and with notification only on the morning of the test. In addition to heroin metabolites and cocaine, she was monitored for methamphetamines, phencyclidine, LSD, and 12 other substances. Unknown to Sara, the tested substances were constantly rotated so that new addictive substances were monitored. She tested negative for those as well. She paid for each drug test with the money she earned in her job.

Under the state MediCal (Medicaid) program, Sara received medical treatment that included testing for AIDS, hepatitis, and other drug-related diseases. She received dental care. She attended Alcoholic Anonymous and Narcotics Anonymous meetings four to five times a week for the entirety of her program.

At the December 3, 2002, drug court hearing, Sara successfully graduated from the drug court. She had been clean and sober for 19 months.

Sara participated in the graduation ceremony 3 months later where she showed the audience how her arm and shoulder have healed, although she had very little muscle tissue remaining in that location and limited range of motion. Her last treatment report contains the note, "Client has made tremendous life, behavior, and attitude changes. She has been a positive role model for many people in her life and in recovery. Sara has plans of staying active in the recovering community. Sara has been inspirational to many, including myself." She was asked to speak at the annual community graduation ceremony in October 2003 before an audience of 2,000 people and, although she was scared, she gave an inspiring talk detailing her fight with drug addiction and the fact that she could not have escaped the cycle she was in without the structure of drug court.

Following graduation, Sara completed a 6-month aftercare program that included drug testing, Alcoholics Anonymous meetings, group sessions, and monthly court appearances.

Approximately a year after graduating, Sara wrote a letter to the judge indicating that her husband was addicted to methamphetamine and could not stop using it. She asked if he could be placed in the drug court because he repeatedly returned to prison on parole violations. The judge told her to have him come to court and request to be placed in the drug court. He came with her the following week and an appointment was made with the probation officer. The following week Sara wrote another letter to the judge indicating that her husband had decided not to participate in the drug court and that she was leaving him because she was not willing to live with a drug user and risk returning to the cycle of use.

At the time of this writing Sara has remained clean and sober for over 5 years. She has a job and a much better life. Her story demonstrates that some people with few indicators of probable success can successfully graduate from the drug court and make major, productive life changes. It also demonstrates the need for a judge who understands the addictive cycle and a system that can rapidly respond to changes in the client's lives, recognizing that relapse is a foreseeable part of recovery for many people.

Appendix
Forms Used in Drug Court

Form 1. Probation Intake

Tulare County Probation Department
Drug Court Intake/Suitability Statement

Court Date: ______________________________

Court/Judge: ______________________________

Date Interviewed: _________ Officer: _________ Case #(s)_________

Name: ____

DOB: ___________

Age: _________ Sex: _________ Hair: _________ Eyes: _________

Height: ___________ Weight: ___________

Ethnicity: _________________ Citizenship: _________________

Language: _________________

Address: ____

Resides with: ______________________

Telephone: ______________________

Social Security #: ______________________

CDL# or ID#: ______________________

Employer: ______________________

Income: ______________________

Offenses(s): ______________________

Education: ______________________

Previously in Prop 36/Recovery Court: Yes____ No____

Does the defendant believe he/she has an alcohol/drug problem? No ____

Yes/DOC: _________________

Suitable for Drug Court

Not Suitable for Drug Court based on the following:

Defendant had a prior grant of Drug Court.

Defendant does not wish to participate.

Defendant lacks means of transportation to treatment/drug testing.

Defendant reports he/she cannot comply with program requirements.

Defendant does not have the means to afford treatment.

Defendant has a prior record of violent offenses including: ______.

Defendant has a prior record of sex offenses, including: ______.

Other: ___________

Original: Court Canary: Probation Pink: Public Defender Goldenrod: District Attorney

Form 2. Probation Agreement to Enter Drug Court

SUPERIOR COURT OF THE STATE OF CALIFORNIA
FOR THE COUNTY OF TULARE
LA CORTE SUPERIOR, ESTADO DE CALIFORNIA
PARA EL CONDADO DE TULARE

☐ **DRUG COURT** *(Corte de Droga)*
DEFENDANT *(Acusado)*____________________________

☐ **RECOVERY COURT** *(Tribunal de Recuperación)*
COURT CASE #*(# de caso de Corte)*____________________________

PROBATION AGREEMENT: It is respectfully recommended by the Probation Officer, the above-named defendant agrees and it is hereby ordered that the defendant be granted a term of Formal Probation Revocable Release for a period of __________ years, subject to the following terms and conditions:
***(ACUERDO DE PROBACIÓN:** Es respetablemente recomendado por el Oficial de Probación, el nombrado acusado consiente y es por este medio ordenado que el acusado le seá concedido un termino de Probación Formal Libertad Revocable por el periodo __________ años, sujeto a los siguientes terminos y condiciónes:)*

THE DEFENDANT SHALL: *(EL ACUSADO CUMPLIRÁ:)*

DUI TERMS *(TERMINOS DE MBI—Manejando Bajo Influencia)*

1. ____ (Pay a fine in the amount of $__________. Attend the first offender multiple offender DUI program for 2.0 or higher blood alcohol content. Do not operate a motor vehicle with any measurable amount of alcohol in his/her blood and unless properly licensed and insured.
(Pagar una fianza en la cantidad de $__________. Atender el primer ofendedor programa ofendedor multiple de MBI para 2.0 o mas alto de contenido de alcohol en la sangre. El/ella no debe conducír un vehicúlo motorizado con cualquier cantidad de alcohol en la sangre a menos que esté propiamente licensiado/a y asegurado/a).

2. ____ His/her license is restricted for the next 90 days 18 months to driving to and from employment, within the scope of employment, and to and from the DUI program.
(La licensia de el/ella estará restrictida por los siguientes 90 dias 18 meses para ir y volver del trabajo, y para ir y volver del programa de alcohol.)

OTHER TERMS *(OTROS TERMINOS)*

3. _____ Serve a total of __________ days in the custody of the Tulare County Sheriff, with credit for __________ days actual time plus __________ conduct credit for a total of __________ days served.
(Servir un total de __________ diás en custodia del Sheriff del Condado de Tulare, con crédito por __________ diás actuales mas __________ crédito de conducta por un total de __________ diás servidos.)

4. _____ Return to Court on __________________, 200 _____ at 12:30 p.m. in the Visalia Court 8:00 a.m. in the Porterville Court with proof of enrollment in the treatment program, Global Drug Testing and contact with Probation, and at any other time as directed by the Court or Probation Officer.
(Volver a Corte en __________________, 200 _____ a 12:30 p.m. en la Corte de Visalia 8:00 a.m. en la Corte de Porterville con prueba de inscripción en el programa de tratamiento, con Global Drug Testing, hacer contacto con la oficina de Probación, y a cualquier otro tiempo como dirigído por la Corte o el Oficial de Probación.)

5. __X__ Return to Department _______ in the Visalia Court, in the Porterville Court for Drug Court every ☐ Monday ☐ Wednesday at 8:30 a.m. 1:30 p.m. until otherwise ordered.
(Volver al Departamento _______ en las Corte de Visalia, en la Corte de Porterville para el programa de Corte de Droga cada Lunes Miercoles a las 8:30 a.m. 1:30 p.m., hasta que le ordenen lo contrario.)

6. __X__ Enroll in, participate in and successfully complete the following treatment program(s) as directed:
(Inscribirse en, participar en, y exitosamente completar el siguiente programa de tratamiento:)
Treatment as provided by: ______________________________
(Tratamiento como proveido por:)

7. _____ Pay for the cost of treatment directly to the treatment provider specified above as directed by the treatment provider.
(Pager por el costo de tratamiento directamento al proveedor de tratamiento como specificado anteriormente como dirijido por el proveedor de tratamiento.)

8. __X__ Report to the Probation Office within 72 hours of discharge from treatment. Failure to report will constitute a violation of probation.
(Reportarse a la Oficina de Probación dentro de 72 horas despues de ser dado de alta de tratamiento. Falla de reportarse constituye una violación de su probación.)

9. __X__ Complete any necessary waivers of confidentiality with the Probation Department, Health and Human Services Agency, treatment providers and drug testing services to enable these entities to report to the Court your compliance with your terms and conditions of your probation.
(Completar cualquier renuncia de confidencialidad necesaria con el Departamento de Probacion, Agencia de Servicios de Salubridad y Humanidad, proveedores de tratamiento y servicios de pruebas de detección para autorizar a estas entidades a reportar a la Corte su complaciencia con sus terminos y condiciones de su probación.)

10. _____ Complete 300 hours of community service work through the Tulare Volunteer Bureau, 115 S. "M" Street, Tulare, CA. 100 hours to be suspended upon completion of Phase I; 100 hours to be suspended upon completion of Phase II; and 100 hours to be suspended on completion of Phase III.
(Completar 300 horas de trabajo de servicio a la comunidad con Tulare Volunteer Bureau, 115 calle "M" S., Tulare, CA. 100 horas seran suspendidas al completar Fase I; 100 horas seran suspendidas al completar Fase II; y 100 horas seran suspendidas al completar Fase III.)

11. _____ Attend five (5) self-help meetings such as Alcoholics Anonymous or Narcotics Anonymous per week and provide proof of attendance to the Court and/or Probation Officer upon request. The defendant shall also participate in the 12 step recovery process as outlined by the AA/NA or similar program as may be approved by the treatment program, obtain a sponsor and work through each step in an expeditious manner.
(Attender cinco [5] juntas de esfuerzo propio como Alcohólicos Anónimos o Narcóticos Anónimos por semana y proveer prueba de asistancia a la Corte y/o al Oficial de Probación. El acusado debe de igualmente participar en el proceso de recuperación 12 pasos como trazados por AA/NA o programa similár mientras sea aprobado por el programa de tratamiento, obtener un padrino y trabajar a través de cada paso en una manera apresurada.)

12. __X__ Obey all federal, state, local laws and all orders of the Court.
(Obedecer todas las leyes federales, estatales, locales, y todas ordenes de la Corte.)

13. __X__ Report to the Probation Officer as directed and provide whatever information the Probation Officer requests.
(Reportarse al Oficial de Probación como dirigído y proveer cualquier información que el Oficial de Probación requiera.)

14. __X__ Reside in the State of California, County of Tulare, unless permission is granted by the Court, or the Probation Officer, in writing, to reside elsewhere.
(Residir en el Estado de California, el Condado de Tulare, a menos que la Corte o el Oficial de Probación le de permiso, en escrito, a que resída en otra parte.)

15. _____ Enroll in a program to obtain a high school diploma or its equivalent and continue in such a program until such time a diploma or its equivalent is obtained.
(Inscribírse en un programa para obtener el diploma de la escuela secundaria o su equivalente y continuar en tal programa hasta tal tiempo que se obtenga el diploma o su equivalente.)

16. __X__ Seek and maintain employment or be enrolled in school on a full-time basis.
(Buscar y mantener empleo o estar matriculado en la escuela por tiempo complete.)

17. __X__ Submit to narcotic detection tests/chemical testing at the direction of the Court, treatment provider, Probation Officer or any peace officer during the term of probation at his/her own expense.
(Someterse a pruebas de deteción de narcoticos/pruebas de química a dirección de la Corte, proveedor de tratamiento, Oficial de Probación o cualquier oficial de paz publica durante su término de probación a su propio/a costo.)

☐ The defendant is required to enroll in, telephone daily and submit to testing at Global Drug Testing Services whenever required.
(El acusado es requerido inscribirse, telefonear diariamente a Global Drug Testing Services y someterse a prueba de deteción cuando sea requerido.)

18. __X__ Not use or possess alcoholic beverages and shall not enter a place where alcohol is the primary beverage sold or served.
(No usar o poseer bebidas alcoholicas y no entrar a lugares donde el alcohol es la bebída primaria vendida o servida.)

19. __X__ Not use or possess narcotics or any restricted or controlled substances without a prescription. The defendant shall not use any prescribed or over-the-counter medications without the prior approval of the Judge, Probation Officer or assigned treatment provider.
(No usar o poseer narcoticos o alguna sustancia de control restrictida sin recetá. El acusado no debe poseer medicina recetada o medicina sin recetá médica sin ser antes aprobada por el Juez, Oficial de Probación o proveedor de tratamiento asignado.)

20. __X__ Not falsify or attempt to falsify any drug test. The defendant shall not use any substance for the purpose of attempting to mask, dilute or adulterate drug test results.
(No falsificár o intentar falsificár cualquier prueba de deteción. El acusado no debe de usar alguna sustancia para el proposito de atentar ocultar, diluir, o alterar los resultados de los examenes de droga.)

21. __X__ Not associate with any person(s) using, selling or trafficking in narcotics or dangerous drugs.
(No asociarse con alguna persona(s) usando, vendiendo o traficando narcoticos o drogas peligrosas.)

22. __X__ Submit to a search of his/her person, residence and automobile, at any time by the Probation Officer or any peace officer.
(Someterse a cacheo de su persona, residencia y automobil, a cualquier hora por el Oficial de Probación o cualquier otro oficial de paz publica.)

23. __X__ Not become an undercover agent or confidential operator for any law enforcement agency.
(No convertirse en agente clandestino o operador confidencial para cualquier agencia de enforsamento de ley.)

24. __X__ Register as a narcotic offender pursuant to Section 11590 of the Health and Safety Code within 30 days of this date. Further, the defendant shall register within 30 days of establishing a new residence in any city or county with the law enforcement agency having jurisdiction in that city or county; and shall notify, within 10 days of establishing a new residence, in writing, the law enforcement agency with which he/she last registered. The responsibility to register shall terminate five (5) years after the expiration of the term of probation.
(Registrarse como ofendedor de narcoticos según la Sección 11590 del Código de Salubridad y Seguridad dentro de 30 dias de esta fecha. Ademas, el acusado se registrará dentro de 30 dias de establecer una nueva residencia en cualquier cuidad o condado con la agencia de enforsamento de ley que tenga jurisdicción en esa cuidad o condado; y notificár, dentro de 10 dias de establecer una nueva residencia, en escrito, en la agencia de enforsamento de ley en que el/ella se registro préviamente. La responsabilidad de registrarse se terminará cinco [5] años despues que se termine el término de probación.)

25. _____ His/her license to drive is suspended for a period of 12 months pursuant to Section 13202.5 CVC.
(La licencia de conducir de el/ella sera suspendida por el periodo de 12 meses sequn la Seccion 13202.5 CVC.)

26. __X__ Receive AIDS counseling as mandated by Section 1001.10 of the Penal Code.
(Recibír aconsejamiento de SIDA como mandado por Sección 1001.10 del Código Penal.)

27. __X__ Immediately or upon release from custody, report, in person, to the Tulare County Probation Department, at the address listed below:
(Imediatamente o despues de ser dado de libertad de custodia, reportarse, en persona, al Departamento de Probación Del Condado de Tulare, a la dirección siguiente:)

☐ 3307 South Fairway, Visalia, CA. 93277
Telephone: (559) 730-2610 *(Teléfono)*

☐ 1055 West Henderson, Suite 7, Porterville, CA. 93257
Telephone: (559) 788-1330 *(Teléfono)*

☐ 221 South Mooney Boulevard Room 206, Visalia, CA. 93291
Telephone: (559) 733-6207 *(Teléfono)*

☐ Immediately or upon release from custody, report in person, to the __________________ County Probation Department.
(Imediatamente o cuando seá dado de libertad de custodia, reportarse en persona, a __________________ Departamento de Probación del Condado.)

28. __X__ Not own or possess any weapon. *(No ser propietario o poseér alguna arma.)*

29. __X__ Upon completion of, or termination from, Drug Court or Recovery Court, report in person, to Probation Accounting Services, Room 204, Courthouse, Visalia, California, for a consultation regarding financial obligations.
(Al completar, o terminación de, Corte de Droga, o Corte de Recuperacción, el acusado reportarse, en persona, a Servicios de Cuentas de Probación, Cuarto 204, Casa de Corte, Visalia, California, para una consulta tocante obligaciónes financiales.)

30. __X__ Immediately report any changes of address or telephone number to the Probation Officer.
(Imediatamente reportar cualquier cambio de domicilio o numero de telefono al Oficial de Probación.)

31. __X__ All prior terms and conditions of probation shall remain in full force and effect.
(Todos terminos y condiciónes de probación anteriores seguirán en efecto y validos por completo.)

32. __X__ The defendant is advised that should he/she be found in violation of probation, said finding could result in the imposition of sentence.
(El acusado es advertido que si el/ella es encontrado en violación de probación, tal descubrimiento puede resultar en imposición de sentencia.)

33. _____ The defendant is advised that, pursuant to Section 12021 of the Penal Code, possession of a firearm by a felon is a felony and can result in new charges being filed. The defendant may never again possess a firearm of any kind.
(El acusado es advertido que, según la Sección 12021 del Código Penal, posesión de una arma por un felón es una felonía y puede resultar en nuevos cargos. El acusado nunca mas debe de poseér una arma de cualquier clase.)

34. __X__ Immediately report any contact with law enforcement which results in arrest or citation to the Probation Officer.
(Imediatamente reportar cualquier contacto con algun enforzamiento de ley que pueda resultar en arresto o citación al Oficial de Probación.)

35. _____ ____

FINANCIAL RESPONSIBILITIES

FOR EACH CASE:

36. __X__ The defendant is to pay a $20.00 Court Security Fee within 30 days of this date. Said amount to be paid to the Probation Officer of Tulare County who shall deposit such amounts with the Trial Court Security Fund.
(El acusado pagará $20.00 para Tasa de Seguridad de Corte dentro de 30 dias de esta fecha. Tal cantidad será pagada al Oficial de Probación del Condado de Tulare, que depositará tal cantidad con el Fondo de Seguridad de la Corte Tribunal.)

Case #: ________________ Amount: ________________
(# Caso) *(Cantidad)*

Case #: ________________ Amount: ________________
(# Caso) *(Cantidad)*

Case #: ________________ Amount: ________________
(# Caso) *(Cantidad)*

Case #: ________________ Amount: ________________
(# Caso) *(Cantidad)*

Case #: ________________ Amount: ________________
(# Caso) *(Cantidad)*

Case #: ________________ Amount: ________________
(# Caso) *(Cantidad)*

FOR EACH CASE:

37. __X__ Pay a restitution fine in the amount(s) listed below. Each amount includes a 10% Administrative Fee.
(Pagar una fianza de restitutión en la cantidad(es) que a continuación se mencionan. Cada cantidad incluye 10% adiciónal como Fianza Administrativa.)

Case #: ________________ Amount: ________________
(# Caso) *(Cantidad)*

Case #: ________________ Amount: ________________
(# Caso) *(Cantidad)*

Case #: ________________ Amount: ________________
(# Caso) *(Cantidad)*

Case #: ________________ Amount: ________________
(# Caso) *(Cantidad)*

Case #: ________________ Amount: ________________
(# Caso) *(Cantidad)*

Case #: ________________ Amount: ________________
(# Caso) *(Cantidad)*

FOR EACH CASE:

38. __X__ Pay a probation revocation restitution fine in the amount(s) listed below. Said amount(s) to be suspended pending successful completion of probation. Each amount includes a 10% Administrative Fee.
(Pagar una fianza de restitutión en la cantidad(es) que a continuación se menciona. La cantidad será suspendida al completar probación exitosamente. Cada cantidad incluye 10% adicional como Fianza Administrativa.)

Case #: ________________ Amount: ________________
(# Caso) *(Cantidad)*

Case #: ________________ Amount: ________________
(# Caso) *(Cantidad)*

Case #: ________________ Amount: ________________
(# Caso) *(Cantidad)*

Case #: ________________ Amount: ________________
(# Caso) *(Cantidad)*

Case #: ________________ Amount: ________________
(# Caso) *(Cantidad)*

Case #: ________________ Amount: ________________
(# Caso) *(Cantidad)*

FOR EACH CASE:

39. __X__ Pay the amount of $530.00; $50.00 of this amount to be considered a Criminal Laboratory Analysis Fee pursuant to Section 11372.5 of the Health and Safety Code, $100.00 of this amount to be considered a Drug Program Fee pursuant to Section 11372.7 of the Health and Safety Code and $380.00 to be considered additional fees, penalties and surcharges.
(Pagar la cantidad de $530.00; $50.00 de esta cantidad es considerada una cuota de Analises de Laboratorio Criminal según la Sección 11372.5 del Código de Salubridad y Seguridad, $100.00 de esta cantidad que sea considerada una cuota del Programa de Droga según la Sección 11372.7 del Código de Salubridad y Seguridad, y $380.00 que sean considerados cuotas adiciónales, multas y sobrecargos.)

Case #: ________________ Amount: ________________
(# Caso) *(Cantidad)*

Case #: ________________ Amount: ________________
(# Caso) *(Cantidad)*

Case #: ________________ Amount: ________________
(# Caso) *(Cantidad)*

Case #: ________________ Amount: ________________
(# Caso) *(Cantidad)*

Case #: ________________ Amount: ________________
(# Caso) *(Cantidad)*

Case #: ________________ Amount: ________________
(# Caso) *(Cantidad)*

40. __X__ Pay all fines and fees set forth at the rate of at least $25.00 per month beginning on or before ________________ and $25.00 to be paid on a corresponding date of each month thereafter until the entire amount has been paid. This amount is to be paid to the Tulare County Consolidated Court, Room 124, Courthouse, Visalia, CA Probation Accounting Services, Room 204, Courthouse, Visalia, CA. Porterville Court, 87 East Morton, Porterville, CA.
(Pagar todas las fianzas y cuotas ya establecidas, en la cantidad de $25.00 por mes empezando en o antes de ________________ y $25.00 seán pagados correspondiendo el mismo día de cada mes de allí en adelante hasta que toda la cantidad sea pagada. Esta cantidad que sea pagada a la Corte Consolidada del Condado de Tulare, cuarto 124, Casa de Corte, Visalia, CA Servicios de Cuentas de Probación, Cuarto 204, Casa de Corte, Visalia, CA. Porterville Court, 87 East Morton, Porterville, CA.)

41. __X__ Based upon present/future ability to pay pursuant to Section 1203.1b of the California Penal Code, the defendant shall pay $40.00 for the cost of the pre-sentence investigation, payable to Probation Accounting Services for deposit with the Tulare County Treasurer.
(Basada en la habilidad presente/futura para pagar según la Sección 1203.1b del Código Penal de California, el acusado pagará $40.00 para el costo de preparación del reporte pre-sentencia deiInvestigación, pagado a Servicios de Cuentas de Probación para depósito con el Tesoréro del condado de Tulare.)

42. __X__ Pay $20.00 per month for the cost of supervision pursuant to Section 1203.1b of the Penal Code beginning __________.
(Pagar $20.00 por mes para el costo de supervisión según la Sección 1203.1b del Código Penal empezando __________.)

With my signature, I agree to the foregoing terms and conditions of probation. *(Con mi firma, yo estoy de acuerdo con los anteriores terminos y condiciónes de probación.)*

____________________	________________
DEFENDANT	**DATE**
(EL ACUSADO)	***(FECHA)***
____________________	________________
PROBATION OFFICER	**COURT DATE**

NAME *(NOMBRE):* ______________________________
DATE OF BIRTH *(FECHA DE NACIMIENTO):*________________
ADDRESS *(DOMICILIO):* __________________________
MAILING ADDRESS *(DOMICILIO):* ____________________
TELEPHONE *(TELEFONO):* ________________________
SOCIAL SECURITY NUMBER *(NUMERO DE SEGURO SOCIAL):*
____
DRIVERS LICENSE NUMBER *(NUMERO DE LICENCIA DE MANEJAR):* ____________________________

Pursuant to the provisions of Section 1203 of the Penal Code, I have read and considered the report and recommendation of the Probation Officer. *(Según las provisiónes de la Sección 1203 del Código Penal, he leido y considerado el reporte y recommendación del Oficial de Probación.)*

____

JUDGE OF THE SUPERIOR COURT
(JUEZ DE LA CORTE SUPERIOR)

Form 3. Drug Court Waivers

TULARE COUNTY ADULT
DRUG COURT WAIVERS
(RENUNCIAS DE LA CORTE DE DROGA DE ADULTOS
DEL CONDADO DE TULARE)

As a participant in the Tulare County Adult Drug Court, I agree to the following waivers: *(Como participante en la Corte de Droga de Adultos del Condado de Tulare, yo estoy de acuerdo a las siguientes renuncias:)*

1. **WAIVER OF ATTORNEY:** I have the right to have an attorney represent me at all stages of the criminal proceedings against me, and if I cannot afford one, an attorney will be appointed to represent me at no cost. Once I am sentenced into the Drug Court, ordinarily my attorney will not need to appear with me. Unless I indicate to the court otherwise, I hereby waive and give up my right to have my attorney present with me at subsequent hearings. I understand that if I am represented by the Public Defender, the Public Defender will not appear in court with me unless I am charged with violating the terms of my probation. *(RENUNCIA A UN ABOGADO: Yo tengo el derecho de tener a un abogado que me represente en todas las etapas de los procedimientos criminales en contra mía y si no puedo pagar por uno, un abogado será designado a que me representé sin algún costo. Una vez que sea sentenciado a la Corte de Droga, ordinariamente mi abogado no necesita aparecer conmigo. A menos que yo le indique a la corte de lo contrario, yo por este medio renuncio mi derecho a tener a un abogado presente conmigo a audiencias subsiguientes. Yo comprendo que si soy representado por el Defensor Publico, el Defensor Publico no aparecerá en corte conmigo a menos que yo sea acusado de violar los términos de mi probación.)*

   I agree to this waiver: ____________________ Date: ___________
   (Yo estoy de acuerdo con esta renuncia:) *(Fecha:)*

2. **WAIVER OF COURT REPORTER:** I have the right to have a court reporter take down verbatim everything that is said in court regarding my case. Occasionally, the court reporter may not be present during normal court reviews. If the court reporter is not present when my case is called, I give up my right to have the court reporter present unless I tell the judge that I withdraw this waiver, in which case my matter will be put aside until the court reporter is present. ***(RENUNCIA A REPORTERO DE CORTE:*** *Yo tengo el derecho de tener a un reportero de corte que anote palabra por palabra todo lo que se diga en corte tocante mi caso. Ocasionalmente, el reportero de corte no estará presente durante las revisiones normales de corte. Si el reportero de corte no está presente cuando mi caso es llamado, yo renuncio mi derecho de tener presente al*

reportero de corte a menos que yo le diga al juez que yo retiro esta renuncia, en grado caso, mi cuestión será puesto a un lado hasta que este presente el reportero de corte.)

I agree to this waiver: ____________________ Date: ____________
(Yo estoy de acuerdo con esta renuncia:) *(Fecha:)*

3. **WAIVER OF CUSTODY CREDITS:** If I am required to complete a residential treatment program, I understand that I will not receive any credit for being in custody during the time I am in the residential program. *(**RENUNCIO A CREDITOS DE CUSTODIA:** Si soy requerido a completar un programa de tratamiento residencial, yo entiendo que yo no recibiré ningún crédito por estar en custodia durante el tiempo en que yo estoy en el programa residencial.)*

   I agree to this waiver: ____________________ Date: ____________
   (Yo estoy de acuerdo con esta renuncia:) *(Fecha:)*

4. **TEMPORARY JUDGE:** At times an attorney may preside over the Drug Court as a temporary judge. Unless I indicate otherwise when a temporary judge is assigned, I hereby waive my right to have an elected judge preside over my case and stipulate or agree that a temporary judge can preside. At any time I may withdraw this waiver and have an elected judge preside over my case. *(**JUEZ TEMPORÁNEO:** Hay veces que un abogado pueda presidir sobre la Corte de Droga como un juez temporáneo. A menos que yo indique lo contrario cuando un juez temporáneo es designado, yo por este medio renuncio mi derecho de tener a un juez elegido presidir sobre mi caso y estipular o consentir que un juez temporáneo pueda presidir. A cualquier tiempo, yo puedo retirar esta renuncia y tener a un juez elegido presidir sobre mi caso.)*

   I agree to this waiver: ____________________ Date: ____________
   (Yo estoy de acuerdo con esta renuncia:) *(Fecha:)*

5. **RIGHT TO BAIL:** If I am placed in custody by a judge as a sanction for violating the rules of the Drug Court, I agree that I will not bail out of custody, but will serve the entire sanction in custody. I understand and agree that by posting bail instead of remaining in custody, I will be opting out of the Drug Court and will instead have my sentence imposed. *(**DERECHO A FIANZA:** Si soy puesto en custodia por un juez por una sanción por violar las reglas de la Corte de Droga, yo estoy de acuerdo que yo no pondré fianza para salir de custodia, pero serviré la sanción por entera en custodia. Yo entiendo y estoy de acuerdo que con poner fianza en lugar de permanecer en custodia, yo estoy escogiendo estar fuera de la Corte de Droga, y en lugar, tender mi sentencia impuesta.)*

   I agree to this waiver: ____________________ Date: ____________
   (Yo estoy de acuerdo con esta renuncia:) *(Fecha:)*

Form 4. Disclosure Consent

CONSENT FOR DISCLOSURE OF
CONFIDENTIAL SUBSTANCE ABUSE INFORMATION
TULARE COUNTY ADULT DRUG COURT
[Title 42 USC §290dd-2; 42 CFR §2.20]

I, ________________________, hereby consent to communication between:
Fill in the names of the judges, probation department, treatment providers, drug testing contractor, district attorney's office, public defenders office and anyone else who may be involved in the process
and all of their employees to disclose to all parties listed my participation in the Tulare County Drug Court and my treatment attendance, prognosis, compliance and progress in accordance with the drug court program's monitoring criteria.

Disclosure of this confidential information may be made only as necessary for, and pertinent to, hearings and reports concerning case numbers ________________________.

I understand that this consent will remain in effect and cannot be revoked by me until there has been a formal and effective termination of my involvement with the drug court program for the above referenced case(s), such as the discontinuation of all court and probation supervision upon my successful completion of the drug court requirements or upon sentencing for violating the terms of my drug court involvement and probation.

I understand that any disclosure made is bound by Part 2 of Title 42 of the Code of Federal Regulations, which governs the confidentiality of substance abuse patient records, and that recipients of this information may redisclose it only in connection with their official duties.

Signed: ________________________ Dated: ________________

Defense Counsel signature: ______________________________

Interpreter signature: ________________________________

Form 5. Sample Agreement for the Multi-Jurisdictional Drug Court Officer

THIS AGREEMENT is entered into by and between the following agencies and describes the duties and responsibilities of each agency in respect to assignment of a sworn peace officer as defined by the laws of the State of __________ as a DRUG COURT OFFICER for the __________ DRUG COURT.

I. PURPOSE STATEMENT:

__________ & __________ Counties and the municipalities therein have experienced a substantial increase in drug crimes and drug related crimes. This increase stems not only from the state and nationwide methamphetamine crisis, but also from an increase in population in all areas and in changing drug abuse trends. Law enforcement has historically lacked sufficient resources to maximize drug enforcement efforts. Drug abusers commit a significant number of major crimes, including homicides and residential and commercial burglaries, robberies and assaults. The city/county's experience in this regard is consistent with national trends that reveal a truly staggering number of crimes committed by drug users.

Enforcement efforts directed at reducing drug manufacturing, distribution and trafficking have for the most part been fought by law enforcement agencies working alone and together in multi-jurisdictional drug task forces. There has been little coordinated and concentrated effort directed at drug addicts and their addiction. Significant drug arrests have occurred only to return the addicted offender to the community following probation, community service or incarceration. The cities and counties participating in this agreement must address offender addiction to significantly reduce drug related crime.

II. RECOMMENDATION:

The "District Attorney's" office, in conjunction with the county and city law enforcement agencies, develop a special law enforcement Drug Court officer to work with the __________ Drug Court to enhance offender treatment and when necessary to take law enforcement actions throughout the jurisdictions represented in this agreement.

III. PROJECT DESCRIPTION:

The Drug Court Officer may be assigned from any federal law enforcement agency, any state law enforcement agency or any county or city law enforcement agency or the prosecutor's office having law enforcement jurisdiction. It is agreed that ____ full-time person(s) will be assigned from ____ agency(ies). Supervision of the Drug Court Officer will be shared by __________.

IV. <u>STRUCTURE OF ORGANIZATION:</u>

The Drug Court Director shall act as principal liaison and facilitator between the Drug Court and all participating agencies in all matters relating to the function, accomplishments and problems associated with the Drug Court Officer.

All officers assigned as Drug Court Officers shall work under the immediate supervision and direction of the Drug Court Director and shall adhere to his/her rules and regulations as well as their individual departmental rules, policies and procedures.

For the purposes of indemnification of participating jurisdictions against any losses, damages, or liabilities arising out of the services and activities of the Drug Court Officer, the personnel so assigned by any jurisdiction shall be deemed to be continuing under the employment of the jurisdiction and its policing department.

Each agency contributing manpower to the Drug Court will retain that employee as an employee of the contributing agency and will be solely responsible for that employee.

Any duly sworn peace officer, while assigned to duty with the Drug Court herein provided and working at the direction of the "<u>District Attorney</u>," shall have the same powers, duties, privileges and immunities as are conferred upon him/her as a peace officer in his/her own jurisdiction.

Participating agencies may withdraw from the Drug Court by written statement of termination directed to the "<u>District Attorney</u>." Termination of an agency's participation will take place automatically thirty (30) days after receipt of such written notice.

V. <u>CONTEMPLATED DRUG COURT OFFICER ACTIVITIES:</u>

These may include but are not limited to:

- Provide law enforcement-type training to Drug Court staff
  —Criminal law
  —Criminal procedure
  —Identification and collection of criminal evidence
  —Individual safety procedures
  —Interview and interrogation techniques
- Supervise witnessed urine sample delivery for drug testing
- Participate in Drug Court Client staffing
- Information liaison between Drug Court and Law Enforcement
- Participate in Client home visits
- Act as a Bailiff during Drug Court
- Serve Drug Court warrants and court processes

VI. DRUG COURT OFFICER OBJECTIVES:

This section identifies specific targeted measures to be obtained by the Drug Court Officer while assigned to the Drug Court Program.

1. Disrupt drug organizations including usage, manufacturing and distribution through treatment efforts directed at offender addicts
2. Report appropriate intelligence data relating to illegal drug activities to appropriate law enforcement agencies
3. Conduct searches and make arrests when appropriate
4. Seize and place into law enforcement custody all illegal drugs regardless if criminal charges are sought or therapeutic sanctions are sought through the Drug Court process
5. Promote Drug Court–Law Enforcement cooperation through information and supervision sharing

VII. MANNER OF FINANCING OF DRUG COURT OFFICER:

The Drug Court Officer will be financed by ___________. Continued education and mandated training will be provided by ___________. Uniforms, vehicle and other law enforcement equipment will be provided by ___________.

VIII. DURATION:

This agreement shall be automatically renewed annually hereafter by all members and deemed in full force and effect, except for those members previously terminating upon thirty days' written notice as authorized in this agreement.

IX. CONCLUSION:

Law enforcement and community agencies are faced with the responsibility of drug investigations and enforcement with decreasing resources. Nationwide, multi-agency agreements have proven their ability to make significant impacts on crime as well as other personal and social consequences of addiction. Such cooperation is an extremely efficient use of law enforcement and community resources.

On behalf of my agency, I hereby agree to participate in the Drug Court Officer Program in accordance with the objectives and policies set forth in this agreement.

______________________________ ____________

City Chief of Police Date

______________________________ ____________

County Sheriff Date

______________________________ ____________

Drug Court Director Date

______________________________ ____________

District Attorney Date

Form 6. Sample Job Description for Drug Court Officer

DRUG COURT OFFICER

PURPOSE OF POSITION:

- To perform law enforcement and crime prevention work.
- To enforce Local, State and Federal laws and regulations.
- To work with judicial and treatment professionals within a team to combat drug and substance addiction according to Departmental, Judicial, Drug Court administrative policy and inter-agency agreements.

ESSENTIAL JOB FUNCTIONS:

- Perform all job functions of a Peace Officer for the City/County of ______, State of ______.
- Perform all job functions as assigned by the ______ Drug Court.
- Attend and participate in Drug Court Staffing meetings.
- Attend and function as a Bailiff (Court Officer) for the ______ Drug Court.
- Execute warrants and court orders as ordered by the ______ Drug Court.
- Participate in home visits of clients under supervision of the ______ Drug Court.
- Conduct warrant-less searches as necessary of Drug Court clients.
- Act as an information liaison between the Drug Court and law enforcement agencies within the judicial jurisdiction.
- Collect, process, photograph and present evidence using acceptable forensic techniques either for criminal prosecution or Drug Court therapeutic sanctions.
- Serve as a Public Information Officer on issues of public interest involving law enforcement and the ______ Drug Court.
- Take an active role in educating the public on the philosophy, operation and success of the Drug Court model and program.
- Serve as a Training Officer assisting in training and educating law enforcement officers in Drug Court philosophy and operation.
- Contact and cooperate with law enforcement agencies in matters relating to Drug Court clients and their possible involvement in criminal activity.
- Perform related duties as assigned.

EDUCATION, TRAINING & EXPERIENCE REQUIRED:

- Must be a non-probationary sworn peace officer below the rank of sergeant.
- Must have received at least an overall "above average" rating in his/her last departmental performance evaluation.
- Must have completed and be current on all local, state and federal certifications and licenses required to function as a peace officer with powers of arrest.

- Must not be under disciplinary suspension or probation.
- Must not have had any disciplinary action taken within the past twelve months.
- Must not have used any illegal controlled substances within the past five years.
- Must possess a high school diploma or G.E.D.; college degree preferred.
- Must demonstrate through background investigation, interviews and other tests that he/she is suited for the job of Drug Court Officer.
- Must within the first year of appointment attend specialized Drug Court training such as, but not limited to, the National Drug Court Training Conference.

SPECIAL ABILITIES REQUIRED:

- Ability to read, understand, and interpret treatment plans of clients under his/her supervision.
- Ability to deal effectively with the public and other law enforcement officers, administrators and agencies unaware of the operation of the Drug Court Program.
- Ability to make split second decisions that could affect the life and property of the client, the officer and Drug Court personnel during court, treatment or home visit situations.
- Ability to be sensitive and responsive to innovations in treatment while working within the criminal justice system in regard to clients' rights and seizure of property/evidence for criminal prosecution or treatment/administrative sanctions.
- Ability to be sensitive and responsive to the needs and feelings of others; sensitive to community values and norms; have knowledge or appreciation of special lingo and slang to communicate with the public, law enforcement or clients; sensitive to alternate life styles and socioeconomic groups in enforcing the law and assisting with treatment.
- Ability to maintain strict confidentiality in regard to restricted treatment, investigative, or medical information and records.
- Ability to immediately respond to high emotional/high stress or physically taxing situations associated with substance abuse, criminal violations, addiction and recovery.
- Ability to handle persons exposed to HIV, hepatitis, or other communicable diseases.

Form 7. Important Data Elements for Drug Court Research

The following list of data elements is recommended for collection by Drug Court programs. While all of these elements might not be readily available at program onset, it is valuable to consider the broad scope of variables that could be useful for program evaluation and research.

Guidelines for Data Collection

1. All events and activities should be tracked by date.
2. Programs can use paper forms to track these variables, but an automated system is preferred.
3. There are both client level and program level data elements that require tracking.
4. Baseline data should be collected on criminal history, drug use (including frequency, duration, and drug[s] of choice), and personal information (including employment, education history, and family relationships). This information should be collected again at program completion to document outcomes.
5. Addiction severity should be measured at program admission as well as intervals during the program and at completion to document improvement.
6. Exit interviews are valuable for both absconders and graduates.

Personal Data at or Near Intake

1. Name (including alias and maiden names)
2. Unique system identifier
3. Age
4. Date of birth
5. Gender
6. Race (as defined by the client)
7. Language the client speaks
8. Coercive factors:
   a. Current offense(s)
   b. Open cases
   c. Open bench warrants
   d. Suspended sentences
9. Risk factors:
   a. Previous offenses (misdemeanors or felonies)
   b. Arrests
   c. Convictions
   d. Total time served in jail and prison
   e. Suspension of driver's license

10. Substance abuse factors
    a. Primary, secondary and tertiary drug of choice
    b. Length of use
    c. Use in last 30 days
    d. Age at first use
    e. Prior treatment history
        1) 12 Step participation
        2) Last treatment
        3) Inpatient treatment
        4) Outpatient treatment
        5) Adult or juvenile treatment
11. Health factors:
    a. Historical services/disabilities
    b. Pregnancy
    c. Detoxification risk factors
    d. Co-occurring disorders (dual diagnosis)
    e. Psychotropic medications
    f. Other prescription medications
12. Education factors:
    a. Years of formal education
    b. GED certificate
    c. High school diploma
    d. College attendance or graduation
13. Family factors:
    a. Marital status
    b. Children
    c. Custody status of children
    d. Welfare status
    e. Family drug and alcohol use history
    f. Current drug use in immediate family
    g. Homelessness
    h. English as a second language

In-Program Documentation

1. Treatment:
    a. Attendance
    b. Type
    c. Provider
    d. Inpatient vs. outpatient
    e. Time spent in treatment (days)
    f. Halfway houses (days)
    g. Outpatient (hours)
    h. Progress through program
    i. Participation (attendance)

2. Court process:
   a. Screening
   b. Assessment
   c. Drug testing:
      1) Positive
      2) Negative
      3) Absent
      4) Stalled
      5) Tampered
      6) Inconclusive
   d. Program start date
   e. Status hearings
   f. Encounters with judge:
      1) Date of contact (used primarily for absconders)
      2) Sanctions and incentives list and date
      3) Advancement and demotion through the phases
3. Services (referral and performance):
   a. Mental health
   b. Medical
   c. Vocational
   d. Educational
   e. Public assistance
   f. Housing
   g. Family
4. New charges or arrests:
   a. Charge
   b. Date of incident
   c. Date of arrest
   d. Conviction
   e. Type of charge

Post-Program and Follow-Up

1. Aftercare:
   a. Continued treatment
   b. 12 Step participation
   c. Support groups
2. Arrests
3. Failure to pass drug tests
4. Convictions
5. Loss of driver's license

Form 8. Opioid Medication Management Agreement

OPIOID MEDICATION MANAGEMENT AGREEMENT

Patient Name: ____________________________
Medical Record Number #: __________________
Physician: ________________________________

1. What are the goals for taking a "pain killer" (opioid medication)? (Mark and initial what applies.)
   a. Control moderate/severe persistent pain
   b. Control breakthrough pain
   c. Improve mobility
   d. Other goals ____________

2. What is/are the medication(s) and how it (they) should be used:
   ____________ (Patient's initials)
   ____________ (Patient's initials)
   ____________ (Patient's initials)

3. What you MUST AGREE TO before getting the medication:
   a. Doctor ____________ is the ONLY doctor who may prescribe "pain killer" (opioid medications) for you.
   b. You agree not to ask for "pain killers" (opioid medications) from any other doctor unless Dr. ____________ is notified and has given his/her assent (a "go ahead").
   c. You agree to keep all scheduled appointments, not just with your doctor, but also with other specialists your doctor recommended. You will be dismissed and the "pain killer" medication prescriptions will not be renewed if you miss ____________ or more appointments. Same day cancellations count as missed appointments.
   d. Prescriptions will NEVER be refilled early. Prescriptions will NEVER be refilled if your medication gets lost or stolen or destroyed in an accident. Prescriptions will be written ONLY during regular office hours.
   f. In case of emergency you MUST go to the nearest emergency room. It will help if you inform the emergency room workers who your doctor(s) is (are).

4. Additional information that you NEED to understand:
   g. To control pain you will need to comply with everything your doctor recommends, including behavioral medicine (psychology/psychiatry), addiction therapy and counseling, and physical therapy, if needed. Failure to comply may lead to discontinuation of your medication and referral to another physician or treatment center.
   h. To control and manage your pain successfully, you will need to use multiple interventions, including participation in physical exercise

and the use of psychological strategies that help coping with pain. A pattern of passive reliance on medications and failure to comply with recommendations of physical therapy, psychological therapy, and counseling may lead to discontinuation of medications and referral to another physician or treatment center.

i. We understand that emergencies do occur and under some circumstances the doctor may decide to allow an exception to this agreement. All cases will be decided on an individual basis. In case you disagree, you may be discharged from Dr ___________'s practice and referred to a different provider.

j. "Pain killers" (opioid medications) have serious side effects, including addiction. Your doctor has explained to you the side effects and the precautions that you need to follow. Some but not all of the important points include the following: opioids may cause drowsiness that can be worsened with alcohol, sleeping pills, and other medications. You should use great care when driving or operating any machinery. Remember that an overdose can cause severe side effects and may kill you or anybody else, especially children.

k. Other common side effects that may go away with time include constipation, nausea, itching, sweating, depression, and a change in hormones (especially in men). Sleep apnea, if present, may be worsened by opioids. You may notice other side effects, and it is impossible to predict which side effects you will notice and which will bother you the most. Having side effects on one opioid does not necessarily mean there will be side effects on another opioid.

l. You must take your medication only as directed. Federal law prohibits giving this medication to anyone else even if they are in pain.

m. If you stop your medication abruptly, a withdrawal syndrome will develop.
The pain relief that your drugs give may decrease over time; HOWEVER, if you are suffering from chronic pain, this may not occur at all and usually develops very slowly.

n. Some pain may be only partially responsive to medication. Total elimination of all pain is an unrealistic goal.

o. If you demand an increase in dosage, your need for medication will be re-evaluated. It has been scientifically proven that escalating dosages indicate either that opioids are not effective or that there is an underlying problem with addiction or psychological dependence.

p. If needed and requested by your care providers, including physicians, therapists, and counselors, you agree to provide samples for drug screens. Positive test for any illegal substance or an indication that you have obtained other pain killers from another doctor will lead to your dismissal and referral to legal authorities for drug abuse and addiction evaluation and treatment.

r. Discontinuation of "pain killers" (opioid medications) is needed if: there is not enough pain relief, or there are serious side effects, or if there is no improvement regarding goals of opioid treatment (described in paragraph 1), or if there is problematic dose escalation, or inability to comply with this treatment agreement.
s. I affirm that specific questions and concerns regarding treatment have been adequately answered.
t. I agree that if I do not follow these guidelines fully, my doctor may taper and stop opioid treatment and refer me elsewhere for care.

I (write your name) ___________, understand all of the requirements of this agreement and agree to follow them. I give permission to my doctor to contact other health care providers, for the purpose of sharing information concerning my situation, as is deemed necessary for coordinated, high quality care.

I have received a copy of this agreement.

Patient signature: ______________ Date: ______________
Witness signature: ______________

Index

T